Temple Bar
p. 146 – Dish
p. 159 – Mermaid
p. 162 – O Sushi
p. 139 – Bad Ass

p. 148 Eden
01 670 5373

Stephen's Green
p. 159 La Mère Zou
p. 170 Unicorn

pp. 139 – 171
01 661 6669
p 159 – La Mère Zou
p. 139 – Bad Ass, Bats
p. 140 – The Bistro
146 – Davy Byrnes
155 – Jacobs Ladder
Ballsbridge
p. 158 – The Lobster Pot
01 668 0025

T&D
TRAVELLERS & DINERS
GUIDES

THE BEST, INDEPENDENTLY ASSESSED

Grafton St.
p. 146 – Davy Byrnes   01 660 0363
p. 139 – Bats Bistro
p. 155 – Jacobs Ladder
p. 170 – Tosca
01 670 9868

South Gt.
George St & S Wicklow St.
p. 140 – The Bistro
p. 181 – The Good World – Dim Sum
p. 154 – Imperial – " "

Georgina Campbell's

Tipperary Water
Guide
Ireland

1999

GW00634862

Travellers & Diners Guides

Editorial Director   Georgina Campbell
Publishing Director   Stephen Prendergast

Travellers & Diners Guides (Ireland) Ltd
PO Box 6173
Dublin 13
Ireland

website: www.ireland-guide.com
email: info@ireland-guide.com
Guide recommendations for the Greater Dublin
area can be found on the Dublin Live section
of the Irish Times On Line: www.irish-times.com

Main text - © Georgina Campbell 1998
County Introductions - © W. M. Nixon 1998
Georgina Campbell has asserted her right to be
identified as the author of this work in accordance
with the Copyright Designs and Patents Act 1988.

The contents of this book are believed to be correct at the time of printing.
Nevertheless, the publisher can accept no responsibility for errors or omissions
or changes in the details given.

All rights reserved. No part of this publication may be reproduced,
stored in a retrieval system or transmitted in any form or by any
means – electronic, mechanical, photocopying, recording or
otherwise – unless the written permission of the publisher has
been given beforehand.

Cover photographs:
Front cover: Ballymaloe House, Shanagarry, Co Cork
(Credit: John Sheehan)
Back cover: Ashford Castle, Cong, Co Mayo;
Moran's Oyster Cottage, Kilcolgan, Co Galway;
La Stampa, Dublin.

Designed and typeset in Great Britain by Carl Panday for Bookman Projects Ltd.
Image Quality and Scanning by John Symonds.
Printed in Italy.

First published 1998 by Bookman Projects Ltd.
Floor 22
1 Canada Square
Canary Wharf
London E14 5AP

ISBN: 1 84043 020 6

Foreword

from the Minister for Tourism, Sport and Recreation

Georgina Campbell's Tipperary Water Guide to Ireland is all about quality and standards. In the highly competitive international leisure and tourism industry there is a compelling need to promote and maintain quality in all sectors. I am delighted therefore that Georgina Campbell, a leading Irish food writer and journalist, has produced a guide dedicated to Ireland, to focus attention on the best hotels, restaurants, cafes, guesthouses and pubs throughout the island, and to reward them.

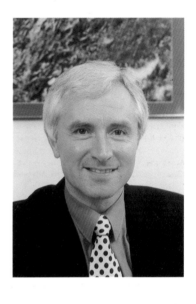

This is an exciting time for Ireland's leisure and tourism industry. Investment in new and existing facilities has reached an all-time high. Successive visitor surveys reveal continuing high levels of satisfaction with the quality of hospitality in all sectors of the industry. *Georgina Campbell's Tipperary Water Guide to Ireland* will help to keep those standards high by rewarding the best and inspiring others to follow the same path.

My congratulations to all the establishments recommended in the Guide. Particular congratulations are also due to those establishments that have been chosen to receive the Guide's special awards.

I am confident that Irish people as well as our international visitors will use and enjoy the establishments listed in the Guide to the full.

Dr. James McDaid, TD

How To Use the Guide

– An entry explained

| 1 | 2 | 3 | 4 | 1 |

Mallow   ★ 🏛 **Longueville House**

HOTEL/RESTAURANT

Mallow Co Cork
Tel: 022 47156   Fax: 022 47459
email: longueville_house_eire@msn.com

Longueville House opened its doors to guests in 1967 – it was one of the first Irish country houses to do so. Its history is wonderfully romantic, "the history of Ireland in miniature", and it is a story with a happy ending. Having lost their lands in the Cromwellian Confiscation ....A fine wine list includes many wines ....
• D£££ & daily light bar L • Acc£££ • Closed 20 Dec-mid Feb • Amex, Diners, MasterCard, Visa •

| 5 | 6 | 7 | 8 |

---

1   **Location/Establishment name**
- Cities, towns and villages arranged in alphabetical order within counties.
- Establishments arranged alphabetically within location.

2   **Category(ies) of establishment**

3   **Address/contact details**
(please phone/fax/email ahead for additional directions if required)
- includes email and website addresses if available.

4   **Rating   – for outstanding cooking and accommodation**
- ⋆   - Demi-Star: restaurant approaching full star status
- ★   - For cooking and service well above average
- ★★   - Consistent excellence, one of the best restaurants in the land
- ★★★   - The highest restaurant grading achievable
- 🏛   - Outstanding Accommodation of its type
- 🏛🏛   - De Luxe Hotel
- 🍺   - Outstanding Pub – good food and atmosphere

       Pub hours in the Republic are 10.30am-11.30pm (summer),
       10.30am-11pm (winter), Sunday 12.30-2pm & 4pm-closing.
       Closed Good Friday & Christmas Day.
       Pub hours in Northern Ireland are 11.30am-11pm (late licence to 1am)
       Sunday 12-4pm and 7-11pm

5   **Food prices – D = dinner, L = lunch**
(average price for a minimum 3 course meal excluding wine/drinks)

£	=	up to £15	per head
££	=	£15 - £25	per head
£££	=	£25 - £40	per head
££££	=	over £40	per head

6   **Accommodation rates – Acc**
(please check with establishments for exact rates, special offers etc)

£	=	up to £25	per night per person sharing
££	=	£25 - £50	per night per person sharing
£££	=	£50 - £75	per night per person sharing
££££	=	over £75	per night per person sharing

7   **Annual closures and holidays**

8   **Credit cards accepted**

Contents

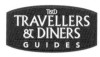

THE BEST, INDEPENDENTLY ASSESSED

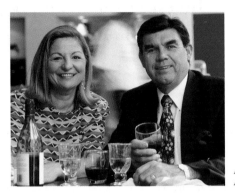

*Patrick and
Marie Cooney*

Where else in the world would you find the simple natural
pleasures that make Ireland so special? The natural warmth
of the welcome. The natural abundance of fresh produce.
The natural beauty of the unspoilt Irish landscape.

As a wholly Irish-owned company we are delighted to sponsor
this new, wholly Irish guide, which highlights and rewards
Ireland's finest hotels, restaurants and other establishments.
As award-winners in our own right (we have three international
gold medals to our name) we are also proud to sponsor the
awards for Ireland's hotel, restaurant and chef of the year.

We are proud too that Tipperary Bottled Waters grace the
very best tables in Ireland and abroad. You will find that our
delicious Sparkling, Still and Naturally Flavoured waters are
the perfect complement to the finest Irish cuisine.

And, because every precious drop is drawn from our source at
Borrisoleigh, in the unspoilt countryside of County Tipperary,
you will find that our natural mineral water is remarkably pure.
Like the natural hospitality, we are confident you will find it
delightfully refreshing.

Marie T. Cooney
Marketing Director

Patrick J. Cooney
Managing Director

Introduction

by Georgina Campbell
Editorial Director

Welcome to the first edition of the first Travellers & Diners Guide, *Georgina Campbell's Tipperary Water Guide to Ireland*. The Guide provides comprehensive, independent recommendations on the best food, accommodation and hospitality throughout Ireland, both North and South.

Local Knowledge

To ensure that we made our recommendations from the widest possible selection of establishments, and that they were assessed to the highest possible standards, we have drawn on a unique combination of in-depth local knowledge complemented by the skills of an experienced international assessment team. These assessors have travelled throughout the country visiting the best hotels, country houses, guesthouses, restaurants, cafes, pubs and farmstays. While our recommendations can never be exhaustive – there are too many new establishments opening up each month – we have tried to be comprehensive, and our web site (www.ireland-guide.com) gives us the opportunity to update entries and include new entries throughout the year.

Business or Leisure

Whatever your reasons for travelling, we aim to help take the guesswork out of choosing the best places to stay, eat, do business or relax. Whether you are visiting Ireland or living in this lovely country, travelling for business or leisure, this guide will help you to find the best places for your purpose.

Food Island

Ireland is at last achieving international recognition for the excellence of its fresh produce from both land and sea – hence the new Bord Bia (Irish Food Board) slogan "The Food Island". It's a joy to see how the production and appreciation of good food has developed in recent years: as well as having superb ingredients, this country's leading chefs now match the best in the world, so eating well has become a major feature of any travel in Ireland. Mediocre meals that disappoint can still be very much a reality, however (as they can in any country). This guide helps you avoid such disappointments by only recommending establishments which operate to a high standard on a consistent basis.

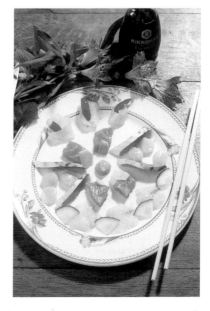

Enjoyable experience at a fair price

No matter how grand or simple an establishment, we have sought the same qualities on behalf of you, the consumer – professionalism, genuine hospitality, high standards and value for money. So, whether you are looking for a venue for a conference or a wedding, planning a business trip or a holiday, booking a meal in a restaurant or simply looking for a pleasant stop on a journey, this guide will inform you of the places most likely to provide enjoyable experiences at a fair price.

Raising Standard – Awards

As well as giving recognition to the best establishments through the Guide's recommendations, Travellers & Diners Guides help raise standards in a number of other important ways. The prestigious Bord Bia Irish Awards of Excellence cover a wide range of categories, including major awards for the leading establishments and individuals, but also awards carefully tailored to highlight excellence in specialist areas: the creative use of the best Irish produce, whether it be seafood, farmhouse cheeses, beef, lamb or pork; the provision of outstanding facilities for business and pleasure; and recognition for those who can make an establishment truly memorable – exceptional hosts or sommeliers giving advice on wines. We even have an award for hotels where not only the guests but also their pets are made welcome!

Recognising excellence – Stars, Accommodation and Pub awards

Recognition of outstanding standards of excellence achieved on a consistent basis is also given through the allocation of 'stars', for food. Restaurant stars are awarded sparingly, up to a maximum of three full stars, with demi-stars given to indicate an establishment approaching full star status. The most luxuriously appointed accommodation is listed as De Luxe (two 'hotels') and especially comfortable and well-run establishments around the country have been highlighted with a single symbol. The number of good pubs in Ireland is legendary, but this is also an area where inconsistent standards are most problematic, so starred 'pub signs' have been awarded sparingly to pubs offering an exceptional combination of hospitality and reliably good (although not necessarily sophisticated) food. Travellers & Diners Guides, Bord Bia and the other bodies and companies supporting the Awards and Stars are delighted to have the honour of recognising and highlighting the achievements of Ireland's leading establishments in food, hospitality and accommodation.

Trends – Chef-Proprietors

The trends in food, drink and hospitality in Ireland are in many ways following a similar pattern to the rest of Europe. A glance at our starred restaurants shows the new generation of seriously talented chefs coming of age; as a result the chef-proprietor restaurants continue to play their very special role as leaders, demonstrating that the great strength of Irish kitchens lies in the partnership of excellent local produce and confident creativity.

Trends – Hotel Restaurants

Parallel to this – and reflecting the current pattern in London and other European cities – we are seeing the re-emergence of the hotel kitchen as a force to be reckoned with. While this is not a new phenomenon – after all our Hotel of the Year, Sheen Falls Lodge in Kenmare, has had one of the country's finest chefs, Fergus Moore, in the kitchen since the hotel opened in 1991, and the same is true of others, including Michel Flamme at The Kildare Hotel & Country Club at Straffan – it is a growing one. This year has seen Restaurant Patrick Guilbaud, Dublin's – and indeed Ireland's – leading restaurant since its inception in 1981, move up to the new Merrion Hotel; not quite as a hotel restaurant, admittedly (they do things differently at RPG), but a very close neighbour indeed – complete with head chef Guillaume LeBrun, who has been the toast of the town throughout. At the time of going to press another momentous move was in progress, as Conrad Gallagher prepared to move his restaurant Peacock Alley into the new Fitzwilliam Hotel, our Newcomer of the Year. Significantly, there were also signs that a new, younger generation of chefs may be preparing to take on the challenge, as the Waterfront Restaurant at the Stakis Hotel suddenly took on an extra dimension with the arrival of head chef Gavin McDonagh, a previous winner of the Baileys/ Euro-Toques Young Chef Competition. This bodes well for a middle market hotel and it will be interesting to watch this area over the coming year.

"Food fashions come and go – mostly in the cities – but the growth of wonderful "culinary clusters" around the country continues regardless. Here we find the great strength of contemporary Irish food: seriously good eating places that note the influence of fashion without taking it too seriously..."

Trends – Informality

Alongside the simultaneous trends towards owner-chefs and committed hotel restaurant chefs, other main developments also reflect the pattern in other countries. A younger, more affluent, dining public is eating out more often and, by voting with their credit cards, dictating a general shift towards brighter, buzzier, more informal restaurants, cafes and bars serving lighter, colourful, cosmopolitan fare. Bistros, cafes, brasseries – call them what we may, they are lively, efficiently run places that provide real value for money – places like Isaac's in Cork and Roly's in Dublin.

New Irish Cuisine

In Irish restaurants, as elsewhere, Cal-Ital, Pacific Rim, Fusion Food and World Cuisine jostle for space alongside every other exotic combination known to food fashion. Young people love it – it's fun, colourful and, when well-executed, full of flavour. But as all the world's once highly individual cuisines blend ever more frenetically – sometimes not just on the same menu but on the same plate – it begins to look more like a crash than a merger. Whatever next? New Irish Cuisine, we hope. This, as you can see from the Bord Bia recipe pages (See pages 32-41) is a concept some of Ireland's top chefs are working on, creating a lighter modern Irish cookery style that aims to please today's palates but is based on traditional themes and ingredients.

Around the Country – Culinary Clusters

Food fashions come and go – mostly in the cities – but the growth of wonderful "culinary clusters" around the country continues regardless. Here we find the great strength of contemporary Irish food: seriously good eating places that note the influence of fashion without taking it too seriously, places where hospitality is paramount and fine chefs concentrate their talents on making the best use of the best local produce. Kinsale was the pioneer and has marketed its Good Food Circle vigorously since the early '70s; although their claim to the title "culinary capital" no longer goes unchallenged, food and hospitality are still major attractions to that pretty seaside town. Over the last 10 or 15 years other similar culinary clusters have developed all around the country, each with its own special way of doing things, and many arc not only thriving but contributing enormously to regional development. If the Guide had an award for Most Hospitable Town it would have to go to Kenmare, home to our Hotel of the Year, Sheen Falls Lodge, and the town with the country's highest concentration of fine restaurants, top grade accommodation and good pubs all working together to offer an exceptionally high standard right across the board, regardless of style or price. Other places where not only lovely locations but also good food and hospitality are a major attraction include: Dingle; Moycullen, just outside Galway where there are several fine restaurateurs, including our Irish Food Award recipient, Gerry Galvin of Drimcong House, and the Clifden area, including Ballyconneely, home to our Beef Award recipient Stefan Matz of Erriseask House. On the east coast, the tiny historic town of Carlingford seems to be developing cautiously (but wisely, to avoid over-commercialisation) and now offers a very nice cross-section of food, drink and accommodation styles. But perhaps the most exciting development is that in the midlands, so recently seen as little more than an area to be travelled through as quickly as possible in order to reach the coast. Here they have produced a real culinary hotspot in the shape of the Shannonside town of Athlone, where readers will find our Atmospheric Restaurant, Le Chateau and also, just outside the town at Glasson, our award-winning Hosts, Jane English and Ray Byrne, at their lovely lakeside restaurant, Wineport.

Food Circles

Another welcome development over the last few years has been the emergence of independently assessed food groups. These started with the Limerick Good Food Circle in 1996 and the concept has now been developed in other areas around the country to include North Tipperary, Tralee, Ennis/Shannon, West Waterford and most recently Meath. Independent assessment, rather than marketing, is the key element in these groups and this, together with a healthy emphasis on the produce of each area, is doing much to improve standards in hotels and restaurants around the country and to highlight areas which might not enjoy the benefits of major tourist attractions.

Service Charges

On a more prosaic note, the question of Service Charges still remains to be addressed. Is service included in prices or added on by the establishment? If so is it 10%, 12$\frac{1}{2}$% or a thumping 15%? If "discretionary" how much should be added? The row about this muddle has been rumbling on for years and there seems to be no end in sight. It can make a big difference to the price you pay, so it is wise to check on policy at the time of booking. Otherwise, check the bill very carefully before paying – unscrupulous establishments have been known to accept an extra payment made in confusion, even when service was already added on to the bill.

Temple Bar

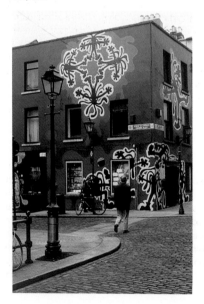

We would like to see more establishments follow the admirable lead of the well-known Dublin restaurant L'Ecrivain, where the service charge is added to food only, before wine is added to the bill. Best of all, we would like to see a national policy adopted so that the confusion could be ended once and for all.

Temple Bar
– The Highs and the Lows

Rewarding excellence is very important in any area of endeavour and certainly helps to improve standards. But sometimes a more direct approach is required in urgent problem areas. Take Temple Bar, for example, an area hailed only a few years ago as "Dublin's Left Bank" but now, in typically colourful Dublin style, dubbed simply "Temple Barf". Despite admirable attempts to upgrade its image as a food destination through an imaginative awards scheme, many Temple Bar eating places are not only not nice, but are also not even cheap. Passing (especially tourist) trade obviously makes it easy for such places to survive, but they're not just a rip-off – they undermine the efforts of the genuinely good establishments the area has to offer.

Staff Shortages

Temple Bar tat is mostly in the restaurant sector, but another serious problem which is emerging throughout the country (and is particularly worrying in Dublin) is the huge number of new hotels which have either been recently built or are due to open shortly without properly trained staff. This problem is likely to cause particular dissatisfaction at the budget and middle-market level and we would welcome comments from readers – whether favourable or unfavourable – regarding the standard of service experienced in all types of accommodation.

New Hotels – Not Always a Pretty Sight

Serious as the thorny problem of staff training is, another aspect of the hotel boom that cannot pass without comment is the extraordinary (and inexplicable) ugliness of many recently opened hotels. Without naming names, let it be said that a new hotel in Limerick has bested even the sitting titleholder in that city for gratuitous

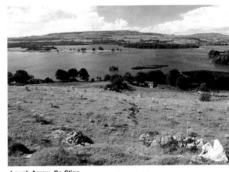
Lough Arrow, Co Sligo

ugliness, although there are plenty of contenders in other areas including Oranmore, Westport and Connemara. Why a new hotel should be an eyesore is a mystery, especially when built on a greenfield site. Once inside things tend to look up and the facilities are often particularly good – but how many people with reasonably normal critical faculties will ever go in to find that out for themselves? On the other hand, there are some inspired new hotels. The Shannon Oaks Hotel & Country Club at Portumna, on the north end of Lough Derg, is a good example – interesting without being ostentatiously over-designed or overdecorated – and the Maryborough in Douglas, Cork city, is imaginatively designed around an old house but without giving in to the "country house concept". There are also some cheering examples of imaginative owners doing well with awesome remnants from the 1960s and '70s, such as Aghadoe Heights, near Killarney, which has recently changed hands and the Ardagh, near Clifden, which has always had an attractive interior (and a wonderful view) but now, with a softer shade of paint, looks much better from the road.

Standards and Consistency

The guide is aware that inconsistent standards are a problem in many areas, resulting in disappointment for customers. In restaurants it may be "chef's night off" (do we ever see reduced prices?) while pubs are particularly prone to difficulties because of varying numbers and types of custom on different days and different times. Putting proper procedures in place would ease many of these problems – in pubs, for example, it is all too rare to find a system in operation for the regular checking of toilets. This fundamental requirement was a consideration when compiling our list of starred pubs; while it should not need comment, only the very best pubs seem to recognise its importance and even these can be subject to occasional lapses.

"No matter how grand or simple an establishment, we have sought the same qualities on behalf of you, the consumer – professionalism, genuine hospitality, high standards and value for money."

Complaints and Recommendations

Even establishments that are normally well-run can occasionally give cause for complaint. How complaints are handled can affect the customer's view of an establishment far more than the original problem. Consumer groups consistently recommend that customers should make their dissatisfaction known to the management at the time if at all possible. The Guide recognises that this can be difficult, especially for a host when there are other guests present, and having to make a complaint can ruin an otherwise enjoyable outing. Also, although this is inexcusable, it is not unusual for complaints to be handled in such a way as to make guests feel very uncomfortable. A complaint in writing, made as soon as possible after the event, requires an effort but is more likely to receive the serious consideration it deserves. Please also let us know if there are problems regarding establishments which are recommended in the guide. Equally, we would also very much like to hear about places which you feel deserve assessment for the next edition.

Prices and Opening Hours

Please note that prices and opening hours may have changed since the Guide went to press. Times and price bands are given as a guideline only and should be checked before travelling or when making a reservation.

Please note also that prices in the Republic of Ireland are given in Irish punts and those in Northern Ireland in pounds sterling.

– Georgina Campbell
Editorial Director

Thanks and Acknowledgements

No project as large as a new guide would be possible without the invaluable support of the many organisations and companies who have sponsored awards within the Guide or assisted in other ways. In addition, there have been many individuals within the food, drink and hospitality industries throughout Ireland who have helped us in many different and practical ways. Their support has helped greatly, and on behalf of Travellers and Diners Guides we would like to thank them all. Thanks also to Nick Kent at Bookman Publishers for having faith in the project, Carl Panday for rescuing us from potential disasters and producing the book design, Angela Tindall, Una McEvoy and her colleagues at The Irish Times On Line, Tom Skinner at Parallel, the Euro-Toques organisation, William Nixon for the county introductions, The Irish Architectural Archive for historic photographs and Ray Henry of Fairway Course Guides for the computer simulation of the K Club course.

– Georgina Campbell, Editorial Director
– Stephen Prendergast, Publishing Director

Irish Food in the 20th Century

by Myrtle Allen

The second world war with its shortages put an end to fine dining in Britain and throughout Europe. It marked the end of the Edwardian and post Great War period when the art of the great chefs had flourished.

Almost all the ingredients needed for fine dishes were unobtainable or severely rationed, and it was made illegal to charge more than five shillings for a meal in Britain, no matter whether you dined at a famous restaurant or in a very ordinary one. The great hotels and restaurants were crowded with young service people grasping a few hours of pleasure away from the war, but the food was wretched everywhere.

"For years after Jammets had closed I played a little game in Dublin restaurants trying to spot the courteous and polished waiters who had been trained in Jammets and had since moved to other dining rooms. Amongst the trainees from the Russell kitchen was Declan Ryan, afterwards to make Arbutus Lodge a famous name in Cork."

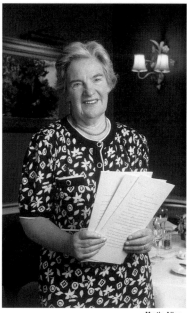

Myrtle Allen

In Ireland, where basic foods were produced for export, only tea and coffee and to some extent sugar were real problems, and so our finest restaurant, Jammets in Dublin, sailed on without great disruption, as did other good restaurants such as the Red Bank and the dining room of the old Royal Hibernian Hotel. Once the war was over, Irish restaurants did a roaring trade serving steaks to British visitors deprived of them since before the war.

Gradually, throughout the 1950s, Great Britain and Europe began to re-establish better restaurants. The Good Food Guide gave encouragement by publishing their first edition in 1951, but throughout Ireland the scene was dismal. Dull menus and badly cooked food were almost universal. Only in some private houses, especially in country houses with their glass-houses and walled gardens still intact, could one find innovative food, perfectly cooked, for private entertaining.

During this period, lasting a decade, scampi or prawn cocktail followed by steak and chips was the required fare for diners out. To ignore this demand was to put a

13

restaurant business at risk. Then the arrival of the food guides opened the customers' eyes to other possibilities, and freed chefs from a tyranny. By the '60s there was light on the horizon and some pioneering restaurants had brought a new excitement to the scene. I believe it had taken these fifteen years for all of Europe, Ireland included, to throw off the trauma of war and concentrate on food as an art once more.

The Russell Hotel and Jammets had a wonderfully good influence on other Irish establishments. For years after Jammets had closed I played a little game in Dublin restaurants trying to spot the courteous and polished waiters who had been trained in Jammets and had since moved to other dining rooms. Amongst the trainees from the Russell kitchen was Declan Ryan, afterwards to make Arbutus Lodge a famous name in Cork.

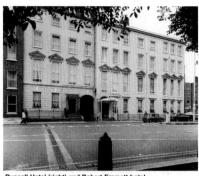

Russell Hotel (right) and Robert Emmett hotel
courtesy of The Irish Architectural Archive

By the '60s some hitherto unlikely people had opened interesting and sometimes eccentric hostelries all over the country. This was the start of a new fashion in catering which has developed strongly since. Let me run through some names.

In Dublin we had Snaffles, the Soup Bowl and The Unicorn.

In the West, in Mayo and Galway, two good fishing lodges, Mount Falcon and Currarevagh came on stream and are still going.

There was Ernie Evans who ran the family hotel in Glenbeigh in County Kerry. His mother ran a smaller and prettier hotel further down the street. They transformed a small, sleepy village into a thriving tourist centre.

In the South-West Ardinagashel House and Ballylickey House had fine wine and good food. The former was informal, fun and sometimes disorganised, the latter French orientated and elegant with superb food. Here one could idle away a wet day in Robert Graves' library. Sadly, Ardinagashel burned down, but the Graves' family still run Ballylickey.

Mrs Good, a Danish lady, owned a small elegant house overlooking Glandore Bay. Presiding over drinks and dinner she made this the most interesting and civilised of all the houses.

But for me, the real mould-breaker was the Spinnaker Restaurant in Kinsale, run by Hedley McNeice. Maybe the cooking was not consistently good but the menu was exciting, the fish was fresh, Hedley was a great character and the soft, catchy music haunted me long after leaving.

The '70s were a disaster. Troubles in the North left the island empty of visitors. Rising costs of fuel and wages did the rest. Dublin had lost the Red Bank Restaurant and the Russell; the Royal Hibernian and Snaffles were soon to follow. Smaller and less ambitious establishments weathered the storm and slowly climbed back to normality.

One positive feature of those early years was that you could at least obtain good native ingredients. Fresh, unpasteurised cream and eggs from unhurried hens made great dishes. It was also easier then to get good potatoes and rashers. In any midlands hotel you would get wonderful beef – well done. But there were no farmhouse cheeses, and fish could be very stale. The present array of tropical fruits was unknown to us. Peppers started to come during the '60s but it was another thing to know how to use them. Life was straightforward; nobody was frightened of eating. Good food was

"Good food was good for you and pictures were for walls, not plates."

good for you and pictures were for walls, not plates. The good restaurants and hotels strived for perfection in the old days. They strive to exist now and are much more orientated towards perfection in the balance sheet.

From the late '60s to the mid-80s, Bord Failte (the Irish Tourist Board) had a particularly brilliant representative in Paris, in Barry Maybury. He perfectly understood those qualities in Ireland which were of interest to the French. He envisaged a grouping of owners who had opened their beautiful country houses to paying guests, running them themselves to a high standard. In 1970 the dream came true with the launching of "The Irish Country House & Restaurant Association", now known as "The Blue Book". This was soon followed by "Hidden Ireland", a similar group of especially beautiful old country houses, and many other groupings followed on. This ensured a quality, variety and vitality in the accommodation sector not found in many other countries.

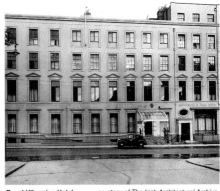

Royal Hibernian Hotel *courtesy of The Irish Architectural Archive*

In 1987 a noted Belgian chef, Pierre Romeyer, backed strongly by Paul Bocuse of France, approached a chef in each country to help to "defend" the quality of European food against the tide of cheap production methods and declining flavours and textures. This movement (the Euro-Toques) took off strongly in Ireland and has helped us greatly in retaining the quality and individuality of Irish food.

Thus Ireland offers a wide range of places to go to, from the eccentric, amusing and brilliantly good, to the charming, old, small-town hotels, not forgetting also the more conventional chain and city hotels. It is impossible to name all the people and organisations that contributed to this rich variety. That would take a book in itself.

– Myrtle Allen

Myrtle Allen is the doyenne of Irish food and hospitality. By food we mean not only cooking (at which she has excelled since opening Ireland's first country house restaurant, The Yeats Room, with her husband, the late Ivan Allen, at Ballymaloe House in County Cork in 1964), but also as a champion of the best of native Irish produce. Her unique understanding of the vulnerability of food artisans and quality produce (long before these issues were popular) made her the ideal founding Irish Commissioner General of Euro-Toques, the professional cooks' association which aims to defend what Paul Bocuse called "these vital building blocks of cooking".

Myrtle has recently completed a 2-year term as International President of Euro-Toques. She continues to fight tirelessly to protect the treasury of Ireland's food, its small producers and purveyors, against the threats of market conformity, European bureaucracy and complacency. She is also an active member of the Irish Food Writers Guild and has written extensively about food, published several books and appeared in countless television programmes.

The Best of the Best

Bord Bía

Irish Food Board

★★ / ★ / ⋆   BORD BIA STARRED RESTAURANTS

Republic of Ireland

2 Star:

Dublin	Thornton's

1 Star:

Dublin	Le Coq Hardi
Dublin	Restaurant Patrick Guilbaud
Cork	Arbutus Lodge
Co Cork	Assolas Country House, Kanturk
Co Cork	Ballymaloe House, Shanagarry
Co Cork	Longueville House, Mallow
Co Galway	Drimcong House, Moycullen
Co Galway	Erriseask House, Ballyconneely
Co Kerry	Park Hotel, Kenmare
Co Kerry	Sheen Falls Lodge, Kenmare
Co Kildare	Kildare Hotel, Straffan,
Co Sligo	Cromleach Lodge, Castlebaldwin

Demi-Star:

Dublin	L'Ecrivain
Dublin	Lloyd's Brasserie
Dublin	One Pico
Dublin	Roly's Bistro

Dublin	The Clarence Hotel, The Tea Room
Cork	Isaacs
Cork	Michael's
Co Cavan	MacNean Bistro, Blacklion
Co Clare	Dromoland Castle, Newmarket-on-Fergus
Co Kerry	d'Arcy's, Kenmare
Co Limerick	The Mustard Seed at Echo Lodge, Ballingarry
Co Mayo	Ashford Castle, Cong
Co Westmeath	Crookedwood House

Northern Ireland

1 Star:

Belfast	Deane's
Belfast	Roscoff
Co Down	Shanks, Bangor

Demi- Star:

Co Antrim,	Ramore, Portrush
Co Londonderry,	Trompets, Magherafelt
Co Down,	The Yellow Door, Gilford

🏛 🏛   DE LUXE HOTELS

Republic of Ireland

Dublin	The Berkeley Court, Ballsbridge
Dublin	The Clarence Hotel, Temple Bar
Dublin	The Merrion Hotel, Merrion Street
Dublin	The Shelbourne Hotel, St Stephen's Green
Dublin	The Doyle Westbury, Grafton Street
Cork	Hayfield Manor Hotel
Co Clare	Dromoland Castle, Newmarket-on Fergus

Co Kerry	Park Hotel Kenmare
Co Kerry	Sheen Falls Lodge Hotel, Kenmare
Co Kildare	Kildare Hotel, Straffan
Co Kilkenny	Mount Juliet, Thomastown
Co Limerick	Adare Manor, Adare
Co Mayo	Ashford Castle, Cong,
Co Wexford	Marlfield House, Gorey

Northern Ireland

Co Down	Culloden Hotel, Holywood

🏛   OUTSTANDING ACCOMMODATION

Republic of Ireland

Dublin,	Conrad International Hotel
Dublin,	Fitzwilliam Park Hotel
Dublin,	Jurys Hotel & Towers, Ballsbridge
Dublin,	Number 31
Co Dublin,	Portmarnock Hotel & Golf Links
Cork city,	Maryborough Hotel
Co Cork,	Aherne's, Youghal
Co Cork,	Assolas Country House, Kanturk,
Co Cork,	Ballymaloe House, Shanagarry
Co Cork,	Ballyvolane House, Castlelyons,
Co Cork,	Longueville House, Mallow
Co Cork,	Perryville House, Kinsale
Co Clare,	Carnelly House, Clarecastle,
Co Clare,	Gregans Castle Hotel, Ballyvaughan
Galway city,	Killeen House, Bushypark
Co Galway,	Cashel House Hotel, Connemara
Co Galway,	Fermoyle Lodge, Costello
Co Galway	St Cleran's, Craughwell

Co Galway	The Quay House, Clifden
Co Kerry	Caragh Lodge, Caragh Lake
Co Kerry	Shelburne Lodge, Kenmare
Co Kildare	Barberstown Castle, Straffan
Co Kildare	Moyglare Manor, Maynooth
Co Limerick	Dunraven Arms Hotel, Adare
Co Limerick	Echo Lodge, Ballingarry
Co Limerick	Glin Castle, Glin
Co Mayo	Newport House, Newport
Co Monaghan	Hilton Park, Clones
Co Offaly	Kinnity Castle, Kinnity
Co Sligo	Coopershill House, Riverstown
Co Wicklow	Humewood Castle, Kiltegan
Co Wicklow	Rathsallagh House
Co Wicklow	Tinakilly House

Northern Ireland

Co Antrim	Galgorm Manor, Ballymena
Co Londonderry	Ardtara House, Upperlands

✚   OUTSTANDING PUBS (for good food & atmosphere)

Republic of Ireland

Dublin	The Porterhouse, Temple Bar
Co Dublin	Johnnie Fox's Pub, Glencullen
Co Clare	Monk's Bar, Ballyvaughan
Co Cork	Mary Ann's, Castletownshend
Co Galway	Moran's Oyster Cottage, Kilcolgan
Co Kerry	The Point Bar, Caherciveen
Co Kildare	The Ballymore Inn, Ballymore Eustace

Co Offaly	The Thatch, Crinkle
Co Tipperary	Sean Tierney's, Clonmel
Co Waterford	Buggy's Glencairn Inn, Lismore
Co Wexford	The Lobster Pot, Carne
Co Wicklow	Roundwood Inn, Roundwood

Northern Ireland

Co Down	The Hillside Bar, Hillsborough

Awards of Excellence

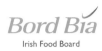

Irish Food Board

Bord Bia
Irish Awards of Excellence

Annual awards for the best establishments and staff in a variety of categories, sponsored by leading Irish companies and organisations

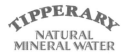

Hotel of the Year

Sheen Falls Lodge

Kenmare, Co Kerry

This stunning hotel made an immediate impact from the day it opened in April 1991, and it has continued to develop and mature most impressively since then, taking advantage of its beautiful location in a manner which is both discreet and focussed. A welcoming fire always burns in the elegant foyer, luxurious rooms all overlook the waterfalls or Kenmare Bay and exceptional facilities for business and private guests include state-of-the-art conference facilities, a fine library, an equestrian centre and a recently completed Health Spa. This, together with an informal bar/bistro, has been so carefully landscaped and integrated with the older building that it feels as if it has always been there. But it is the staff, under the guidance of the exceptionally warm and hospitable General Manager, Adriaan Bartels, who make this luxurious and stylish international hotel the home from home that it quickly becomes for each new guest. One of Ireland's most talented chefs, Fergus Moore, has been executive chef since the hotel opened, and the main restaurant, "La Cascade" has always been a major attraction for its consistently high standards of food and service.

1999

Bord Bia Irish Awards of Excellence

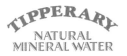

Sheen Falls Lodge

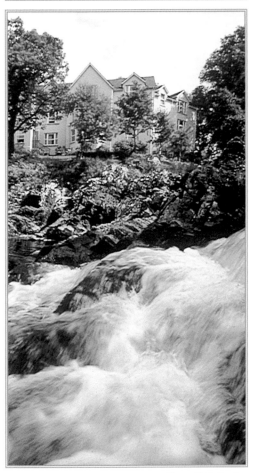

Sheen Falls Lodge

Tipperary Water congratulates

SHEEN FALLS LODGE

winner of
Hotel of the Year

Bord Bia Irish Awards of Excellence

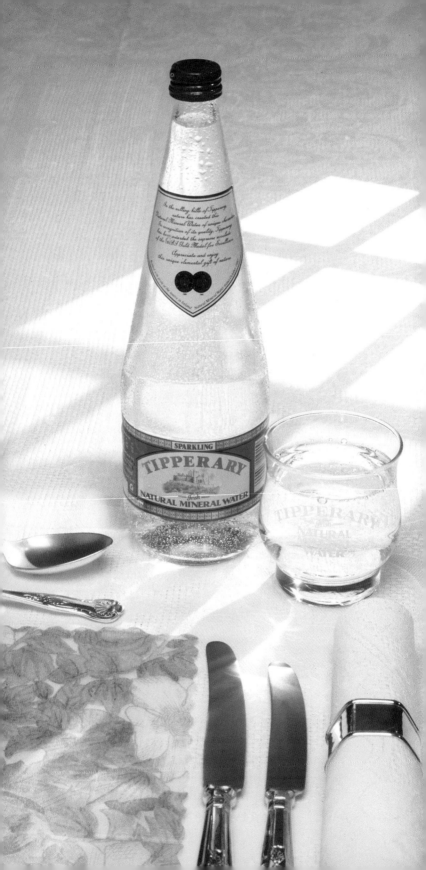

TO THE

c o n n o i s s e u r

IT'S THE

p u r i s t

WATER

IT'S NOT WHAT IS IN A MINERAL WATER

THAT DETERMINES ITS QUALITY,

IT'S WHAT IS ABSENT. IN THAT RESPECT,

TIPPERARY NATURAL MINERAL WATER

IS OF THE HIGHEST QUALITY.

IT HAS THE LOWEST MINERALISATION

OF ANY IRISH MINERAL WATER

AND A PERFECT PH BALANCE.

—

FROM THE PUREST ENVIRONMENT,

THE PURIST'S WATER.

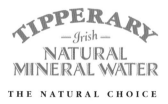

THE NATURAL CHOICE

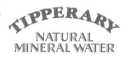

TIPPERARY
NATURAL
MINERAL WATER

Bord Bia Irish Awards of Excellence

Restaurant of the Year

Deane's

Belfast

Since moving from his small but characterful Helen's Bay railway station restaurant to spacious city centre premises in May 1997, Michael Deane has become a serious force to be reckoned with on the Irish (and British) restaurant scene. The main restaurant is an elegant first-floor room with an other-worldly atmosphere that is in total contrast to the bustle of the all-day baroque-meets-modern-cafe-style brasserie downstairs. Theatre in the restaurant is provided by the chef-patron himself, cooking in a small open kitchen which, thanks to the thoughtful positioning of mirrors, is also visible to diners. The ferociously energetic Deane has been described as "propelled by his pure passion for food and its possibilities", and although he has made it clear that this restaurant intends to "set trends, rather than follow them", Deane's talents are particularly well-suited to currently fashionable "fusion food" – an eclectic mix of world cuisines that can only succeed in the surest of hands. Service is excellent, staff soft-footed and discreet, and since Deane doesn't 'do' TV, he can be relied on to be in his own kitchen. No wonder Deane's has taken Belfast by storm.

1999

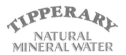

TIPPERARY
NATURAL
MINERAL WATER

Deane's

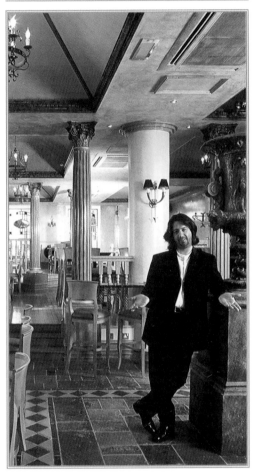

Michael Deane in the brasserie

Tipperary Water congratulates

DEANE'S

winner of
Restaurant of the Year

Bord Bia Irish Awards of Excellence

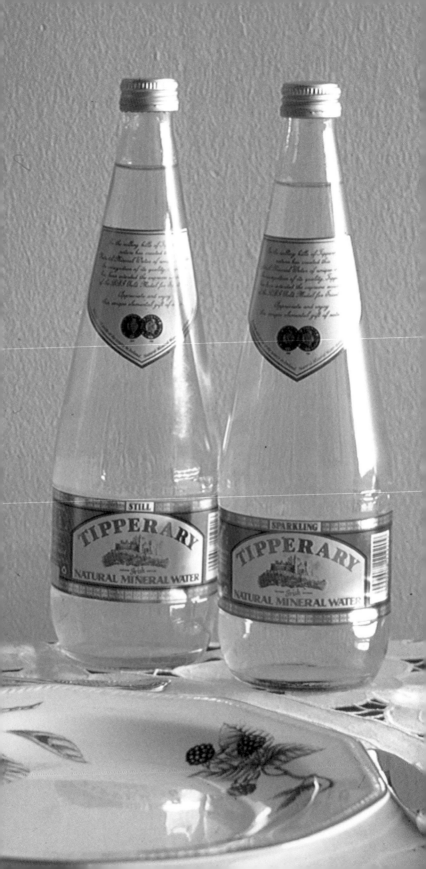

TO THE

connoisseur

IT'S THE

purist

WATER

IT'S NOT WHAT IS IN A MINERAL WATER

THAT DETERMINES ITS QUALITY,

IT'S WHAT IS ABSENT. IN THAT RESPECT,

TIPPERARY NATURAL MINERAL WATER

IS OF THE HIGHEST QUALITY.

IT HAS THE LOWEST MINERALISATION

OF ANY IRISH MINERAL WATER

AND A PERFECT PH BALANCE.

—

FROM THE PUREST ENVIRONMENT,

THE PURIST'S WATER.

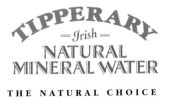

TIPPERARY
=== *Irish* ===
NATURAL
MINERAL WATER

THE NATURAL CHOICE

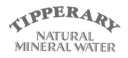

Chef of the Year

Kevin Thornton, Thornton's Restaurant

Dublin

Kevin Thornton is the only chef throughout Ireland to be awarded two stars in this guide. Having attracted a loyal following at his first restaurant, The Wine Epergne, which he ran from 1990-1992, Kevin went on to teach and gain international experience, including time at the renowned Restaurant Paul Bocuse in Lyons. But it was the opening of this 40-seater canal-side restaurant in 1995 that brought wider recognition to this outstandingly talented and dedicated chef. No trouble is too great for him when it comes to sourcing the very best of ingredients, and this philosophy regarding produce is continued in the kitchen, where he "treats it with respect and coaxes out the flavours to create dishes he is proud of"; and what dishes they are – stylish and totally in tune with the current approach to food, yet in no way subservient to fashion. The two-storey restaurant is sparingly decorated, providing a simple, but chic background for the food. Typically, Kevin gives much of the credit for his success at Thornton's to his staff, notably restaurant manager Olivier Meisonnave and his partner, Muriel, as well as those who give such sterling assistance behind the scenes.

1999

Bord Bia Irish Awards of Excellence

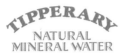

TIPPERARY
NATURAL
MINERAL WATER

Kevin Thornton

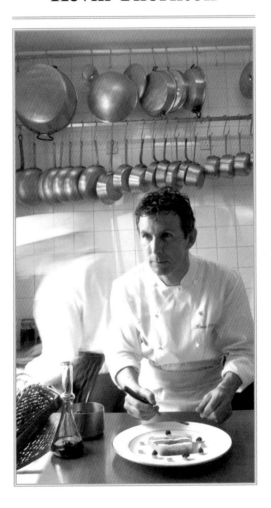

Bord Bia Irish Awards of Excellence

Tipperary Water congratulates

KEVIN THORNTON

winner of
Chef of the Year

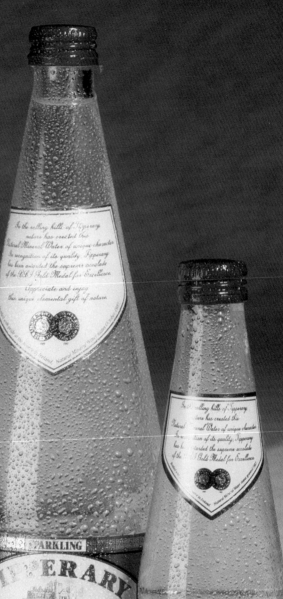

In the rolling hills of Tipperary
nature has erected this
Natural Mineral Water of unique character.
In recognition of its quality, Tipperary
has been awarded the supreme accolade
of the C.G.I Gold Medal for Excellence.

Appreciate and enjoy
this unique elemental gift of nature.

SPARKLING

TIPPERARY

Irish

NATURAL MINERAL WATER

TO THE

connoisseur

IT'S THE

purist

WATER

IT'S NOT WHAT IS IN A MINERAL WATER

THAT DETERMINES ITS QUALITY,

IT'S WHAT IS ABSENT. IN THAT RESPECT,

TIPPERARY NATURAL MINERAL WATER

IS OF THE HIGHEST QUALITY.

IT HAS THE LOWEST MINERALISATION

OF ANY IRISH MINERAL WATER

AND A PERFECT PH BALANCE.

=

FROM THE PUREST ENVIRONMENT,

THE PURIST'S WATER.

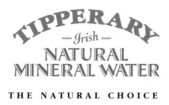

TIPPERARY
—Irish—
NATURAL
MINERAL WATER

THE NATURAL CHOICE

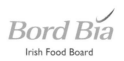

Bord Bía
Irish Food Board

Irish Food Award

Gerry Galvin,
Drimcong House Hotel

Moycullen, Co Galway

Gerry Galvin is one of Ireland's culinary pioneers – indeed he has been described as the father of modern Irish cuisine. Since the 1970s, when he and his wife Marie ran their famous Kinsale restaurant, The Vintage, Gerry has been outstandingly innovative in his development of original dishes (and a consistently dedicated supporter of the best local produce and its suppliers). Always ahead of his time, he has not only developed some stunningly original concepts in his own restaurants, but as a Commissioner was also among the first to nurture Euro-Toques, the European association of chefs dedicated to protecting the integrity of their ingredients. Always a great enthusiast for local suppliers ("the less ingredients have to travel, the fresher they are on the table"), Gerry delights in sharing the details. Many of the ingredients on his menus - the salads, herbs and apples - are grown in the garden at Drimcong, while Connacht Organic Growers supply other vegetables, the dillisk comes from Cara Seaweeds, the pork from local butcher John Palmer and free range eggs from Mark Faherty (all in or around Moycullen), the mussels from Kellys of Oranmore and the smoked eel from Willem at Galway market. Gerry Galvin was the first 'New Irish Cuisine Chef of the Year' in 1996.

1999

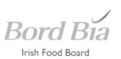

Irish Food Board

Gerry Galvin

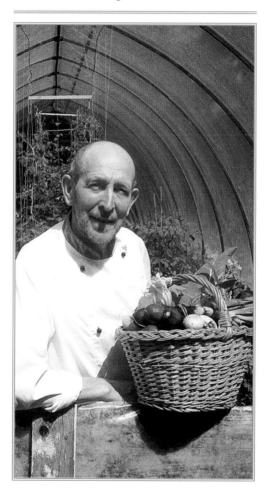

Bord Bia congratulates

GERRY GALVIN

winner of
The Irish Food Award

Irish food & drink...

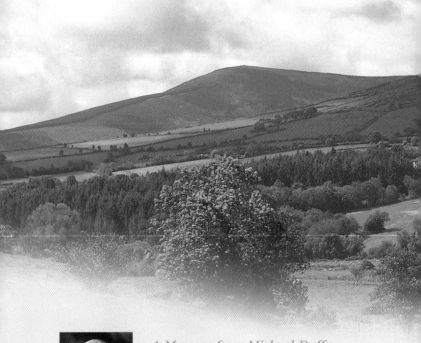

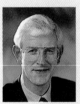

A Message from Michael Duffy,

Chief Executive, Bord Bia.

Bord Bia, Irish Food Board was set up to promote
and develop markets for Irish food and drink.
We have found that the very best way to promote
Irish food is to have people taste it – personal
experience of the flavour, quality and range of
Irish products is certain to leave a lasting and
positive impression.

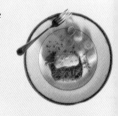

Most visitors experience Irish food in hotels, pubs and restaurants,
and they have an important role to play in developing the image of
Irish cuisine. They act as showcases for the very best in Irish food
and drink. This is why Bord Bia is choosing to highlight those
using fine Irish ingredients with distinction and creativity through
our Irish food awards of excellence.

...naturally good

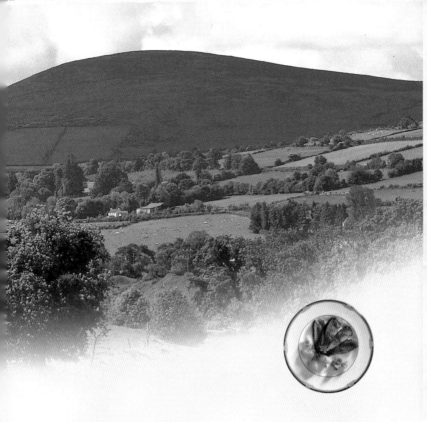

Bord Bia encourages Irish suppliers to recognise the importance of, and maximise the opportunities offered by, the food service sector, by meeting the high standards demanded by restaurateurs and consumers alike.

This guide will show you the way to some of the finest cuisine on offer in Ireland – and to experiences that will stay with you.

Enjoy Ireland – the food island.

Michael Duffy

Michael Duffy,
Chief Executive.

Irish Food Board

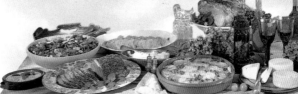

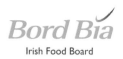

Irish Food Board

Irish Beef Award

Stefan Matz, Erriseask House Hotel

Ballyconneely, Co Galway

Stefan Matz is head chef and, together with his brother Christian, co-owner of the remote Connemara hideaway Erriseask House Hotel, near Clifden. Using the best of local ingredients, Stefan enjoys working on the traditional themes of his adoptive country. He brings a continental sophistication to the dishes he creates, lending a deceptive air of elegant simplicity to meals made memorable by his scrupulous attention to detail. Stefan's menus are always beautifully balanced and regularly feature Irish beef and Connemara lamb as well as an abundance of local seafood. This wonderful dish owes its inspiration to the Connemara landscape and was part of a menu that earned this talented and dedicated chef the title 'New Irish Cuisine Chef of the Year' in 1997.

1999

Bord Bia Irish Awards of Excellence

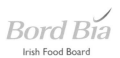
Stefan Matz

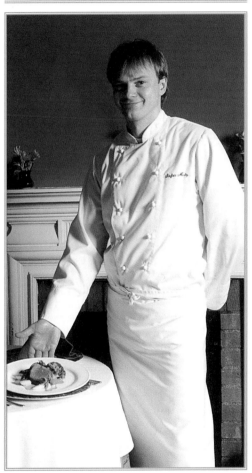

Fillet of Beef Freshly Smoked on Turf, served with
Potato Pancakes & Glazed Autumn Vegetables

Bord Bia congratulates

Stefan Matz

winner of
The Irish Beef Award

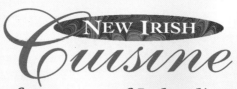

NEW IRISH Cuisine

Recipes from some of Ireland's top chefs

STEFAN MATZ OF ERRISEASK HOUSE HOTEL

Ballyconneely, Connemara, Co Galway.

"New Irish Cuisine"
Chef of the Year 1997
Stefan Matz is head chef and, together with his brother Christian, co-owner of Erriseask House Hotel, near Clifden. Using the best of local ingredients, Stefan enjoys working on the traditional themes of his adopted country and brings a continental sophistication to the dishes he creates.

STARTER

Pan-Grilled Scallops
on a Potato & Carrot Salad

4 potatoes, boiled, refreshed under cold water, peeled and thinly sliced
8 scallops, shelled and thoroughly cleaned
3 carrots peeled, 1 sliced lengthways with peeler, blanched and refreshed (purée remaining carrots and trimmings very finely for sauce)
60ml/2 fl oz oil, mixed with puréed carrot
1 head frisée lettuce, trimmed, washed and dried
2 shallots, peeled and finely diced
75ml/3 fl oz oil and 30ml/1 fl oz white wine vinegar
Seasoning, fresh chives, chervil sprigs

Dry the potato slices and grill in a hot, oiled griddle pan; season with salt and pepper; keep warm. Halve scallops, cook very briefly in the griddle pan; season; keep warm. Reserving a little dressing for the salad, mix the blanched carrot slices and potatoes in the oil and vinegar mixture, adding a few chopped chives. Arrange, with the dressed frisée lettuce and shallots, on four serving plates. Place scallops on top and garnish each with four sprigs of chervil. Pour the carrot oil around the salad and serve the dish warm.

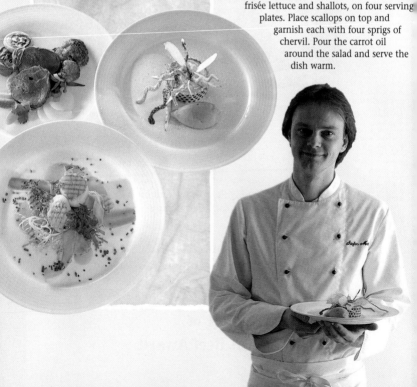

Fillet of Beef Freshly Smoked on Turf
served with Potato Pancakes & Glazed Autumn Vegetables

Smoking equipment is required to make this visually simple but inspired dish as it is done in the restaurant but, although not quite as subtle, char-grilled beef fillet would be a delicious alternative to the turf-smoked original.

POTATO PANCAKES:

250g/9 oz potatoes, cooked
50g/2 oz flour
1 egg
Salt, Pepper, Nutmeg

Blend potatoes with flour, egg and seasoning to taste; use this thick purée to make eight small pancakes, frying on both sides until golden brown; keep warm.

VEGETABLES:

2 heads broccoli, cleaned and trimmed
2 white turnips, turned (neatly shaped with vegetable knife)
1 courgette, turned

Blanch and refresh prepared vegetables, glaze in a little chicken stock and 50g/2 oz butter; season with salt and pepper; keep warm.

SAUCE:

4 shallots, finely diced
200ml/7 fl oz chicken stock
100ml/4 fl oz white wine
200ml/7 fl oz cream
Herbs, eg flat parsley, tarragon, chervil, basil, chopped

Cook shallots, stock, wine and half the cream to reduce by two-thirds. Blend and strain. Mix in enough herbs to turn the sauce grass-green. Before serving, whip the remaining cream and fold into the sauce, adjusting the flavour with salt, pepper and lemon juice if required.

MEAT:

600g/1¼ lb trimmed beef fillet, seasoned
A little smoking powder, small chip of turf

In a heavy, preheated pan, seal the meat on all sides over medium heat, then place in a smoker for about 10 minutes until cooked medium rare. Keep warm.

To serve: Pour the sauce onto the centre of four heated plates, slice the fillet into eight, place two slices each on the sauce and arrange vegetables and potato pancakes around the meat. Garnish with sprigs of herbs.

Mousse of Bramley Apples
with a Sorbet of Apples, Ginger & Spinach

APPLE MOUSSE:

150g/5 oz Bramley purée (cooked with 30g/1 oz sugar, juice of ½ lemon, 1 clove and 1 bay leaf)
1 tsp. powdered gelatine, soaked in a little cold water
25g/1 oz butter
40ml/1½ fl oz whiskey
150ml/5 fl oz cream, whipped

Blend the warm apple purée with the soaked gelatine, butter and whiskey, then fold in the whipped cream and leave to set.

SORBET:

3 Bramley apples, peeled and cored
50g/2 oz spinach leaves
10g/2 tsp. root ginger, freshly grated
120ml/4½ fl oz stock syrup
½ lemon

Liquidise the apples, ginger and spinach leaves, sieve and mix with the stock syrup. Adjust the sweetness with lemon juice if necessary. Freeze in a sorbetière, or in a domestic freezer, whisking occasionally during freezing.

Crisp Apple Slices: Slice an eating apple, such as Golden Delicious, very thinly with an electric slicer and dry in a very cool oven (about 200°F/100°C/gas mark ½) until crisp and golden brown.

WARM WHISKEY SAUCE:

Mix 2 egg yolks with 25g/1 oz caster sugar, 1 tbsp. water and 4 tbsp. of whiskey. Whisk over hot water until light and fluffy.

To serve: Fill a crisp pastry or meringue case with the apple mousse, arrange the crisp apple slices on top and the sorbet alongside, pour the sauce around and garnish the plate with mint leaves.

Irish Food Board

Clanwilliam Court, Lower Mount St.
Dublin 2, Ireland
Tel+353-1- 668 5155
Tel+353-1- 668 7521

Taken from the Bord Bia Booklet
New Irish Cuisine II

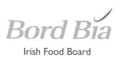

Irish Food Board

Irish Lamb Award

Phil McAfee, Restaurant St Johns

Fahan, Co Donegal

Together with her partner Reggie Ryan, Phil McAfee owns and runs the waterside Restaurant St John's at Fahan on the Inishowen Peninsula. Here their lovely location and joint skills – hers in the kitchen, his front of house – have been delighting guests (including many distinguished visitors to Ireland) since 1980. Phil's cooking combines a respect for tradition and understanding of the value of simplicity with a willingness to experiment, ensuring that the many guests who regularly return always have a meal that is both stimulating and relaxing. Given the location, seafood is very popular at Restaurant St John's but Phil's menus are always based on a wide range of local ingredients and Donegal mountain lamb, which she cooks in many different ways, is an established favourite.

1999

Bord Bia Irish Awards of Excellence

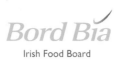

Bord Bia

Irish Food Board

Phil McAfee

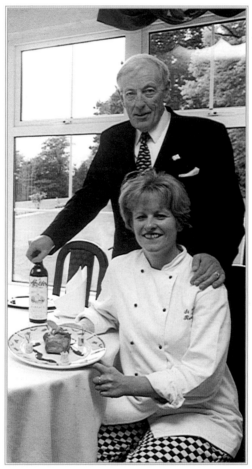

Rack of Donegal Mountain Lamb with
Rosemary and Mascarpone Risotto

Bord Bia congratulates

Phil McAfee

---

winner of
The Irish Lamb Award

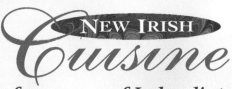

New Irish Cuisine

Recipes from some of Ireland's top chefs

Derry Clarke of L'Ecrivain Restaurant,

Lower Baggot Street, Dublin, 2. Tel: 01-661 1919.

Derry is head chef and, together with his wife Sallyanne, co-owner of L'Ecrivain, where they have built up a remarkably solid reputation in just a few years. Despite its French name it is for modern Irish cooking that Derry is becoming especially well known. Derry takes evident pleasure in using local Irish ingredients, interpreting traditional Irish themes with verve, originality and warmth.

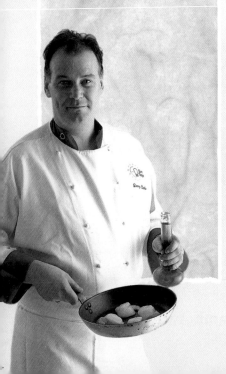

STARTER

Seared Bere Island Scallops

with Regato Crisps, Buttermilk & Cucumber Dressing, Pepper & Tomato Chutney

8 good-sized scallops - ask the fishmonger to clean and trim them.

PEPPER & TOMATO CHUTNEY:

½ onion, diced
4 peppers, deseeded and chopped
1 bay leaf
125g/5 oz brown sugar
100ml/4 fl oz vinegar
4 tomatoes, peeled and chopped
1 clove garlic, finely chopped
450g/1 lb tinned tomatoes
5g/1 tsp. root ginger, grated

Combine all the above ingredients together in a stainless steel pan and simmer very gently, uncovered, for two hours until fairly thick, stirring occasionally to prevent sticking. Cool a little then pour into small clean, warmed jars; seal and label when cold. Use as required.

REGATO CRISPS:

50g/2 oz Regato cheese, grated
25g/1 oz flour
2 egg whites, lightly beaten
Seasoning

Mix cheese, flour, egg whites and seasoning with a wooden spoon until smooth. Preheat oven to 400°F/200°C/gas mark 6. Line a baking sheet with greaseproof paper. Place small balls of the mixture onto the paper and flatten gently with a spatula or fork to make thin discs, allowing at least two per portion. Bake for about seven minutes, until golden brown. Remove carefully when cool and crisp.

BUTTERMILK & CUCUMBER DRESSING:

Lightly whip 150ml/¼ pint cream add 150ml/¼ pint buttermilk, season with salt and freshly ground pepper, then add ½ cucumber, peeled and finely chopped.

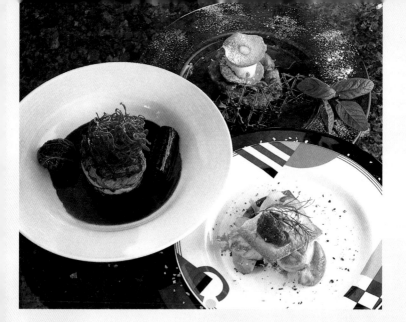

Cook the scallops and assemble the dish:

Heat a little olive oil in a large non-stick frying pan. Slice scallops and quickly sear until golden brown, about 30 seconds on each side. (Do not overcook or they will be tough.) Transfer from the pan onto greaseproof paper and keep warm.

To assemble: Place one Regato Crisp on each plate, spoon some buttermilk and cucumber mixture on top, arrange the scallops on the dressing, place a spoon of chutney on top of the scallops and cover with another Regato Crisp. Garnish with a crisp salad of your choice and some fresh bread.

MAIN COURSE

Char-Grilled Rib Eye of Beef

Prawn & Bacon Sausage, Champ Potato & Cabbage with Porter Jus

First get your butcher to select and trim four rib eye beef steaks, then leave them to marinate in a mixture of thyme and rosemary (leaves stripped from one bunch each), one tbsp. crushed black pepper an half tbsp. sea salt. Sprinkle the mixture over the steaks and leave them to chill while preparing the other ingredients.

PRAWN & BACON SAUSAGE:

100g/4 oz cooked prawns, minced
100g/4 oz cooked chicken breast, minced
25g/1 oz smoked bacon, minced
2 egg whites
270ml/Scant ½ pint cream
Salt and freshly ground pepper

Put prawns, chicken and bacon into a mixing bowl, blend in egg whites and slowly add the cream, without over-mixing. Season. To make four sausages, spoon a quarter of the mixture along the centre of a square of clingfilm, roll and tie each end, making a sausage shape; repeat to use all the mixture. Poach, preferably in a stock, for 10 minutes. To serve, remove clingfilm and lightly sauté in butter and oil.

CHAMP POTATOES:

Boil and mash six peeled potatoes. Trim and thoroughly wash one leek, then chop and simmer in 500ml/a good ½ pint cream until tender. Blend into the mashed potatoes and season well.

Finally, sear the steaks on a char-grill pan (cook to your liking) and assemble the dish on four warmed plates.

Irish Food Board

Clanwilliam Court, Lower Mount St.
Dublin 2, Ireland
Tel+353-1- 668 5155
Tel+353-1- 668 7521

Taken from the Bord Bia Booklet
New Irish Cuisine II

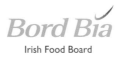

Bord Bía
Irish Food Board

Irish Pork Award

John Howard,
Le Coq Hardi

Dublin

John Howard is chef-patron of Le Coq Hardi, the fine Ballsbridge restaurant that he has been running with his wife Catherine since 1977. It is one of the most highly regarded restaurants in the land. This wonderful dish tells us a great deal about John Howard and his philosophy of food. First the kassler, trademark of that great pork butcher Ed Hick of Sallynoggin, indicates the care John takes with sourcing the best ingredients. The overall theme of the dish shows a great respect for traditional Irish food, yet this is definitely a contemporary creation, lighter and fresher than its traditional predecessors. Then, in its attention to detail – the saucing, the presentation – we see a background of classical French cooking. This surprisingly complex creation looks deceptively simple – and it is certainly presented without undue artifice. But it is in the eating that its true depths are revealed – it proves to be a memorable dish indeed.

1999

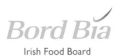

Bord Bia

Irish Food Board

John Howard

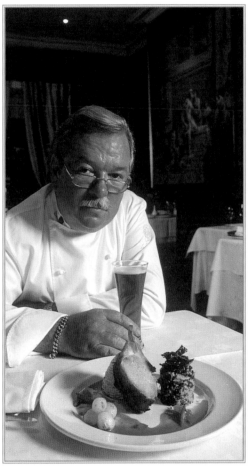

Roast Loin of Kassler with Green Cabbage
& Fresh Herb Mash, Calvados Jus

Bord Bia congratulates

JOHN HOWARD

**winner of
The Irish Pork award**

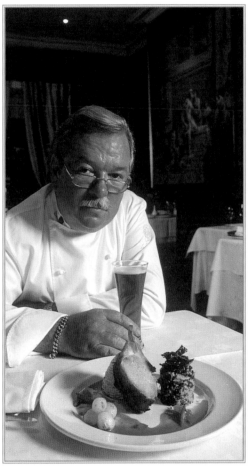

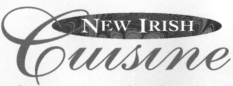

NEW IRISH Cuisine

Recipes from some of Ireland's top chefs

FREDA WOLFE OF EDEN RESTAURANT,

Temple Bar, Dublin.
Tel: 01-670 5372.

Pastry chef at Eden, one of Dublin's most talked-about modern restaurants in the bustling "Left Bank" area of Temple Bar. Always innovative, Freda is currently working on a recipe booklet of progressive Irish fare for the European Irish pub market where, she says, the combination of traditional Irish flavours and New Irish Cuisine style is proving very popular.

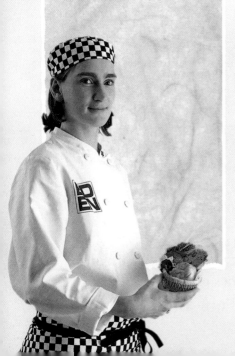

STARTER

Dubliner Cheese, Leek & Cashel Blue Tartlet

These tasty little tartlets use a farmhouse style cheese which is made right in the heart of Dublin, as well as the famous Cashel Blue. Given here as a starter, the same idea could be applied to make a delicious light vegetarian main course.

PASTRY:

In a food processor, mix together 100g/4 oz plain flour, 100g/4 oz wholemeal flour, a pinch of salt and 125g/4½ oz chilled unsalted butter, diced. Blend in two egg yolks and three tbsp. chilled water until the mixture binds to form a dough. Wrap in clingfilm and chill for one hour, then use to line four individual tartlet tins and bake blind at 400°F/200°C/gas mark 6.

FILLING:

In a lidded pan, sweat 25g/1 oz finely chopped onion in 25g/1 oz butter to soften, add one small leek, finely chopped and fry until barely tender; divide mixture plus 100g/4 oz grated Dubliner cheese between the four tartlet cases. Whisk together 100ml/4 fl oz cream, one crushed clove roasted garlic, a good pinch of paprika, and salt and freshly ground white pepper to taste. Cream 100g/4 oz Cashel Blue and add to the mixture.

Divide the filling between the four tartlet cases. Bake in the hot oven for about 15 minutes until set.

Just before serving, make this **Pear Sabayon** sauce by whisking together in a bowl over hot water: 2 egg yolks, 7g/¼ oz caster sugar, 2 tbsp. puréed pear and 3 tbsp. Poire William (liqueur), until frothy. Coat the warm tartlets liberally with the sabayon and glaze under a hot grill, allowing the leeks to caramelise slightly. Garnish with fresh chives and serve the tartlets with a salad of baby leaves.

Bord Bia

Irish Food Board

Clanwilliam Court, Lower Mount St.
Dublin 2, Ireland
Tel +353-1- 668 5155
Tel +353-1- 668 7521

Taken from the Bord Bia Booklet
New Irish Cuisine II

Simple Roast Peppery Beef

A variation on the popular concept of peppered steak, this pleasingly straightforward roast has a dark spicy crust that contrasts deliciously with the juicy, pink meat within.

900g/2 lb rib eye of beef, rolled and tied

1 tbsp. lard, to baste

Preheat oven to 475°F/240°C/gas mark 9. Mix two tbsp. coarsely crushed white peppercorns with one tbsp. sea salt and scatter on a roasting tin. Brush the joint with 1½ tbsp. mustard, then roll meat in the pepper and salt to coat evenly. Place joint on a trivet in the roasting tin. Cook in the hot oven for 15 minutes to seal, then baste, reduce temperature to 400°F/200°C/gas mark 6, and cook for a further 15 minutes (or longer if preferred). Remove and leave to rest on its rack for 20 minutes.

Freda served her roast beef with crisp onion rings, dipped in buttermilk and bran before deep-frying, and these tasty **Gingered Potato & Turnip Cakes** - an interesting development of the traditional Irish potato cake:

Peel and chop 400g/14 oz potatoes, boil in salted water until tender then drain and mash with 25g/1 oz unsalted butter, 25g/1 oz grated Regato cheese and 15g/½ oz grated root ginger. Add 250g/9 oz grated turnip to the potato mixture, season to taste, then leave to cool. To cook, shape the mixture into 12 balls, coat lightly in flour, then flatten into rounds. Heat a little oil in a frying pan and cook the cakes for two to three minutes on each side, until crisp and golden. Drain on kitchen paper.

To serve: Place the Gingered Potato & Turnip Cakes on four heated plates, arrange the thickly sliced beef on top and spoon over sauce of your choice - Freda used an unusual Thyme & Gorse Wine Jus but a simple gravy made with the beef juices would be fine. Garnish with seasonal vegetables and a sprig of fresh herbs.

Gooseberry & Mead Swiss Roll

Freda chose gooseberries, one of our most under-used and easily-grown cottage garden fruits, for this homely dessert. She also made an unusual Honey & Lavender Ice Cream to accompany it, but the swiss roll really needs no other embellishment except, perhaps a little whipped cream and a sprig of lavender.

Line a swiss roll tin (20 x 25cm/8"x10") with baking parchment. Preheat oven to 400°F/200°C/gas mark 6. Whisk three eggs with 75g/3 oz caster sugar until thick and creamy, then gently fold in 75g/3 oz sifted flour. Turn into the prepared tin and bake for 10 minutes until well-risen and firm to the touch, then turn onto greaseproof paper scattered with caster sugar. Gently peel off lining paper and loosely roll up the sponge and paper together; leave to cool. Stew 225g/8 oz gooseberries (topped and tailed) with 50g/2 oz sugar and one tbsp. water; mash to a purée and add one tbsp. Mead; leave to cool. Whip 150ml/¼ pint cream and fold in the gooseberry purée. Unroll the cold swiss roll, spread evenly with the gooseberry cream and re-roll carefully. Just before serving, sprinkle another two tbsp. Mead over the swiss roll and dust it with icing sugar. Serve sliced, possibly with a home-made ice cream.

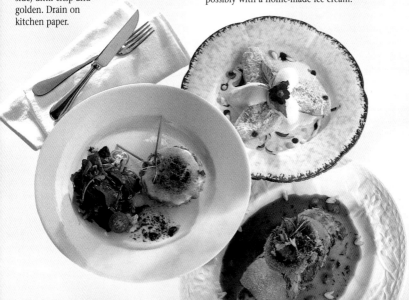

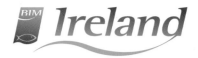

Seafood Restaurant of the Year

Lawrence Cove House Seafood Restaurant

Bere Island, Co Cork

Surprise and delight are the usual reactions from first time visitors to the seafood restaurant that Mike and Mary Sullivan have run on Bere Island since 1995: surprise that a restaurant could succeed at all in this unlikely spot – it's just a short ferry ride from Castletownbere, but there certainly isn't too much passing trade – and delight at its professionalism and the warmth of the Sullivan's hospitality. But a loyal following is building up, and the new marina on the island encourages sailors to tailor their cruising plans to fit in a comfortable and well-fed overnight stay. Perhaps it isn't quite so surprising that this restaurant has come into being, when you realise that Mike is the fisherman who supplies many of the country's top restaurants with fresh West Cork fish and shellfish. The menu is not over-long, yet it embraces a wide range of fish and seafood, including some unusual varieties unlikely to be found elsewhere, such as grouper and coryphene ("sunfish") when in season. Mike will even bring guests over to the restaurant in his fishing boat and deliver them back to the mainland after dinner if the ferry times aren't convenient.

1999

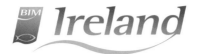

Lawrence Cove House
Seafood Restaurant

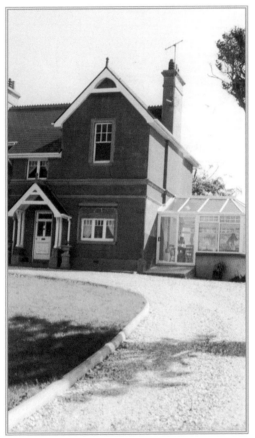

Lawrence Cove House Seafood Restaurant

BIM congratulates

LAWRENCE COVE HOUSE

winner of
Seafood Restaurant of the Year

BIM Ireland

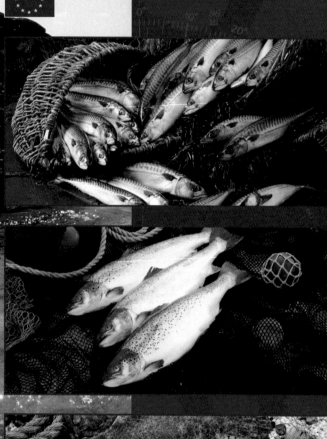

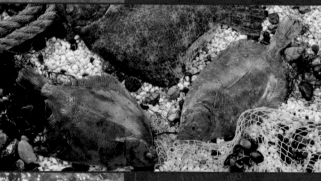

IRISH SEA FISHERIES BOARD/BIM, P.O. BOX 12
CROFTON RD, DUN LAOGHAIRE, CO. DUBLIN, IRELAND
TEL: + 353 1 2841544   FAX: + 353 1 2841123

Get hooked on seafood !

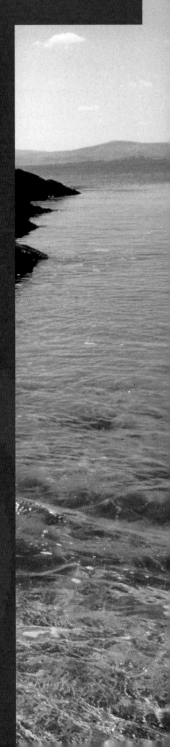

Explore . . .

Simply grilled or combined with exotic ingredients seafood tempts the taste buds. Was it luck or a kind Creator that placed Ireland so strategically on this planet ? Geographically, we're rather unique and though very much part of Europe, we do live on the edge.

Being on the edge has its advantages when it comes to seafood. There's an Irish song that goes "Thank God we're surrounded by water", with our beautiful and indented coastline stretching for 2,000 miles around the island and more rivers and lakes per square mile than any other country in Europe. Naturally then it's not surprising that we enjoy an abundance of seafood from our surrounding waters. It's versatile, easy to prepare, quick to cook and the perfect choice for every dining occasion.

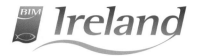

Seafood Dish
of the Year

Caviston's of
Sandycove

Sandycove, Co Dublin

Caviston's of Sandycove has long been a mecca for lovers of good food. Here you will find everything that is good, from organic vegetables to farmhouse cheeses, cooked meats to specialist oils (and other more exotic items). But it was always for fish and shellfish that Caviston's was especially renowned – even providing a collection of well-thumbed recipe books for on-the-spot reference. So what could be more natural than to cook their fish on the spot and open a little restaurant next door – which is just what they did in 1996. Here they do two sittings in their tiny restaurant at lunchtime, serving an imaginative range of seafood dishes influenced by various traditions (and all washed down by a glass or two from a very tempting little wine list). Our lovely dish is not too complicated but speaks volumes for how good seafood can be: a trio of golden brown, crisp monkfish pieces arranged bonfire style, along with strips of juicy, meltingly soft roast red pepper, all surrounded by a very lightly spiced dressing of olive oil and fresh herbs. Simple, colourful, perfectly cooked.

1999

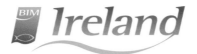

Caviston's
of Sandycove

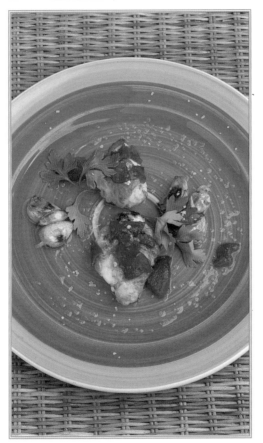

Roast Monkfish Fillets, Roast Red Pepper
& Olive Oil Dressing

BIM congratulates

LAWRENCE COVE HOUSE

winner of
Seafood Dish of the Year

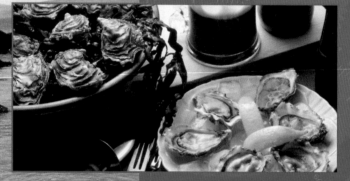

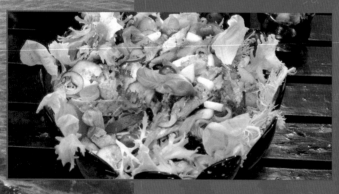

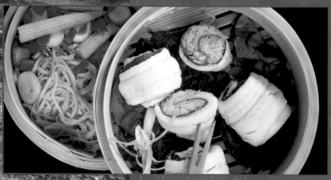

IRISH SEA FISHERIES BOARD/BIM, P.O. BOX 12
CROFTON RD, DUN LAOGHAIRE, CO. DUBLIN, IRELAND
TEL: + 353 1 2841544   FAX: + 353 1 2841123

Get hooked on seafood !

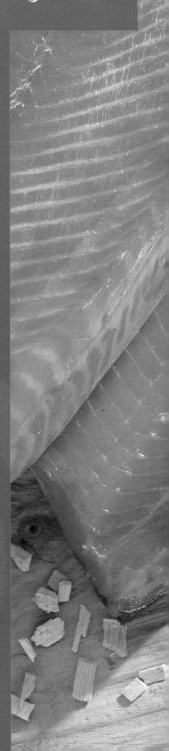

Inspirational . .

Our pubs and inns will serve you freshly smoked salmon, Irish fisherman's chowder or great bowls of sumptuous mussels from Bantry Bay or Connemara.

You can taste ten different oysters from Lough Foyle in the North of Ireland to Roaring Water Bay in the South, and due to the advances in aquaculture you'll soon be dining out on abalone and urchins, scallops or turbot, eel or halibut.

Keep your heart healthy and feast on fresh mackerel, silvery herring or some lively trout from the crystal clear mountain streams of Wicklow or Wexford.

If you're European, Asian or American you'll no doubt have tasted our seafood at the best tables in your country. And if you're lucky enough to live on or visit this green island in 1999, you'll have the chance once more. Go on . . . get hooked on our Seafood !

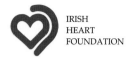

Happy Heart
Eat Out Award

101 Talbot

Dublin

Ever since opening 101 Talbot in 1991, Margaret Duffy and Pascal Bradley have created a real buzz around this groundbreaking northside restaurant. Its proximity to the Abbey and Gate theatres, and the constantly changing art exhibitions in the restaurant, have been partly responsible for drawing an interesting artistic/theatrical crowd, but its popularity with this discerning clientele is also due to the joyfully creative healthy food. Always interested in experimentation, and very obviously willing to help with any particular dietary requirements (even down to the chef coming out to discuss the options with guests), the Mediterranean and Middle Eastern influences at work in the kitchen here explain why there are so many dishes that meet the Irish Heart Foundation's definition of a Healthy Choice, ie dishes with lots of fruit and vegetables that are high in fibre and low in fat, especially saturated fat. Vegetarians also get a strong selection of dishes to choose from.

1999

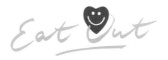

101 Talbot

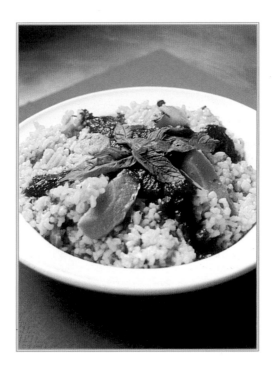

**The Irish Heart
Foundation congratulates**

101 TALBOT

winner of
The Happy Heart Eat Out Award

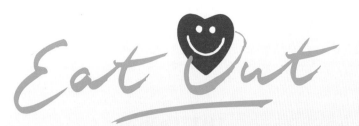

Eat Out

For a Happy Heart ...
Go For Low Fat Healthy Eating

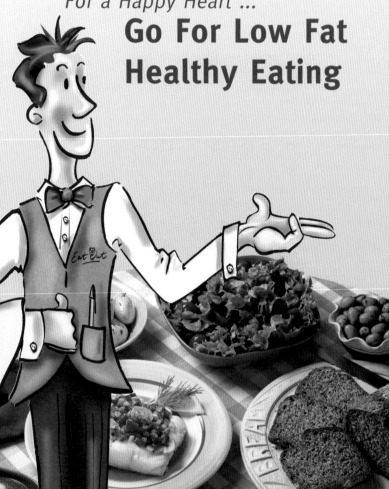

Just Ask

More and more people are interested in healthy eating when eating out, and yet still want to enjoy delicious food. A recent customer survey conducted by the Irish Heart Foundation indicated that over three-quarters of people ask for the healthier choice.

Many chefs and restaurants are responding to this demand for lighter cuisine. To help you offer your customers a wider and more creative range of healthy choices, the Irish Heart Foundation and the Health Promotion Unit in the Department of Health and Children organise **HAPPY HEART EAT OUT** for the month of June each year.

The theme for 1999 is **'Go For Low Fat Healthy Eating'** and customers are encouraged to *Just Ask* for the low fat healthy choice. Our evaluations show that many establishments continue to provide low fat choices all year round.

For information and suggestions on healthy choices and recipes contact the Irish Heart Foundation, Telephone: 01 668 5001.

NATIONAL HEALTHY EATING CAMPAIGN

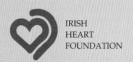
IRISH
HEART
FOUNDATION

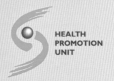
HEALTH
PROMOTION
UNIT

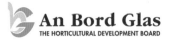

An Bord Glas
THE HORTICULTURAL DEVELOPMENT BOARD

Vegetarian Dish of the Year

Ballymore Inn
Ballymore Eustace, Co Kildare

The O'Sullivan's pub looks unassuming enough from the outside, but word about the food has definitely "got out" and people are coming from all over to get a taste of the wonderful things this country kitchen has to offer. One of the best things they've done recently is to install a really good pizza oven, so there's always a choice of pizzas on their varied but unpretentious menus – and what pizzas they are. Not only are the bases wonderfully light, thin and crisply cooked, but every ingredient is in tip-top condition. The range includes some wonderful combinations, most of which happen to be vegetarian. No ordinary pizzas these; you can choose from the likes of Pepperoni, Tomato, Chilli & Mozzarella or Grilled Peppers with Olives & Pesto, or dither between Spinach, Oyster Mushroom & Goat's Cheese and Anchovy, Black Olives, Capers, Red Onion & Cooleeney Cheese. They're all wonderful but best of all, we think, is the Grilled Fennel, Roasted Peppers, Basil & Ardrahan Cheese – a pizza worth travelling miles for.

1999

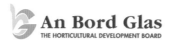

An Bord Glas

THE HORTICULTURAL DEVELOPMENT BOARD

Ballymore Inn

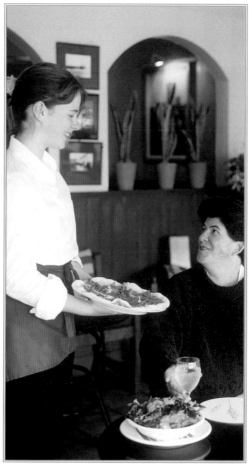

Grilled Fennel, Roasted Peppers,
Basil & Ardrahan Pizza

An Bord Glas congratulates

BALLYMORE INN

winner of
Vegetarian Dish of the Year

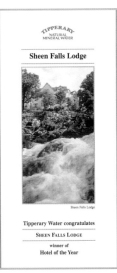

Sheen Falls Lodge

Tipperary Water congratulates

SHEEN FALLS LODGE

winner of
Hotel of the Year

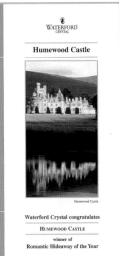

Humewood Castle

Waterford Crystal congratulates

HUMEWOOD CASTLE

winner of
Romantic Hideaway of the Year

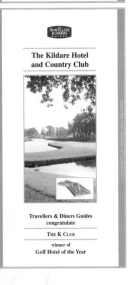

The Kildare Hotel and Country Club

Travellers & Diners Guides
congratulate

THE K CLUB

winner of
Golf Hotel of the Year

Good Company?

Annual **Travellers and Diners Guides** awards are given to the best food, drink and hospitality establishments throughout Ireland, rewarding excellence in a wide variety of categories.

Copies of the Guide are sold and distibuted to business and leisure tourists and local travellers and diners (including a high proportion of business people and decision makers). The Guide also has its own website and provides establishment reviews for the Irish Times On Line.

If you feel your company or organisation could profit from the promotional benefits – public relations, advertising and internet – associated with sponsorship of awards, or you wish to purchase goldbocked, leather-bound copies of the Guide, please contact Travellers and Diners Guides to arrange a presentation or discuss our award sponsorship packages and special bound copy prices.

The Best.

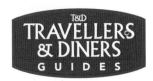

Contact:
Stephen Prendergast
Publishing Director
Travellers and Diners Guides
PO Box 6173, Dublin 13, Ireland
Tel/Fax : +44 (0) 1730 821 995
email: stevep@ireland-guide.com

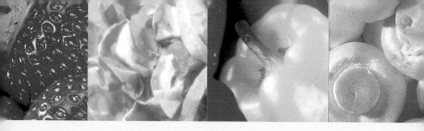

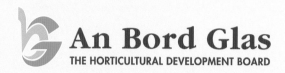

An Bord Glas
THE HORTICULTURAL DEVELOPMENT BOARD

Developing all aspects of Horticulture

SERVICES

Quality Programme

Provision of Market Information

Business Development Programme

Generic Promotion of Horticultural Produce

8-11 Lower Baggot Street   Dublin 2   Ireland

Tel: +353 1 6763567   Fax: +353 1 6767347   Email: Info@BordGlas.ie

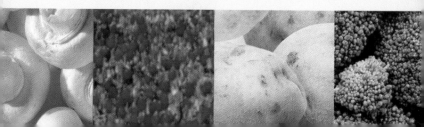

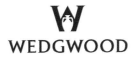

WEDGWOOD

Dessert of the Year

Restaurant
Patrick Guilbaud

Dublin

Since moving to their new premises next door to the
Merrion Hotel in 1998, Restaurant Patrick Guilbaud
has the advantage of more space – including larger
reception and private dining areas and the pleasant
option of opening the main restaurant onto a quiet
sunny terrace in fine summer weather. But behind it all
lies the same highly professional team, headed up by
Patrick himself with the able front of house support of
Restaurant Manager Stephane Robin – and, of course,
the ever-modest Guillaume Lebrun in the kitchen. Our
Dessert of the Year is the kind of dish that could have
originated nowhere else: who but Guillaume could
make a stunning success out of such an unlikely
ingredient as fennel, served in partnership with a classic
nougatine millefeuille? Stranger successes may yet be
to come – meanwhile we applaud Guillaume for this
brilliantly audacious (and utterly delicious) dish.

1999

Bord Bia Irish Awards of Excellence

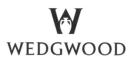

WEDGWOOD

Restaurant Patrick Guilbaud

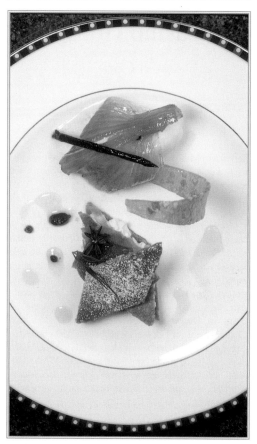

Nougatine Millefeuille served with a Fennel Confit

Wedgwood congratulates

RESTAURANT PATRICK GUILBAUD

winner of
Dessert of the Year

Bord Bia Irish Awards of Excellence

Farmhouse Cheese Award

Casino House

Co Cork

Kerrin and Michael Relja's delightful restaurant is just a few miles west of Kinsale – and yet it's one of the country's best kept secrets. The couple's cool continental style makes a pleasing contrast to their lovely old house, and the warmth of Kerrin's hospitality is matched only by the excellence of Michael's food. Their attention to detail in every aspect of the restaurant is admirable, as is shown by the way they handle cheese. The selection is far from comprehensive, but it is perfectly tailored to the scale of their operation and presented with great care: on the Guide's most recent visit we found a quartet of farmhouse cheeses – Desmond, Durrus and Gubbeen from west Cork plus Cashel Blue from Tipperary – all in excellent condition, served plated with herb-sprinkled sliced tomatoes and a choice of home made bread and crackers. While Irish farmhouse cheeses are now well known and widely available, it is still all to rare to find them handled with such respect.

1999

Bord Bia Irish Awards of Excellence

Casino House

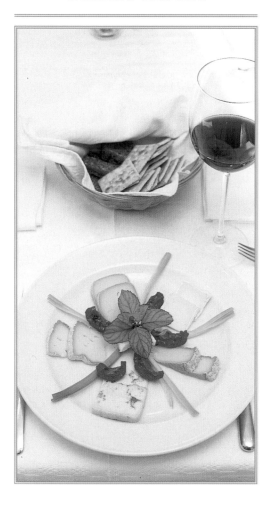

Jacobs congratulates

CASINO HOUSE

winner of
The Farmhouse Cheese Award

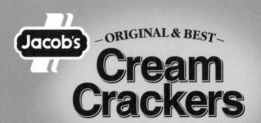

Jacob's — ORIGINAL & BEST — Cream Crackers ~ SINCE 1885 ~

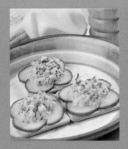

TUNA CRUNCH

Mix a tin of tuna with some sweetcorn. Add in a tablespoon of mayonnaise and a teaspoon of tomato ketchup. Spread thickly on to a Jacob's Cream Cracker topped with a couple of slices of cucumber. Season with black pepper before eating.

SPICY PRAWN

Mix some cottage cheese with finely chopped spring onion. Spread on to a Jacob's Cream Cracker. Place three or four fresh peeled prawns on to the mix and season with paprika.

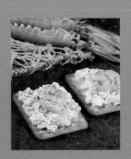

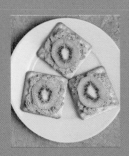

FRUIT PATE

A thick spread of your favourite pate topped off with a slice of succulent kiwi. A savoury and sweet Jacob's Cream Cracker suitable for any time.

MINI PIZZA

Ideal for entertaining or a tasty lunch. Spread some tomato puree onto a Jacob's Cream Cracker. Add a little mozzarella and then top with your favourite pizza toppings. For example, we chose salami and ham. Place under a moderately heated grill until the cheese is melted. Serve hot.

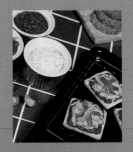

TOP THEM WITH YOUR IMAGINATION

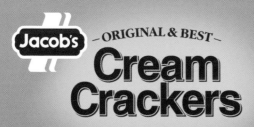

Jacob's — ORIGINAL & BEST — Cream Crackers — SINCE 1885 —

CREAM OF THE SEA

Thickly spread cream cheese on to a Jacob's Cream Cracker. Then place a generous slice of smoked salmon neatly on top. Finish off with a squeeze of fresh lemon juice and serve.

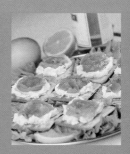

MEXICAN MIX

An exciting way to spice up a party! Peel and slice half an avocado on to a buttered Jacob's Cream Cracker. Chop some spring onion and a green pepper and sprinkle on top of the avocado. Add a small pinch of chilli powder and a squeeze of lemon juice to taste.

BLUE ORCHARD

Slices of green apple arranged alternatively with some slices of blue cheese on a Jacob's Cream Cracker. A tasteful way to finish a pleasant meal.

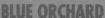

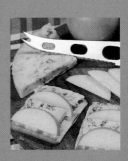

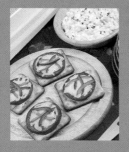

MOZZARELLA MUNCHIE

Top a Jacob's Cream Cracker with a large slice of juicy tomato. Grate some mozzarella cheese and sprinkle it on top. Add some slices of green and red pepper and pop into the microwave for 15-20 seconds (per cracker). Eat hot served with coleslaw.

TOP THEM WITH YOUR IMAGINATION

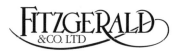

Wine List of the Year

Moyglare Manor
Maynooth, Co Kildare

Wine is the particular passion of Shay Curran, Manager at Moyglare Manor – he takes great pride in ensuring that his list is kept up to date and that everything listed is always available. No mean feat this, with 335 bins to maintain. Deep pockets are required for many of the best vintages (some of them now rare) as is to be expected. But connoisseurs will be happy to have the choice of shelling out, say £1050.00 for a 1961 Chateau Mouton Rothschild Premier Grand Cru Classe ("the gold dust of the wine world") and close reading reveals a fair selection under £20 and even a sprinkling under £15 (including some from the special selection of ten or so Wines of the Month). The list runs to some 16 pages and is clearly laid out with informative notes on regions and vintages. World wines are represented, but the great strength of the list is its classic French wines, particularly Bordeaux. Lovers of Sauternes will be delighted by the choice of no less than thirty vintages of Chateau d'Yquem Grand Crus Classe!

1999

Bord Bia Irish Awards of Excellence

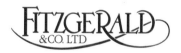

Moyglare Manor

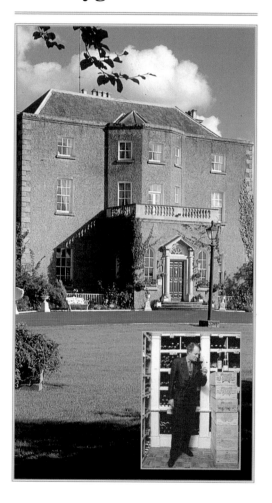

Fitzgerald & Co. congratulates

MOYGLARE MANOR

winner of
Wine List of the Year

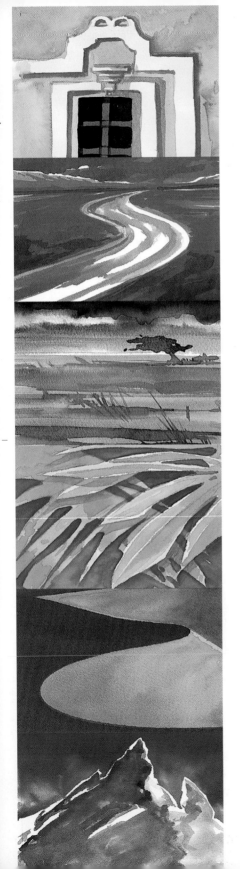

Stril
in A

There was a time whe

all came from South A

in the opposite directio

was the only Argentine

Wine Magazine's Inter

It's just one of a delici

style wines from one o

premium wine produc

Enjoy the taste of Etch

Chardonnay, Cabernet

and see for yourself w

return to South Ameri

RI
PL

DISTRIBUTED BY: FITZG

ng Gold

gentina

most precious gold items in the world

a. These days, they're travelling

o de Plata Cabernet Sauvignon

to be awarded a Gold Medal in

al Wine Challenge 1997.

nge of New World

entina's best known

o de Plata

gnon and Malbec soon

much gold is set to

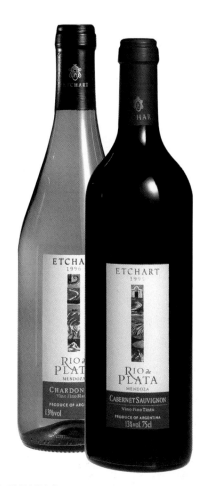

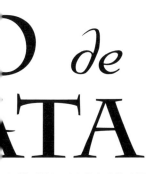

& CO. LTD., 11/12 BOW STREET, DUBLIN 7.

Cork Dry Gin

Hosts of the Year

Ray Byrne
& Jane English,
Wineport Restaurant
Co Westmeath

Ray Byrne and Jane English opened their wonderful lakeside restaurant Wineport in the dark days of February, 1993. Since then they have worked tirelessly on improvements – the restaurant is now much bigger and includes a private dining room, The Chart Room – but, most of all, they have made many friends who now see Wineport almost as a second home. For, as well as its stunning location, it is the hospitality at Wineport that draws guests back time and again – guests who return with additions to the now famous Wineport collections (nauticalia, cats), guests who just feel like spending time with their friends Ray and Jane and their terrific staff. Although easily reached by road, guests often arrive at Wineport by boat, or even by seaplane. But it says a lot about the hospitality at Wineport that Ray and Jane will make sure people get home safely too – by arranging a complimentary taxi service in the Athlone area.

1999

Bord Bia Irish Awards of Excellence

Cork Dry Gin

Ray Byrne
& Jane English

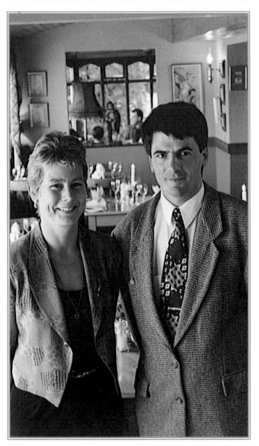

Jane English and Ray Byrne

Cork Dry Gin congratulates

RAY BYRNE & JANE ENGLISH

joint winners of
Hosts of the Year

Bord Bia Irish Awards of Excellence

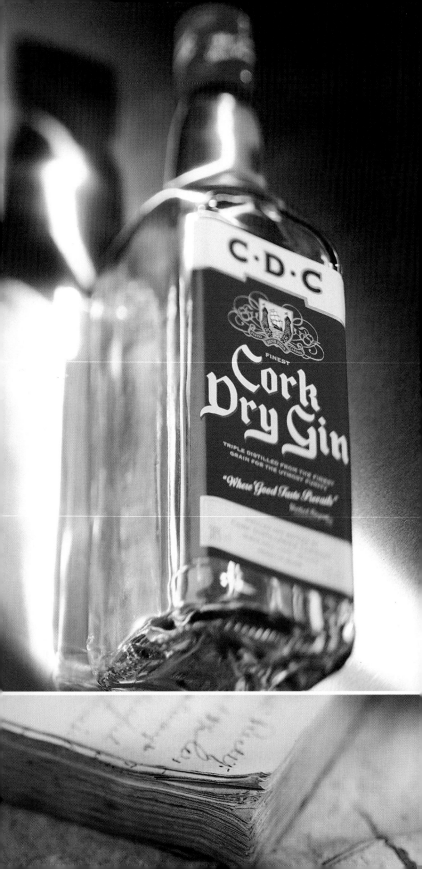

When It Comes To Perfecting A Unique Tasting Gin, Mr Coldwell Wrote The Book.

In 1799, a distiller at Old Watercourse, William Coldwell, began recording the development of a recipe for a fine gin. His recipe book, which has been handed down through eight generations of Cork distillers, was the inspiration for one of the finest tasting gins in the world - Cork Dry Gin.

Today, that book is jealously guarded at the offices of the Cork Distilleries Company. However, if you want to know how the story ends - simply taste a Cork Dry Gin. We think you'll agree, it's a rather thrilling climax.

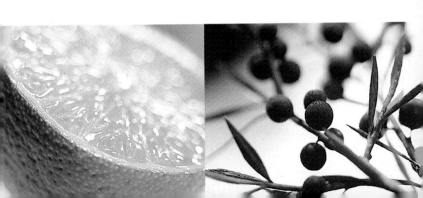

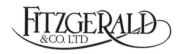

Sommelier of the Year

Breda McSweeney
Lacken House Restaurant
Kilkenny

Breda McSweeney has taken a special interest in wine since 1983 when she and her husband Eugene bought Lacken House in Kilkenny, setting up the establishment that was soon to become the leading restaurant in the area. Since passing her first professional examination with distinction in 1984, Breda has progressed steadily through a long and distinguished series of examinations and competitions. 1994 was a particularly good year for her, as she was winner of both the Sopexa Grand Prix in Ireland and the Irish Guild of Sommeliers' Wine Waiter of the Year. Breda has also represented Ireland on many occasions, notably at the 'Association Sommelier International' World Sommelier final in Paris in 1989 and, most exciting of all, at the same competition final in Tokyo in 1995. She also passes on her extensive knowledge of wine to others in her role as a lecturer. All of which means that guests at her Lacken House Restaurant are exceptionally fortunate, benefitting from her exceptional expertise in wine (and her enthusiasm and dedication) on a daily basis.

1999

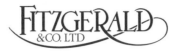

Breda McSweeney

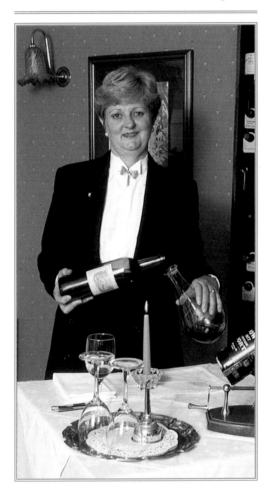

Fitzgerald & Co. congratulates

BREDA MCSWEENEY

winner of
Sommelier of the Year

Bord Bia Irish Awards of Excellence

RATHBORNES
ESTABLISHED 1488

Table Presentation of the Year

The Bakery Restaurant

Wicklow

This lovely restaurant has great character, partly because the fine stone building has retained some of its old bakery artefacts, including the original ovens in the café downstairs. But most of the credit must go to the artistic endeavours of owner Sally Stevens, who has a keen eye for detail and an understanding of the strength of understatement. Lots of candles in the reception area and restaurant set a warm tone which is then complemented by an admirably restrained theme – stone walls and beams provide a dark background for quite austere table settings. These feature white linen tablecloths with the napkins laid simply folded in a square in the place setting; beside it there might typically be two sets of white flowers, a large and a small vase, on each table – all lit by white candles.

1999

Bord Bia Irish Awards of Excellence

RATHBORNES
ESTABLISHED 1488

The Bakery
Restaurant

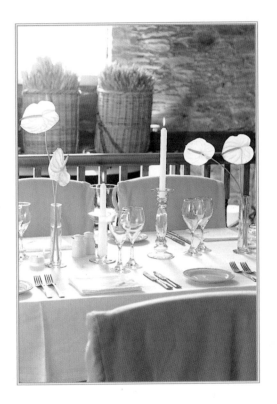

Rathbornes Candles congratulates

THE BAKERY RESTAURANT

winner of
Table Presentation of the Year

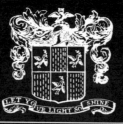

RATHBORNES

ESTABLISHED 1488

Turn

the

evening

into

an

occasion

RATHBORNE CANDLES
132 EAST WALL ROAD, DUBLIN 3, IRELAND,
TEL: + 353 1 8743515, FAX: + 353 1 8365987

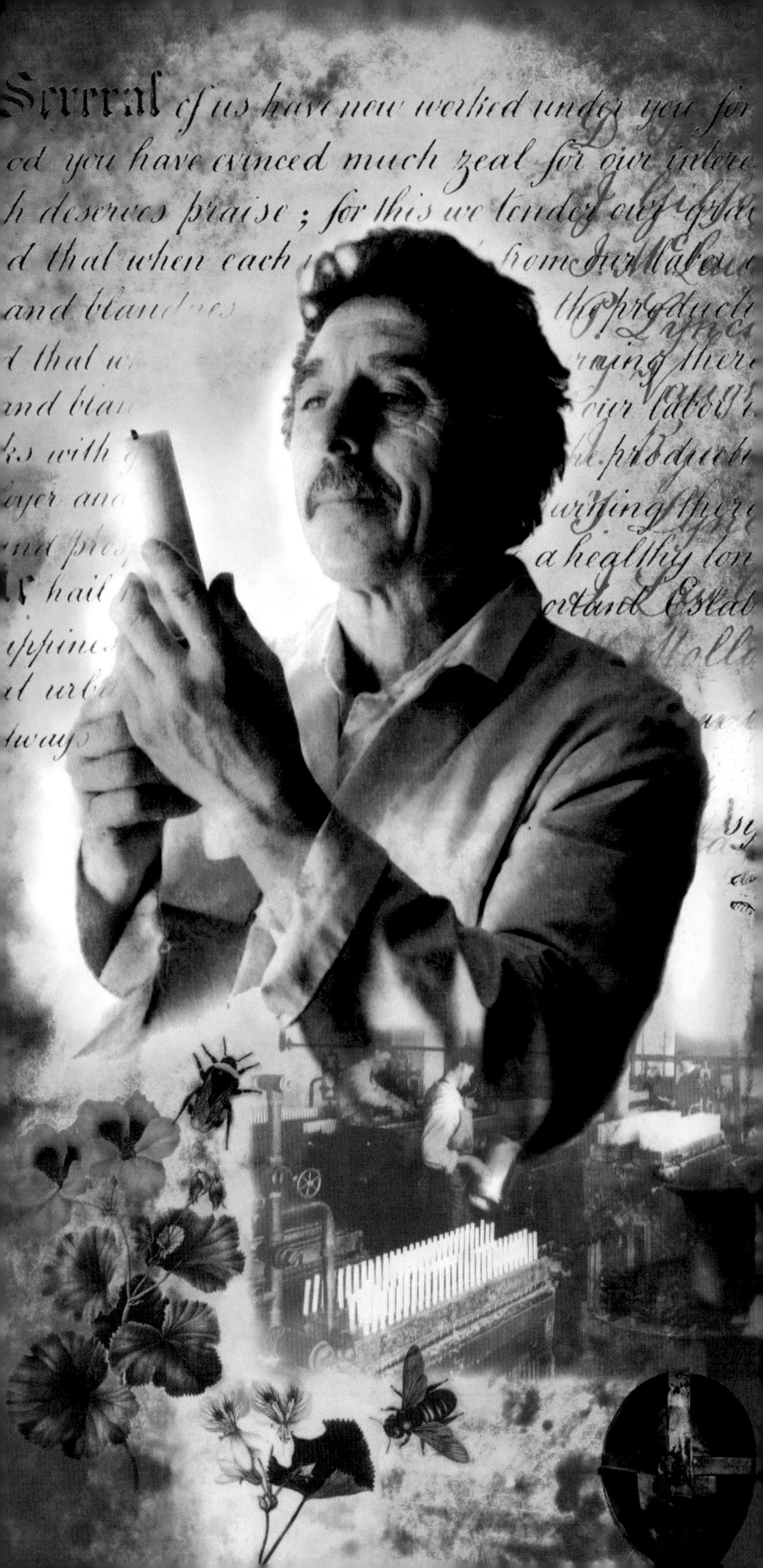
Several of us have now worked under you for
ed you have evinced much zeal for our intere
h deserves praise ; for this we tender our

RATHBORNES
ESTABLISHED 1488

Atmospheric Restaurant of the Year

Restaurant Le Chateau

Athlone, Co Westmeath

A Presbyterian church in Athlone has recently taken on a new lease of life since Steven and Martina Linehan moved Le Chateau – the restaurant they first opened in 1989 – a couple of hundred yards down the hill to its present quayside location. The church, which was closed in the early 1970s, has been magnificently transformed to provide a two-storey restaurant of great character. As well as the couple's established reputation for excellent food and hospitality – and facilities ranging from wheelchair access and air conditioning to a full bar – the restaurant's main attraction is now the atmosphere created by this dramatic conversion. Designed around the joint themes of church and river, the upstairs section has raised, galleon-like floors at each end, while the church theme is reflected in the windows – notably an original "Star of David" at the back of the restaurant – and the general ambience, which is very atmospheric. Candles are used generously to create a relaxed, romantic atmosphere, as they were also in the old Restaurant le Chateau (where the Linehans established the Candlelight Dinner Menu for which they are now renowned).

1999

RATHBORNES
ESTABLISHED 1488

Restaurant
Le Chateau

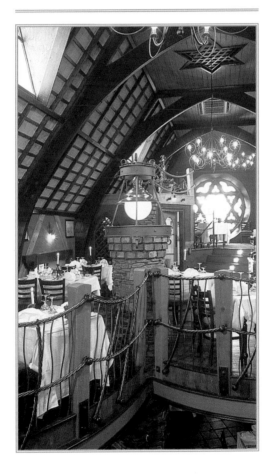

Rathbornes Candles congratulates

RESTAURANT LE CHATEAU

winner of
Atmospheric Restaurant of the Year

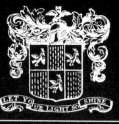

RATHBORNES
ESTABLISHED 1488

Turn
the
evening
into
an
occasion

RATHBORNE CANDLES
132 EAST WALL ROAD, DUBLIN 3, IRELAND,
TEL: + 353 1 8743515, FAX: + 353 1 8365987

Several of us have now worked under you for
...od you have evinced much zeal for our intere...
...h deserves praise; for this we tender our grat...
...d that when each ... from ...labour...
...and blandnes... the product...
...d that w... raying there...
...nd blan... our labour...
ks with ... product...
...yer and ... writing there...
...nd pro... a healthy ton...
...r hail ... ortant Estab...
...ppines... Volla...
...t urb...
...tways

Pub of the Year

The Porterhouse

Dublin

When The Porterhouse opened in 1996, it changed Dubliners' perception of what "a good pub" should be and opened up a whole new range of possibilities that hadn't been considered before. It was, for a start, Ireland's first micro-brewery, and although several others have set up since and are doing an excellent job, it was The Porterhouse that started this new trend in the brewing of real ale. They make a selection of ten beers on the premises, several of which have won international awards, and beer connoisseurs can sample a special "tasting tray" selection. But you don't even have to like beer to love The Porterhouse. The loving attention to detail which has gone into the design is a constant source of pleasure to visitors – the bottles in glass cases that line the walls, the brewing-related displays in glass-topped tables – and the food, while definitely not gourmet, is a cut above the usual bar food and, like the pub itself, combines elements of tradition with innovation. This is a real Irish pub in the modern idiom and we applaud it.

1999

Bord Bia Irish Awards of Excellence

JAMESON The Spirit of Ireland

The Porterhouse

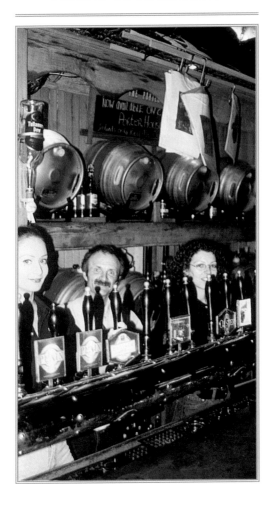

Jameson congratulates

THE PORTERHOUSE

**winner of
Pub of the Year**

Bord Bia Irish Awards of Excellence

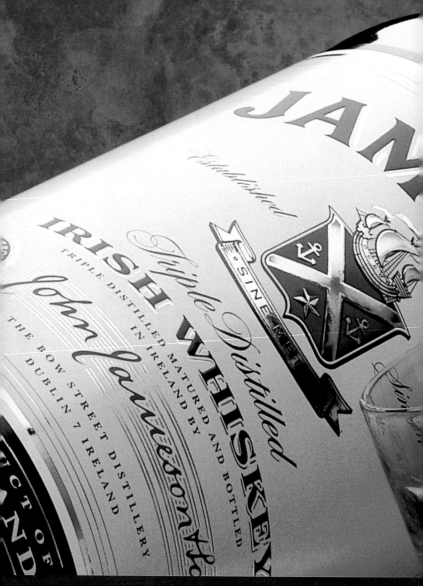

Smoothest

Before maturing our whiske
distil it a third time. We think you'
gives our whiskey a

JAMESON® The

Whiskey.

or many years, we like to
ind this rather unique finishing touch
xceptional smoothness.

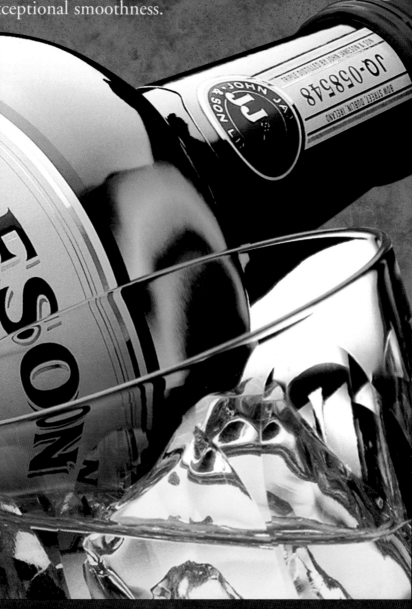

Spirit of Ireland

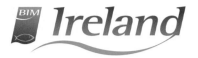

BIM *Ireland*

Seafood Pub
of the Year

Moran's Oyster Cottage
Kilcolgan, Co Galway

This is just the kind of Irish pub that people everywhere dream about. It's as pretty as a picture with a well-kept thatched roof and a lovely waterside location with plenty of seats outside (where you can while away the time and watch the swans floating by). It's brilliantly well-run by the Moran family – and so it should be, after all they've had six generations to practice – who are famed throughout the country for their wonderful local seafood, especially the native oysters (from their own oyster beds) which are in season from September to April. Willie Moran is an ace oyster opener, a regular champion in the famous annual competitions held in the locality, and they have the farmed Gigas oysters on the menu all year. Then there's chowder and smoked salmon and seafood cocktail and mussels – and, perhaps best of all – delicious crab sandwiches and salads.

1999

Bord Bia Irish Awards of Excellence

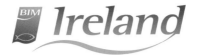

Moran's
Oyster Cottage

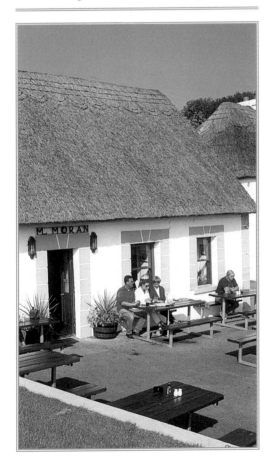

BIM congratulates

MORAN'S OYSTER COTTAGE

winner of
Seafood Pub of the Year

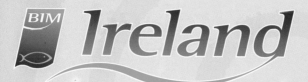

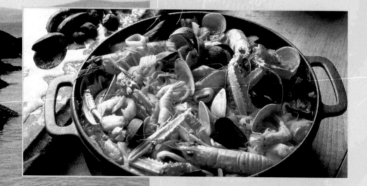

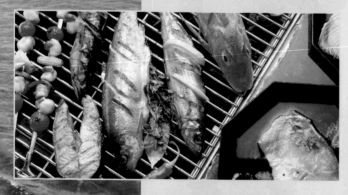

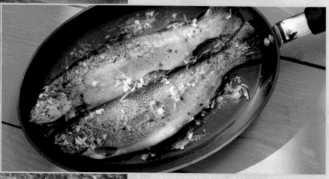

IRISH SEA FISHERIES BOARD/BIM, P.O. BOX 12
CROFTON RD, DUN LAOGHAIRE, CO. DUBLIN, IRELAND
TEL: + 353 1 2841544   FAX: + 353 1 2841123

Get hooked on seafood !

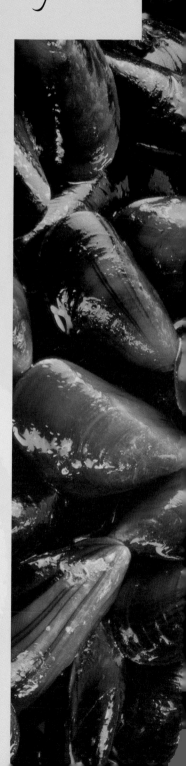

Gastronomic . .

The food of a country is part of its history and civilisation and if you haven't tasted the salmon of knowledge or sang Ireland's second national anthem "Crying cockles and mussels alive alive o" then do so before you leave this emerald isle.

Take a gastronomic sea adventure around Ireland and taste the fruits of its seas and rivers. Get hooked on seafood on any of the 28 inhabited islands around the coast. Visit and see up to sixty varieties of fish being landed at any of Ireland's ten main ports or more than one hundred smaller fishing ports whose fishermen send high quality fish, the freshest in the world on a daily basis to the kitchens of the country.

Try turbot, brill, sole and salmon, lobster, prawns, swordfish and tuna in some of our renowned restaurants or breakfast on a symphony of seafood in some of our country homes and friendly B&Bs.

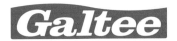

Irish Breakfast Award

Anglesea Town House
Dublin

Bord Bia Irish Awards of Excellence

Helen Kirrane's Anglesea Town House brings all the best "country" qualities to urban Dublin – a delightful building and pleasant location near Herbert Park, Ballsbridge; comfortable, attractive bedrooms with a very high standard of daily housekeeping; and a warm, welcoming drawingroom with a real period flavour (with books of art on display). But no-one who stays at the Anglesea Town House can forget perhaps its most distinctive feature – the delicious, generous breakfasts that prepare guests for the rigours of the most arduous of days, whether as a tourist or a business traveller. A request for fruit brings several cut glass bowls with different varieties, which may include delicious stewed rhubarb, along with the Anglesea's own baked cereal with cream (thoroughly recommended); the cooked breakfast can vary between variations on such favourites as kedgeree, omelettes or a full Irish breakfast, all of which are excellent. As if this were not enough, a genius in the kitchen conjures up delicious, delicate pastries which are brought to one's table just when it seemed things were as good as they could get. Thoroughly recommended for its creativity and perfectionism in re-defining what a good breakfast can be, and a very worthy winner.

1999

Galtee

Anglesea Town House

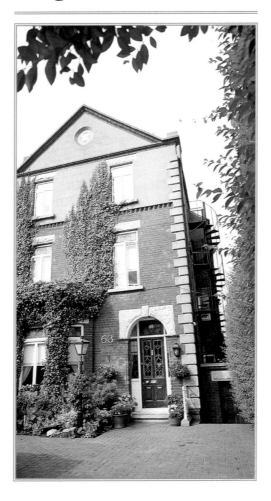

Galtee congratulates

ANGLESEA TOWN HOUSE

winner of
The Galtee Irish Breakfast Award

Bord Bia Irish Awards of Excellence

Taste the Galtee Difference!

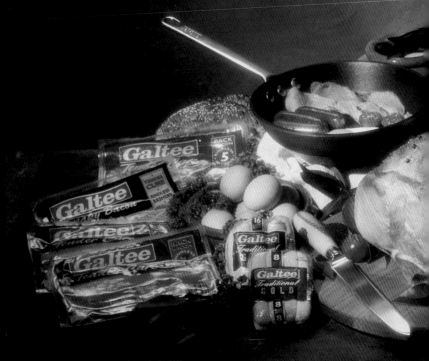

Enjoy the traditional Irish breakfast at its best

Galtee have always been synonymous with traditional cooked breakfasts. Irish people both at home and abroad insist on the unique taste of Galtee, which is unequalled anywhere in the world!

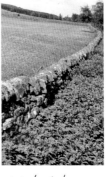

There's no doubt that we're very fussy about what we want in a traditional Irish breakfast, no matter where we are.

Breakfast has always been an important part of Irish everyday life and Galtee is an essential part of that tradition. For generations it has been the fuel which helps a nation start the day and is still every bit as popular today.

It's hard to beat the taste and aroma of cooked bacon and sausages in the morning or, at any other time of the day! That's why Galtee rashers are the best selling brand in Ireland and are one of the 3 most requested food products by Irish people living abroad.

We insist on Galtee when we want the best taste and turn to home when we want the guarantee of one of Irelands best known and loved brands. After all, home is where the Galtee is!!

Galtee

BUSHMILLS

International Hospitality Award

Johnny & Lucy Madden
Hilton Park

Clones, Co Monaghan

Johnny and Lucy Madden's wonderful 18th century mansion Hilton Park has been described as a "capsule of social history" because of its collection of family portraits and memorabilia going back 250 years or more. On 200 acres of woodland and farmland (home to Johnny's champion rare breed sheep) with lakes, Pleasure Grounds and a Lovers' Walk to set the right tone, the house is magnificent in every sense, and the experience of visiting it a rare treat indeed. Johnny and Lucy are natural hosts, and as the house and its contents go back for so many generations, there is a strong feeling of being a privileged family guest as you wander through grandly-proportioned, beautifully furnished rooms, A special pleasure is sitting in the dining room watching the light fading over the garden (after enjoying the produce from the lakes or the organic garden), but it's the warmth of Johnny and Lucy's welcome that lends that extra magic.

1999

Bord Bia Irish Awards of Excellence

BUSHMILLS

Johnny & Lucy Madden

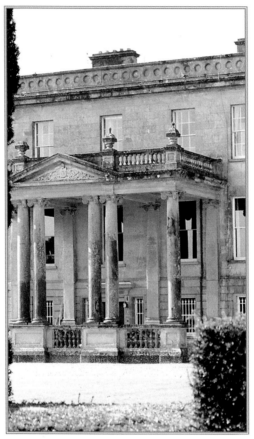

Hilton Park

Bushmills congratulates

JOHNNY & LUCY MADDEN

winners of
The International Hospitality Award

Our Days Are often Soft, Our Malt Is always Mellow.

Close by the stunning Antrim coast, nestles the time-touched village of Bushmills.

There, in a distillery licenced since 1608, we first ferment and then triple-distil Irish malted barley. Ten maturing years follows in American oak bourbon barrels and European oak sherry casks creating the unique mellowness that characterises Bushmills Single Malt Irish Whiskey.

In just one smooth sip, you'll discover why Bushmills Malt was a Gold Medal Winner at the World Spirits Championships and noted as having:

"A silky mouthfeel; a soft, elegant finish with expanding warmth."

Above all, you'll savour a rare softness and mellowness that reflects a quiet land and a warm people.

Come softly to Bushmills Malt. Come softly.

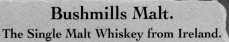

Bushmills Malt.
The Single Malt Whiskey from Ireland.

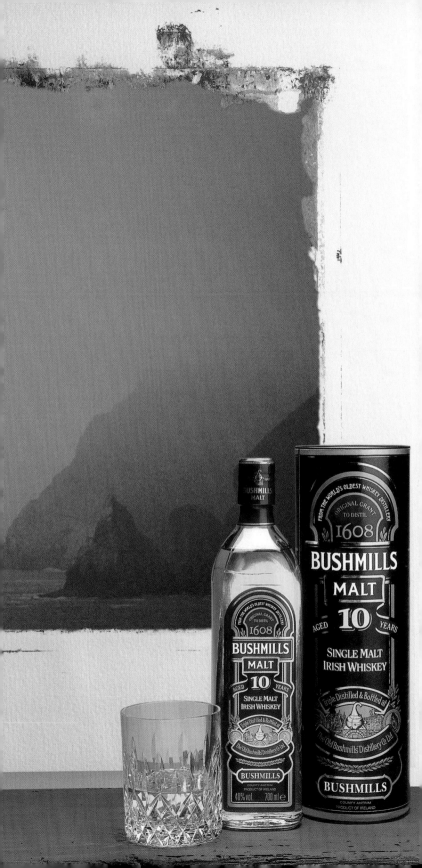

We've got Ireland covered

www.irish-times.com

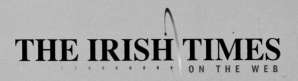

THE IRISH TIMES
ON THE WEB

Bord Bia Irish Awards of Excellence

Business&Finance

Business Hotel
of the Year

Jurys Hotel
and Towers

Dublin

The demands that businesses and business people make on hotels can vary enormously. Business centres, secretarial services, conference and meeting rooms, banqueting, entertaining, computing, presentation, internet and other facilities – all of these features are essential ingredients for any hotel hoping to compete in this highly competitive and specialised market. Both Jurys (currently undergoing a major refurbishment and modernisation) and its associated hotel The Towers provide them all, consistently, and to a very high standard. There have been many new hotels built for the business market in Dublin in recent years, and Jurys has had to ensure that, while it has long been held in high regard as a Dublin institution, it also continued to upgrade its facilities and levels of service to match the increasingly tough competition. This has been done, and perhaps one reason for its continued success is the commitment on the part of all levels of staff to high quality service for its customers, delivered with a friendly and relaxed helpfulness. Added to this are the facilities provided for business (and non-business) guests to relax and unwind after the most demanding of days – complimentary early evening drinks for Towers guests and a pub, cocktail bar and restaurants offering genuine Dublin hospitality, variety and local colour.

1999

Business & Finance

Jurys Hotel
and Towers

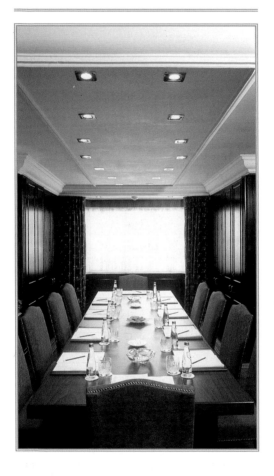

**Business & Finance Magazine
congratulates**

JURYS HOTEL AND TOWERS

**winner of
Business Hotel of the Year**

Bord Bia Irish Awards of Excellence

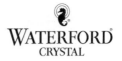

WATERFORD
CRYSTAL

Romantic Hideaway of the Year

Humewood Castle

Co Wicklow

It's impossible to imagine anywhere more romantic to stay than Humewood Castle. A fairytale 19th-century Gothic Revival castle in private ownership, set in beautiful parkland in the Wicklow Hills, it has been extensively renovated and stunningly decorated. While the castle is very large by any standards, many of the rooms are of surprisingly human proportions. Thus, for example, while the main dining room provides a fine setting for some two dozen or more guests, there are more intimate rooms suitable for smaller numbers. Similarly, the luxuriously appointed bedrooms and bathrooms, while indisputably grand, are also very comfortable. Under the professional management of Chris Vos, formerly of The Stafford at St James's Place London, Humewood Castle can also offer fine food prepared by Peter Barfoot, a talented chef who has already made a mark elsewhere in Ireland. Country pursuits are an important part of life at Humewood, but even if you do nothing more energetic than just relax beside the fire, this is a really special place for a weekend for two.

1999

Bord Bia Irish Awards of Excellence

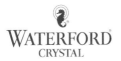

Humewood Castle

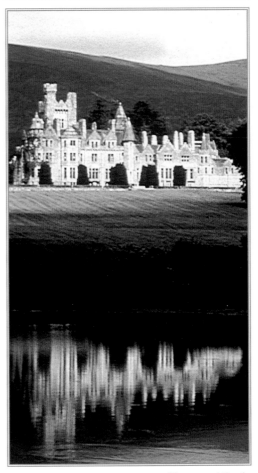

Humewood Castle

Waterford Crystal congratulates

HUMEWOOD CASTLE

winner of
Romantic Hideaway of the Year

Newcomer of the Year

Fitzwilliam Hotel

Dublin

This stylish contemporary hotel enjoys a superb location overlooking St Stephen's Green and close to one of Dublin's main shopping areas. Behind its deceptively low-key frontage lies an impressively sleek interior created by CD Partnership, Sir Terence Conran's design group. Public areas combine elegant minimalism with luxury fabrics and finishes, notably leather upholstery and an unusual pewter bar counter – and, although only open a short time before we went to press, the bar was already becoming established as a chic place to meet in the Grafton Street area. Bedrooms, while quite compact for a luxury hotel, are finished to a high standard with fax/modem points, stereo CD players and mini bars. Care has been lavished on the bathrooms, too, down to details such as a good choice of toiletries. As we went to press Conrad Gallagher's "Peacock Alley" restaurant was poised to move from its South William Street premises to become "Peacock Alley at The Fitzwilliam" (in an upper floor location, close to the roof garden) while the all-day brasserie-style mezzanine restaurant "Christopher's", which is also operated by Gallagher, was already up and running. Although it had not quite settled down at the time of writing, the Guide admires the statement made by The Fitzwilliam; this impressive, confidently modern hotel may well mark the beginning of a new era in Irish hotel design.

1999

Fitzwilliam Hotel

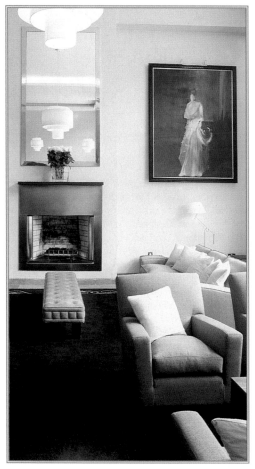

Fitzwilliam Hotel

Travellers & Diners Guides
congratulate

FITZWILLIAM HOTEL

winner of
Newcomer of the Year

Bord Bia Irish Awards of Excellence

Pet Friendly Establishment of the Year

Kylenoe

Co Tipperary

Located close to Lough Derg, in the rolling Tipperary countryside, Virginia Moeran's lovely old stone house on 150 acres of farm and woodland offers home comforts and real country pleasures. The farm includes an international stud and the woodlands provide a haven for an abundance of wildlife including deer, red squirrel, badgers, rabbits and foxes. With beautiful walks, riding (with or without tuition), golf and water sports available on the premises or close by, "Kylenoe" provides a most relaxing base for a break. What's more – and this will be of special interest to visitors from the United Kingdom and Ireland who like to travel with their dogs – this is a place where man's best friend is also made welcome. Dogs may come into the house with their owners and there is a loose box for larger dogs if required at night.

1999

Kylenoe

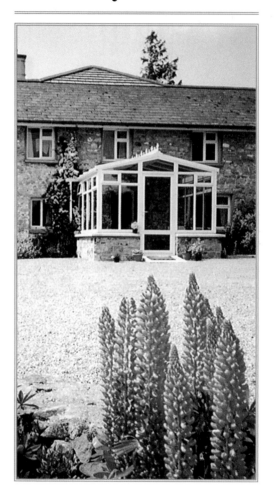

Pedigree & Whiskas congratulate

KYLENOE

winner of
Pet Friendly Establishment of the Year

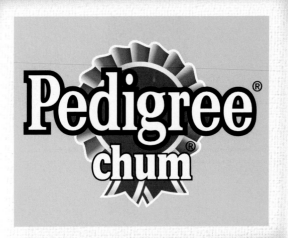

Supporting
Pet Friendly
Accommodation

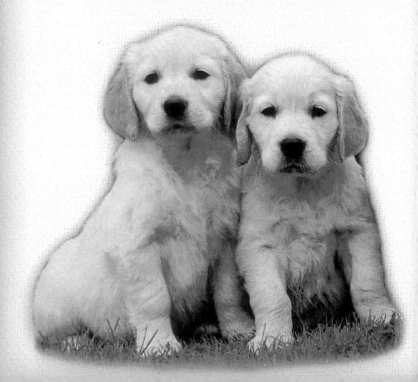

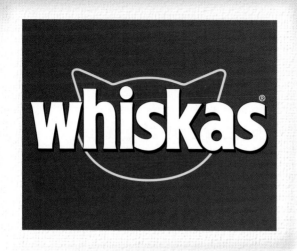

Don't leave home
without your pet!

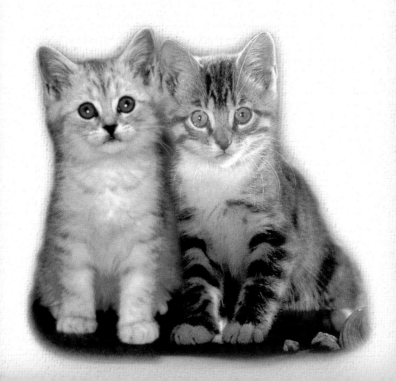

Café of the Year

Michael's Restaurant

Cork

Above Boots the Chemist in the city's main shopping
street, Michael Clifford makes a welcome return,
though in much less formal surroundings than his
previous restaurant. Here you can relax in a large and
bright first-floor room without frills – indeed, there's
even a blackboard above a couple of simple pine
dressers along one wall, indicating daily specials
additional to the menu. However, what has not changed
is his enthusiasm for cooking (he still crosses over to
France to undertake unpaid 'stages' and learn new
techniques from the hands of some of France's greatest
chefs). The menu is not overly long – start with a chili
and sweetcorn chowder, local smoked salmon or
chicken (deep-fried pieces) with Milleens cheese and a
red onion marmalade, to be followed by roast monkfish
with a carrot and orange risotto, sirloin of beef with a
whiskey cream, or oven-baked baby chicken with a
bread and clove sauce. Lunchtime sees simpler dishes
at bargain prices, so it's no surprise to see the place
packed with a lively crowd of workers and shoppers
alike. Service, too, is the business: swift, friendly and
professional. The wine list reflects the atmosphere of
the place, neither pretentious nor expensive.

1999

Michael's Restaurant

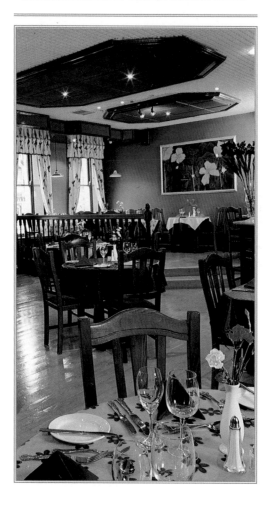

**Travellers & Diners Guides
congratulate**

MICHAEL'S RESTAURANT

winner of
Café of the Year

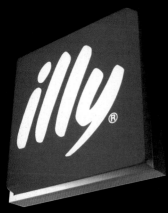

How reassuring that in Ireland too, the illy coffee sign tells coffee lovers where they can indulge their passion.

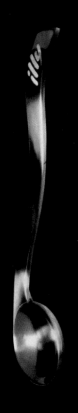

Whether you are a frequent visitor to Ireland or you're here for the very first time, you're always on a quest for the perfect Italian espresso and cappuccino. How reassuring, then, that wherever you travel and wherever you dine throughout Ireland, you know you're in the right place if they serve illy.

Ever since Francesco Illy founded the family company in Trieste 65 years ago, illy's mission has been to offer the entire world the best coffee on earth. The company's passion to produce the perfect, aromatic and rich espresso is evident in every delicious cup of illy coffee in over 40 countries.

illy is dedicated exclusively to espresso. Literally every single coffee bean is checked and sorted twice before blending and roasting. Within 20 minutes of roasting, the beans are pressure sealed with inert gas and matured for 15 days to allow the full flavour to develop.

EXCLUSIVE DISTRIBUTOR IN IRELAND AND NORTHERN IRELAND:
FOOD SOLUTIONS LTD.

Here in Ireland, our Italian-trained illy experts
personally share their expertise with espresso
bartenders, helping them develop and maintain
illy standards. The result: you will always benefit
from the highest Italian level of skill in
preparing impeccable espresso, cappuccino
and other exciting variations.

Many establishments have installed illy's
exclusive l'espresso system - ground, pressed
coffee pods between 2 layers of filter paper
that ensure a simple, fail-safe method of
preparing the perfect espresso in seconds.

To further add to your enjoyment of the
illy experience during your Irish travels,
look for the distinctive illy Designer
Collection. These cups are inspired by a
desire to unite pure creativity with the
time-honoured traditions of a company
that has a mission and a passion for
good coffee.

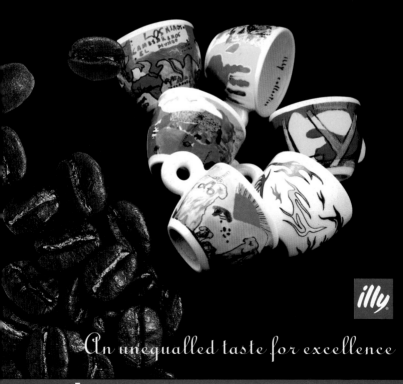

illy

An unequalled taste for excellence

FOR TRADE ENQUIRES ABOUT ILLY COFFEE, THE DESIGNER CUP COLLECTION
AND ESPRESSO EQUIPMENT, CALL RICHARD MARTIN ON CALLSAVE 1850 33 33 22
(FROM NORTHERN IRELAND PLEASE PHONE 00353 42 9322922)

Golf Hotel of the Year

The Kildare Hotel and Country Club

Straffan, Co Kildare

A beautiful, deceptively seductive but extremely demanding 18 hole course, designed by a golfing legend, plus all the back-up facilities and support, in both the hotel and the clubhouse, that may be required to provide succour after defeat or refreshment after victory – what more challenge or reward could a dedicated golfer want? The Kildare Hotel and Country Club, known more commonly as 'The K Club', is a golfer's paradise, providing drama, excitement, beauty and luxury in the context of a 220 acre, Arnold Palmer-designed, par 72, 7,159 yard course. With the same perfectionism and dedication to their guests' pleasure that are associated with everything connected with the K Club itself, the golf course and associated facilities (golf shop, The Legends Bar and Restaurant and the Arnold Palmer Room for private entertaining) are all world class and a pleasure to experience. Some indication of the course's status is indicated by the fact that it regularly hosts a major international tournament, the Smurfit European Open. All these factors combined make the K Club a most worthy winner of the first Travellers and Diners Guides Golf Hotel of the Year award.

1999

Bord Bia Irish Awards of Excellence

TRAVELLERS & DINERS GUIDES

The Kildare Hotel and Country Club

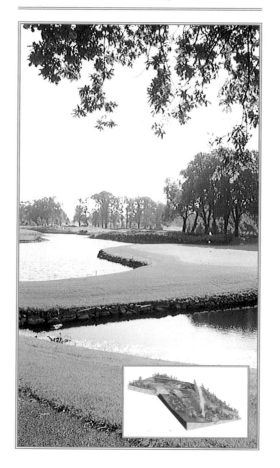

**Travellers & Diners Guides
congratulate**

THE K CLUB

**winner of
Golf Hotel of the Year**

Bord Bia Irish Awards of Excellence

Bord Bia Irish Awards of Excellence

Oriental Restaurant of the Year

The Imperial Chinese Restaurant

Dublin

The rich variety and exoticism of the regional cuisines of China sometimes seem to be "lost in translation" when reproduced in Chinese restaurants in the West. Concessions to blandness are often made to increase the appeal of Chinese food to Western palates. Sadly, the compromises made can result in some dishes becoming uniformly dull, the more exotic ones not appearing at all, and Chinese cuisine in general acquiring a reputation for not being as innovative as, say, the food from Thailand. The Imperial has bucked this trend and presents a menu of both regular favourites, done with a real concern for the authenticity of dishes (even with such modest dishes as spring rolls), along with an extensive special menu of more obscure dishes. Fixed-price three-course lunches are very good value, as is Sunday dim sum. It should come as no surprise therefore that the restaurant, run by Mrs Cheung and her team, is strongly supported by perhaps that most demanding group of customers, the local Chinese community.

1999

The Imperial Chinese Restaurant

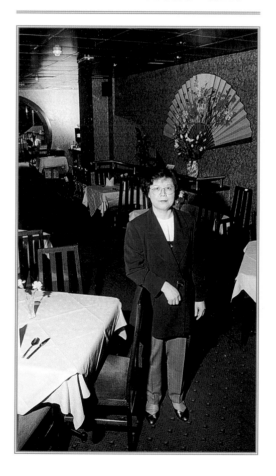

**Travellers & Diners Guides
congratulate**

THE IMPERIAL CHINESE RESTAURANT

**winner of
Oriental Restaurant of the Year**

Bord Bia Irish Awards of Excellence

Bord Bia Irish Awards of Excellence

**Travellers & Diners Guides
congratulate**

Ballymakeigh House
Killeagh, Co Cork
Farmhouse of the Year

Newport House
Newport, Co Mayo
Country House of the Year

Hanora's Cottage
Clonmel, Co Waterford
Guesthouse of the Year

1999

1999 Winners

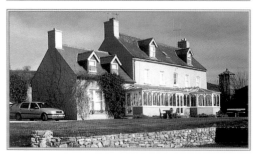

Ballymakeigh House

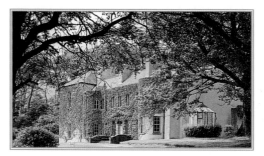

Newport House

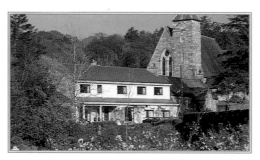

Hanora's Cottage

Bord Bia Irish Awards of Excellence

Euro-Toques

Guardians of European Food

Euro-Toques is a 2,500 strong association of chefs throughout Europe who have banded together in order to preserve the quality of natural and traditional foods. They are committed to supporting producers of the best foods in Europe, so that the fine quality and flavour of ingredients can be maintained. By the same token, they also wish to maintain the traditional dishes and the traditional ways of preparing and cooking the regional foods of Europe.

Euro-Toques sees itself as guardian of European cultures of good food and of a good quality of life. It is not an elitist organisation but open to members who wish to follow a code of honour which includes a commitment to promote the use of fine quality and traditional artisan foods and to avoid convenience products.

Each country operates a Chapter through a group of commissioners led by a Commissioner-General – Ireland's is currently Derry Clarke of L'Ecrivain, Dublin – supported by a Founder Member and regional Commissioners. For a small country the Irish Chapter is very strong, with over a hundred members. This is largely due to the inspired leadership and energy of the Irish Commissioners, notably Mrs Myrtle Allen of Ballymaloe House, Cork. She was the Founder Member for Ireland when Euro-Toques was established in 1986 by its first

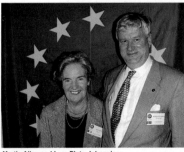

Myrtle Allen and Lars Pluto Johannison

President M Pierre Romeyer, chef-patron of the Brussels restaurant Maison de Bouche. In 1994, Mrs Allen succeeded the famous French chef Paul Bocuse as President. The current President is Lars Pluto Johannison of Sweden

Euro-Toques' foundation was supported by the then President of the EC, M Jacques Delor, who welcomed this "European Community of Cooks". The Brussels connection is extremely important to Euro-Toques, as it is the only organisation of chefs recognised by the EU as a lobbying group on European Food Legislation, and it is in this area that much of the group's most urgent work is done. They have lobbied successfully on topics such as defending the sale of unpasteurised milk cheese and ensuring that the quality aspect of food be a factor in food legislation, rather than simply safety. Current lobbying areas include genetic engineering of food, additives and labelling.

Euro-Toques is responsible for selecting an Irish representative to the world's most prestigious cooking competition, the Bocuse d'Or, which is held in Lyons, France, every two years. Within Ireland they have also nurtured young talent through the Baileys Young Chef Competition which, since 1990, has given some of Ireland's most promising young chefs the opportunity to gain experience under leading chefs in some of Europe's finest kitchens.

There is also a lighter side to the organisation, as each branch organises activities such as mushroom hunts, visits to food producers and a European Day of Taste, when members visit schools to teach young children about taste. In true chef style, Euro-Toques outings involve much bonhomie and, through enjoyment, commitment to their common goal is strengthened.

European Partners

Electrolux and Euro-Toques

Electrolux, the world's largest manufacturer of household appliances, is currently committed to a three year European sponsorship of Euro-Toques. Citing Euro-Toques as "a partner for the new millenium", Electrolux is building on its traditional areas of strength with added concentration on all aspects of Food Care, from safe refrigeration to sophisticated cookery. Euro-Toques and Electrolux share many values and the two organisations are highly compatible: both are concerned to serve their customers good, healthy and exciting food. Restaurateurs need the

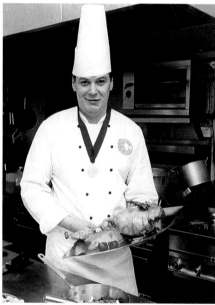

Derry Clarke, Irish Commissioner-General of Euro-Toques

best equipment and Electrolux, with advice from Euro-Toques chefs, will also be well placed to provide home cooks with the best products for preparing top quality meals.

Electrolux aims to position the brand as the authority and leader in food preservation and cooking in Europe. According to Matsola Palm, Head of Global Marketing: "We will be having fun doing what we do best: bringing a stream of innovative and great new products onto the market at competitive prices to help us all to be Europe's favourite chefs."

For a free copy of the booklet listing
Euro-Toques Chefs and Restaurants
of Ireland contact:

Euro-Toques Irish Branch
11 Bridge Court
City Gate
Dublin 8
Tel: + 353 1 677 9999

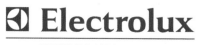

ELECTROLUX GROUP (IRELAND) LTD.

127

supreme in this town, should look in on the Palace Bar on Fleet Street, Doheny's & Nesbitt's 5 Lr Baggot St and Toners of 139 Lr Baggot Street.

Traditional Irish music haunts include O' Donoghues pub 15 Merrion Row (01 676 2807), The Brazen Head on 20 Lr Bridge Street (01) 679 5186 (the oldest pub in Dublin), and The Merchant 12 Bridge Street (01) 679 3797.

Remember, last orders are at 11.00pm during the winter months and 11.30pm during the summer. However, many of the larger pubs have extended licences at the weekend and serve until 2.00am.

Music Venues

The most popular late night live music venues featuring Irish and international artists include the Mean Fiddler on 26 Wexford Street (01) 475 8555, Break for the Border at Johnson's Place (01) 478 0300, Whelan's of 25 Wexford St (01) 478 0766, DA(Dublin Arts) Club 3 Clarendon Market (01) 671 1130 and The Red Box in the old railway station on Harcourt Street (01) 478 0210. The Red Box also hosts some late night zany club nights with internationally acclaimed DJs.

Shortly before midnight most Fridays and Saturdays, The Gaiety Theatre South King St (01) 677 1717 and The Olympia Theatre 72 Dame St (01) 677 7744 are transformed into lively warrens of late night music with full bar licences. The Olympia tends to feature upbeat live music acts while the Gaiety hosts club nights – a Latin and salsa theme night called Salsa Palace on Fridays and a jazz, rhythm and blues-flavoured night called The Soul Stage on Saturdays. A live jazz and blues supper club is held from 9.30pm until 2.00am on Monday to Wednesday night in Renards of South Frederick Street (01) 677 8876.

The National Concert Hall on Earlsfort Terrace provides a great setting for classical musicians, jazz, folk and dance groups too. An events listing can be obtained by calling (01) 475 1666.

For traditional Irish music haunts, see above in the pub section.

Clubs

Top of the nightclub scene is Lillie's Bordello, Adam's Court off Grafton Street (01) 679 9204, which is a favourite of every tycoon and highflier in town. Its VIP area and members' enclave – The Library – is where anyone who's anyone has to be seen. A phone call to an influential friend in Dublin or to the management beforehand might secure a table in this exclusive area of the club. Also popular among those who like more mainstream music is Renards of South Frederick Street (01) 677 8876. The club features a nightclub in the basement, a live music and bar venue on the ground floor and a stylish members or VIP lounge on the first floor.

Popular among younger, trendy dance lovers is the U2-owned club, The Kitchen, East Essex St (01) 677 6635 which is located in the basement of their Clarence Hotel. Dublin's equivalent of New York's Twilo or London's Ministry of Sound is PoD (Place of Dance) on Harcourt Street (01) 478 0225. The dress code is trendy – if you're wearing a suit, forget it. This emporium of dance is also connected to the trendy Chocolate Bar and the equally trendy live music venue and nightclub haunt, The Red Box.

Many older Champagne Charlies around town head for the piano bar in Buck Whaley's on Leeson Street. Below it is the old wine bar which, like several other basement haunts on this street, is known as "The Strip". There's no cover charge but wines prices are on the high side. "The Strip" is well past its heyday but very late at night in the weekends it can be a lively experience, and if the police don't arrive the parties have been known to go on until sun-up.

Late Night Cafes

Cappuccino and espresso culture has yet to make the impact on nightlife in Dublin that it is making elsewhere. The city's favourite coffee houses, Bewleys of Grafton Street and Westmoreland Street, experimented for a while with late night openings but now shut their doors most nights at 8pm. Check out Tosca in Suffolk Street, a great place to eat or while away the hours people-watching in the front window.

Cybernerds will find internet cafes are now springing up around the city. Cyberia on Temple Lane South in Temple Bar and The Beta Cafe located at the Arthouse Multimedia Centre on Curved Street. Both remain open until 10.00pm weekdays and 11pm weekends. Juice on South Great George's Street will appeal to the health food inclined, with macrobiotic and vegetarian fare, and is open until 11.00pm.

Theatre

Dublin's theatre life is bustling, with dozens of mainstream, fringe and visiting theatre companies jostling for space in the city. The Abbey Theatre on Abbey Street (01) 878 7222 is internationally renowned as a venue for productions of older Irish plays. The Gate Theatre on 1 Cavendish Row (01) 874 4045 is known for staging more modern Irish plays. The Gaiety Theatre South King St (01) 6771717 and The Olympia Theatre 72 Dame St (01) 677 7744 stage mainstream theatre, comedy, musicals, ballets and even pantomimes. Experimental theatre and exhibitions are more the staple of The Project Arts Centre on East Essex Street in Temple Bar (01) 679 6622. Comedy lovers need look no further than Murphy's Laughter Lounge (01) 8744611 on Dublin's Eden Quay. Here they will find local and international stand-up talent on stage from Thursdays through to Sundays.

GALWAY

Galway is something of a hedonist's paradise. Its youthful ambience comes from the large number of students at its University and Regional Technical College, who together comprise a fifth of the city's population. Summer festivals, especially the Galway Arts Festival and the Galway Races, ensure this frantically partying town becomes even more hectic during the high season. Galway boasts a very free-spirited, energetic nightlife which is particularly attractive to younger travellers. The hubs of the action are Shop Street and Quay Street, which are full of pubs, clubs and late night revelry.

Pubs

The biggest and possibly the most popular drinking emporium in the city is Busker Brownes of Cross Street, which is connected to The Slate House of Kirwan's Lane around the corner. This three storey bar situated in a medieval convent will provide a lively introduction to the city. Upstairs in The Slate House will provide some respite from the milling crowds downstairs and a better look at the sixteenth century stonework. Don't be fooled by the deceptively small frontage to The Quays bar on Quay Street. This is also a huge three storey emporium of drink that can also get uncomfortably full late at night.

The Hole in the Wall pub on Eyre Street is a particular favourite of students. Other popular watering holes include Cooke's Thatch Bar on Cooke's Corner, Freeney's of High Street, McSwiggans of Eyre Street and a favourite of older party people, The Skeff Bar in the Skeffington Arms Hotel on Eyre Square. The anti-smoking brigade may want to take note of the small bar called An Tobar on 11 Mainguard Street. It is the only bar, possibly in the entire country, which is a smoke-free zone. Those looking to enjoy some bacchanalian bliss should head for Le Wine Bar at Spanish Arch. Wine is sold by the glass or the bottle. The food menu is an optional extra. Doors close at midnight.

Popular traditional music haunts include Neachtains of Cross Street which has sessions every night of the week. An Pucan Bar on Forster Street is popular with tourists and has traditional music most nights. You'll also catch traditional music sessions in Taafe's of Shop Street and Taylor's Bar on Dominic Street. The stylish O'Flaherty's pub located in the basement of The Great Southern Hotel on Eyre Square also hosts Irish music nights every evening.

Last drinks are generally served at 11.00pm during the winter, 11.30pm during the summer. However, licensing hours are not always strictly adhered to. Some larger pubs have bar extensions until 2.00am especially at weekends and during festival times.

Music

There's no shortage of music in this town. Everything from funk, ska and soul to traditional Irish music resonates through the city after dark. For traditional Irish music bars, see above in the pubs section. The Quays bar on Quay Street has live music, mostly pop or rock acts in the big music hall upstairs, most nights of the week. Traditional music is played downstairs one night a week, usually Monday or Tuesday nights. The King's Head on High Street, The Red Square Bar on Eyre Square and Roisin Dubh and Monroes, both located on Dominic Street, are popular venues with a mixed bag of live acts – rock, blues, jazz, cajun, rhythm and trad. Also hopping seven nights a week with live bands is Paddy's Bar on Prospect Hill. The groovy Blue Note music bar on William Street West attracts a young and trendy crowd. Older swingers head for the jazz sessions at Brennan's Yard Hotel on Lower Merchant's road every Saturday. They often have a stylish music session on Friday nights too. You can also continue swinging on Sunday mornings with Busker Browne's of Cross Street, featuring a Sunday brunch jazz session.

Clubs

Exclusivity is not a feature of Galway's club scene. Unlike Dublin, there are no VIP enclaves, memberships or hierarchies of clubbers. The club scene is quite vibrant but unspectacular. One of the most popular venues is Central Park on Upper Abbeygate Street, which attracts a slightly older age group. It features chart music and commercial dance seven nights a week. Church Lane Night Club on Church Lane aims for a slightly more mature clubber too. It's open Thursday through to Sunday nights. Open seven nights a week is The Alley Night Club, located behind the Skeff Bar on Eyre Square. This is a fairly standard mainstream club aiming for over 21s. For acid jazz and funk, young hip clubbers flock to the GPO Night Club on Eglinton Street. It's open seven nights a week.

Cafes

Cappuccinos, lattes, mochas and espressos are becoming as much a part of Galway's nightlife as pints of stout and lager. Cybernerds have a home in Galway with the city's internet cafe Netaccess located at The Olde Malt Arcade. It will be an early night, however, as it closes at 7.00pm. One option for those who want to avoid pub life is Java's on Upper Abbeygate Street. This coffee shop, serving dozens of blends as well as salads and grazing food, is a favourite with insomniacs, with doors closing around 4.00am. It also features mellow jazz or trad sessions most nights. Books, backgammon, chess and coffee are all part of the ambience of Apostasy on Dominic Street. This nightlife haven also stays open until 4.00am and features poetry reading sessions on Monday nights around 9.30am and acoustic gigs every Tuesday at 10pm. The Cafe Du Journal on Quay Street is another popular option for coffee and a browse through the day's papers. However, it closes a little earlier, at 10.00pm.

Theatre

The Druid Theatre Company located on Chapel Lane off Quay Street (091) 568617 is internationally renowned for its productions of new Irish works. The company spends a lot of time touring, so its productions are quickly booked up whenever they come to Galway. An Taibhdhearc on Middle Street (091) 563600 stages Irish and Irish language productions. Its annual summer show of traditional song, dance and drama is popular with visitors to the city. The Town Hall Theatre on Eyre Square (091) 569777 stages mainstream productions, including many popular Irish plays. Comedy is also springing up in the city. The Murphy's Comedy Club takes place in the GPO Nightclub on Eglinton Street (091) 563073 every Sunday night kicking off at 8.30pm. Admission is £5.

Kathryn Rogers
Kathryn Rogers is a well known
showbusiness and fashion writer.

Republic
of
Ireland

Entries
1999

DUBLIN
A Town for our Times

Dublin is a city whose time has come. It's an old town whose numerous meandering stories have interacted and combined to create today's busy riverside and coastal metropolis. Through a wide variety of circumstances, it has become an entertaining place, ideally suited for the civilised enjoyment of life as the 21st Century gets into its stride.

Dubliners tend to wear their city's history lightly, despite having in their environment so much of the past: ancient monuments, historic buildings, gracious squares and fine old urban architecture that still manages to be gloriously alive. They may not take it quite for granted, but nevertheless they do have to get on with everyday life. Indeed, these days they've a vigorous appetite for it. So they'll quickly deflate any visitor's excessive enthusiasm about their city's significance with some throwaway line of Dublin wit, or sweep aside highfalutin notions of some figure of established cultural importance by recalling how their grandfathers had the measure of that same character when he was still no more than a pup making a nuisance of himself in the neighbourhood pub.

The origins of the city's name are in keeping with this downbeat approach. From the ancient Irish there came something which derived from a makeshift solution to local inconvenience. Baile Atha Cliath – the official name today – means nothing more exciting than "the townland of the hurdle ford". Ancient Ireland being an open plan sort of place, without towns, the future city was no more than a river crossing.

But where the Irish saw inconvenience, the Vikings saw an opportunity. When they brought their longships up the River Liffey, they found a sheltered berth in a place which the locals of the hurdle ford called Dubh Linn – "the black pool". Although the name was to go through many mutations as the Vikings were succeeded by the Normans (while they in turn were in the business of becoming English), today's name of Dublin is remarkably similar to the one which the Vikings came upon, although the old Irish would have pronounced it as something more like "doo-lin".

The name makes sense, for it was thanks to the existence of the black pool that Dublin became the port and trading base which evolved as the country's natural administrative centre. Thus your Dubliner may well think that the persistent official use of Baile Atha Cliath is an absurdity. But it most emphatically isn't the business of any visitor to say so, for although Dublin came into existence almost by accident, it has now been around for a long time, and Dubliners have developed their own attitudes and their own ways of doing things.

Located by a wide bay with some extraordinarily handsome hills and mountains near at hand, the city has long had as an important part of its makeup the dictates of stylish living, and the need to cater efficiently for individual tastes and requirements. Quite often the facade has been maintained through periods of impoverishment, but even in earliest mediaeval times this was already a major centre of craftsmanship and innovative shop-keeping. Today, the Dublin craftsmen and shop-keepers and their assistants are characterful subjects worthy of respectful academic study. And in an age when "going shopping" has become the world's favourite leisure activity, this old city has reinvented herself in the forefront of international trends.

For Dublin virtually shunned the Industrial Revolution, or at least took some care to ensure that it happened elsewhere. The city's few large enterprises tended to be aimed at personal needs and the consumer market, rather than some aspiration towards heavy industry. Outstanding of them all was of course Guinness's Brewery, founded in 1759. Today, its work-force may be much slimmed in every sense, but it still creates the black nectar, and if a new mash is under way up at the brewery and the wind is coming damply across Ireland from the west, the aroma of Guinness in the making will be wafted right into the city centre, the moist evocative essence of Anna Livia herself.

Although some of the vitality of the city faded in the periods when the focus of power had been taken away, today Dublin thrives as one of Europe's most entertaining capitals, and as a global centre of the computing and communications industries. While it may be trite to suggest that her history has been a fortuitous preparation for the needs of modern urban life in all its variety of work and relaxation, there is no denying Dublin's remarkable capacity to provide the ideal circumstances for the new, fast-moving, people-orientated industries. A civilised city where the importance of education is a central theme in the family ethos has helped make it a place of potent attraction in the age of information technology.

Such an ancient and literary city naturally has much of interest for historians (both amateur and professional) of all kinds, and a vibrant modern cultural and literary life is available for visitors and Dubliners alike. You can immerse yourself in it all as deeply as you wish, but a detailed introduction to the city's museums, art galleries, libraries, theatres and cinemas, not to mention its many sporting clubs, is beyond the scope of this guide. However, if you're someone who hopes to enjoy Dublin as we know Dubliners enjoy it, we think you'll find much of value here. And don't forget that there's much of enjoyment in Dublin well hidden from the familiar tourist trails. Just walking with (or without) a map and a guide can bring many hidden surprises.

When Dublin was expanding to its present size during the mid-20th Century, with people flocking in from all over Ireland to find work, it was said that the only real "Dub" was someone who didn't go home for the weekend. Today, with Dublin so popular with visitors, the more cynical citizens might well comment that the surest test of whether someone is a real Dub or not is whether they make a point of avoiding Temple Bar. It is rather unfair for Dubliners to dismiss that bustling riverside hotbed of musical pubs, ethnic restaurants, cultural happenings and nightclubs as being no more than a tourist ghetto or theme park since it is Temple Bar which maintains the Dubliner's international reputation as a round-the-clock party animal.

Yet more often than not it is the wall-to-wall out of town visitors in Temple Bar who do much of the maintenance work on that particular image. For, come nightfall, your discerning Dubliner is as likely to be found in a pleasant pub or restaurant in one of the city's many urban villages, delightfully-named places such as Ranelagh or Rathmines or Templeogue or Stoneybatter or Phibsborough or Donnybrook or Glasnevin or Ringsend or Dundrum or Clontarf or Drumcondra or Chapelizod, to name but a few. And then there are places like Stepaside or Howth or Glasthule or Foxrock or Dalkey, places which are sufficiently distant from the town centre as scarcely to be thought of as being part of Dublin at all. Yet that's where you'll find today's real Dubs, enjoying their fair city every bit as much as city centre folk. Lucky is the visitor who is able to savour it all, in and around this town for our times.

Local Attractions and Information

Abbey and Peacock Theatres	Lower Abbey Street 01 878 7222
Andrew's Lane Theatre	off Exchequer Street 01 679 5720
Bank of Ireland (historic)	College Green 01 661 5933
Christchurch Cathedral	Christchurch Place D8 01 677 8099
Drimnagh Castle (moat, formal 17th century gardens)	Longmile Road 01 450 2530
Dublin Airport	01 814 4222
Dublin Castle	Dame Street 01 677 7129
Dublin Film Festival (April)	01 679 2937
Dublin Garden Festival, RDS (June)	01 490 0600
Dublin International Organ & Choral Festival (June)	01 677 3066
Dublin Theatre Festival (October)	01 677 8439
Dublin Tourism Centre (restored church)	Suffolk Street. 1850 230 330
Dublin Writer's Museum (food writer Theodora Fitzgibbon's portrait)	Parnell Square 01 872 2077
Dublinia	Christchurch 01 475 8137
Gaiety Theatre	South King Street 01 677 1717
Gate Theatre	Cavendish Row 01 874 4045
Guinness Brewery	St. James's Gate 01 453 6700 ext 5155
Hugh Lane Municipal Gallery	Parnell Square 01 874 1903
Irish Antique Dealers Fair, RDS (October)	01 285 9294
Irish Film Centre	Eustace Street 01 679 3477
Irish Museum of Modern Art/Royal Hospital	Kilmainham 01 671 8666
Irish Rugby Union	01 668 4601
Irish Tourist Board/Bord Failte	Baggot Street Bridge 01 602 4000
Iveagh Gardens	Earlsfort Terrace 01 475 7816
Kilmainham Gaol	Kilmainham 01 453 5984
Landsdowne Road Rugby Ground	Ballsbridge 01 668 4601
Mother Redcaps Market	(nr St Patricks/Christchurch) Fri-Sun 10am-5.30 pm

National Botanic Gardens	Glasnevin 01 837 7596
National Concert Hall	Earlsfort Terrace 01 671 1888
National Gallery of Ireland	Merrion Square West 01 661 5133
National Museum of Ireland	Kildare Street 01 677 7444
National Museum of Ireland	Collins Barracks 01 677 7444
Natural History Museum	Merrion Street 01 661 8811
Newman House	St Stephen's Green 01 475 7255
Northern Ireland Tourist Board	Nassau Street D2 01 679 1977
Number Twenty Nine (18c house)	Lower Fitzwilliam Street 01 702 6165
Olympia Theatre	Dame Street 01 677 7744
Point Depot (Concerts & Exhibitions)	North Wall Quay 01 836 6000
Powerscourt Townhouse	South William Street 01 679 4144
Pro Cathedral	Marlborough Street 01 287 4292
Royal Hospital	Kilmainham 01 671 8666
St Michans Church	Dublin 7 (mummified corpses) 01 872 4154
St Patrick's Cathedral	Patrick's Close 01 475 4817
Temple Bar Food Market	Saturdays 11am – 4 pm (all year)
The Dillon Garden	45 Sandford Rd Ranelagh D6 01 497 1308
The Old Jameson Distillery	Smithfield D7 01 807 2355
Tivoli Theatre	Francis Street 01 454 4472
Trinity College Book of Kells and Dublin Experience	01 677 2941
War Memorial Gardens (Sir Edwin Lutyens)	Islandbridge D8 01 677 0236

Dublin 4   66 Townhouse

66 Northumberland Road Ballsbridge Dublin
HOTEL   **Tel: 01 660 0333/660 0471   Fax: 01 660 1051**
Conveniently located at 66 Northumberland Road, Ballsbridge, close to the RDS exhibition centre and with a limited amount of off-street parking, this comfortable guesthouse is well sited for out-of-town guests attending shows or other guests wanting a relaxed, family home feel in a city setting. Breakfast is excellent. • Acc££ • Closed 23 Dec-2 Jan • MasterCard, Visa •

Dublin 1   101 Talbot Restaurant

101 Talbot Street Dublin
RESTAURANT   **Tel: 01 874 5011**
Happy Heart Eat Out Award Winner
Ever since opening 101 Talbot in 1991, Margaret Duffy and Pascal Bradley have created a real buzz around this groundbreaking northside restaurant. Its proximity to the Abbey and Gate theatres and the constantly changing art exhibitions in the restaurant have been partly responsible for drawing an interesting artistic/theatrical crowd, but its popularity with this discerning clientele is also due to the joyfully creative and healthy food that has earned the 101 such a fine reputation from the start. Always interested in experimentation, and very obviously willing to help with any particular dietary requirements (even down to the chef coming out to discuss options with guests), the Mediterranean and Middle Eastern influences at work in the kitchen here explain why there are so many dishes that meet the Irish Heart Foundation's definition of a Healthy Choice, i.e. dishes with lots of fruit and vegetables that are high in fibre and low in fat, especially saturated fat. Vegetarians always get a strong selection of dishes to choose from and there's a uniquely enjoyable wholesomeness across the complete range of dishes. • Daytime£ & D£ Tues-Sat •

Dublin 2   Adams Trinity Hotel

28 Dame Street Dublin
HOTEL   **Tel: 01 670 7100   Fax: 01 670 7101**
email: adamshtl@indigo.ie   www.holiday-ireland.com
Plum in the centre of the city, within a stone's throw of Trinity College, this compact hotel offers a high standard of accommodation at a reasonable rate. Rooms, which include two suitable for disabled guests and 14 executive rooms (including four designated lady executive), are individually decorated and very well-appointed with well-planned en-suite bathrooms and double glazing to cut out noise from the busy street below. The foyer is actually at the back entrance, from Dame Court, which is much handier for dealing with luggage. The Mercantile Bar & Grill, next door, is part of the same premises. • Acc££ •

Dublin 2 — Alexander Hotel

Merrion Square Dublin

HOTEL   Tel: 01 607 3700   Fax: 01 661 5663

email: alexanderhotel@tinet.ie   www.alexanderhotel.ie

This hotel opened in 1997 and is very well situated at the lower end of Merrion Square. Although large and new it is remarkable for classic design that blends into the surrounding Georgian area quite inconspicuously. In contrast to its subdued public face, the interior is strikingly modern and colourful, both in public areas and bedrooms, which are all to executive standard, spacious and unusual. Good conference and business facilities. • Acc££££ • Open all year •

Dublin 4 — Anglesea Townhouse

63 Anglesea Road Ballsbridge Dublin

ACCOMMODATION   Tel: 01 668 3877   Fax: 01 668 3461

Irish Breakfast Award Winner

Helen Kirrane's Anglesea Town House brings all the best "country" guesthouse qualities to urban Dublin – a delightful building and pleasant location near Herbert Park, Ballsbridge; comfortable, attractive bedrooms with a very high standard of daily housekeeping; a warm, welcoming drawing room with a real period flavour (with books of art on display); and, the pièce de resistance, delicious, generous breakfasts that prepare guests for the rigours of the most arduous of days, whether as a tourist or a business traveller. A request for fruit brings several cut glass bowls with different varieties, including delicious stewed rhubarb, along with the Anglesea's own baked cereal (thoroughly recommended); the cooked breakfast can vary between variations on such favourites as kedgeree, omelettes or a full Irish breakfast, all of which are excellent. As if this were not enough, a genius in the kitchen conjures up delicious, delicate pastries which are brought to one's table just when it seemed things were as good as they could get. Thoroughly recommended for its creativity and perfectionism in re-defining what a guesthouse can be, and a very worthy winner. • Acc££ •

Dublin 6 — Ashtons

Clonskeagh Dublin

PUB   Tel: 01 283 0045

This famous pub fronts onto a busy road and is built on a steep slope reaching down to the River Dodder. It has an interesting interior and an unexpectedly tranquil atmosphere at the back, where the river view is always full of interest. There is a restaurant, but it is the range and quality of the lunchtime buffet – a roast, hot dishes including a wide selection of seafood, cold buffet and salads – that has earned this pub its enviable reputation. • Meals£ •

Dublin 4 — Avenue

Belmont Avenue Donnybrook Dublin

RESTAURANT   Tel: 01 260 3738   Fax: 01 260 2797

In 1998 Tom Williams opened his new Avenue restaurant in premises previously occupied by his Courtyard restaurant. The contrast could not be stronger: in place of the (rather dated) traditional comforts of the old restaurant, he now has a strikingly modern glass-domed 160-seater restaurant with an adjoining café and outdoor eating area in the courtyard. Although the guide visited very soon after Avenue opened (June 1998), we were impressed: hospitality and service were excellent, the design of the restaurant is extremely stylish, but not at the expense of comfort, and head chef David Veal's cooking – global cuisine with more than a polite nod to New Irish Cuisine – proved confident and well-judged. Avenue's menus are also unusual – priced in euros as well as punts. • L£ & D£-££ Mon-Sat •

Dublin 2 — Ayumi-Ya Japanese Steakhouse

132 Lower Baggot Street Dublin

RESTAURANT   Tel: 01 662 2233   Fax: 01 288 0478

email: info@ayumiya.ie www.ayumiya.ie

Located on Lower Baggot Street, not far from one of Dublin's most famous pubs, Doheny & Nesbitts, is one of the city's best little restaurants. A simpler, informal cousin of the original Ayumi-Ya in Blackrock, this unpretentious little place is popular with business people who drop in for a quick bite at lunchtime as well as regular evening diners. It has a busy feel, with an open kitchen preparing ultra fresh Japanese classics –

sushi, teriyaki, Japanese curry. Together with its sister restaurant, these are still the only authentic Japanese restaurants in Dublin. • D£-££ daily L except Sat L •

Dublin 2   Bad Ass Café

9-11 Crown Alley Temple Bar Dublin
RESTAURANT   **Tel/Fax: 01 671 2596**

Original and still the best – the Bad Ass Café has been charming youngsters (and a good few oldsters) with its particular brand of wackiness and good, lively food since 1986, when most people running Temple Bar restaurants were still at school. Kids love the food (the Bad Ass burger is still one of the favourites, and very good too), the warehouse atmosphere, the loopy menu and the cash shuttles (from an old shop) that whizz around the ceiling. Thirteen years after opening it is still described as "trendy"! • L£ & D££ daily •

Dublin 4   Bats Bistro

10 Baggot Lane Dublin
RESTAURANT   **Tel: 01 660 0363   Fax: 01 298 5653**
email: aguy@indigo.ie

In a laneway just across the road from the Hibernian Hotel, owner-chef Leonie Guy has built up a well-deserved reputation for good cooking, based on the best of ingredients, at this unpretentious little restaurant. Her food has an indefinable character, best described as home cooking at its best. • L£ daily, D££ Mon-Sat •

Dublin 4   Bella Cuba Restaurant

11 Ballsbridge Terrace Dublin
RESTAURANT   **Tel/Fax: 01 660 5539**

Bella Cuba provides another welcome addition to the wide range of ethnic cuisines now represented in Dublin. Authentic Cuban cuisine is presented at its very best in this small, intimate restaurant, which demonstrates so well the Spanish, Caribbean and South American influences on this unique country's cooking. Pork dishes are prepared particularly well, and the atmosphere, style of cooking and presentation indicate perhaps a greater degree of culinary formality than is normally associated with the region; the Cajun cooking of Louisiana across the Bay of Mexico, for example. Well worth a visit to experience something genuinely different. • L£ Tues-Fri & Sun, D£ daily •

Dublin 4   Berkeley Court Hotel

Lansdowne Road Ballsbridge Dublin
HOTEL   **Tel: 01 660 1711   Fax: 01 661 7238**
www.doylehotels.com

Set in its own grounds, and within easy distance of the city centre, this luxurious hotel is well-known as a haunt of the rich and famous when in Dublin. It is particularly spacious, with groups of seating areas arranged around an impressive chandeliered foyer, with bars, restaurants and private conference rooms leading off it. The hotel is famous for its high standards of service and accommodation, which includes two rooms especially suitable for disabled guests, six suites and 24 executive rooms; 20 of the bedrooms are designated non-smoking. Bedroom amenities include computer modem, mini-bars and luxurious extras such as robes and slippers. On-site facilities, including a hair salon and boutique, are augmented by an arrangement with the exclusive Riverview Club, for tennis, squash and swimming. Excellent meeting and conference facilities are available for up to 450 delegates.• L££ & D£££ • Acc£££ •

Dublin 22   Bewley's Hotel at Newlands Cross

Newlands Cross Naas Road Dublin
HOTEL/CAFÉ   **Tel: 01 464 0140   Fax: 01 464 0900**
email: res@bewleys www.bewleyshotels.com

The lobby gives a good first impression at this new (and recently expanded) budget hotel just off the N7. Bedrooms will confirm this feeling, especially at the price – a room rate of £49 offers a large room with double, single and sofa-bed, a decent bathroom with bath and shower (except four rooms for disabled guests, which are shower only) and excellent amenities including a trouser press, iron and ironing board and fax/modem lines. Many more expensive hotels might take note of these standards. Good business facilities too (boardrooms for meetings from only £49 per day). The attached Bewley's Café provides very acceptable food and there is free parking for 200 cars. • Acc£ •

➤ ## Dublin 2 — The Bistro

4 & 5 Castle Market Dublin
RESTAURANT   Tel: 01 671 5430   Fax: 01 677 6016

Well located in the pedestrianised walkway between the Powerscourt Centre and George's Street Market, this relaxed, family-run restaurant has attractive warm-toned decor, a friendly atmosphere and good food cooked by co-owner Maire Block. Martin and Robert Block manage and look after front-of-house and it's a formula that brings people back. Expect tasty new-wave international cooking, with a few classics – Tarte Tatin, for example. Daily specials offer especially good value. • L£ & D££ daily •

Dublin 18 — Bistro One

Foxrock Village Dublin
RESTAURANT   Tel: 01 289 7711   Fax: 01 289 9858

Service may be a little slow on a busy night, but the food at this interesting first floor neighbourhood restaurant is worth waiting for – there is a little bar on the way in, where guests are greeted and set up in comfort, and the attitude throughout is laid back but not without care. Tempting menus might include 6 or 8 choices per course, with starters such as seared marinated salmon on a chive potato cake or Bistro One's salad with crispy bacon and croutons. The pasta selection can be starter or main course as preferred – fettucine with smoked chicken and wild mushroom perhaps. Main courses include classics such as veal alla milanaise and updated club fare like lamb's liver with streaky bacon and red onion. There are generous side vegetables and a choice of farmhouse cheese; home made ice creams or classic puddings to finish. • D££ Tues-Sat • MasterCard, Visa •

Dublin 8 — Brazen Head

20 Lower Bridge Street Dublin
PUB   Tel: 01 679 5186   Fax: 01 677 9549
email: info@brazenhead.com www.brazenhead.com

Dublin's (possibly Ireland's) oldest pub was built on the site of a tavern dating back to the 12th century – and it's still going strong. Strong on genuine character, this friendly, well-run pub has lots of different levels and dark corners. Food is wholesome and middle-of-the-road at reasonable prices. Live music every night in the Music Lounge. • L£ & D£ daily •

Dublin 2 — Brooks Hotel

59-62 Drury Street Dublin
HOTEL   Tel: 01 670 4000   Fax: 01 670 4455

A city sister for the Sinnott family's hotels in Galway – the Connemara Gateway and the Connemara Coast – Brooks is very well located, close to the Drury Street multi-storey car park and just a couple of minutes walk from Grafton Street. Described as a "designer/boutique" hotel, it's high on style in a comfortable country house-cum-club fashion and has been furnished and decorated with great attention to detail. There are four rooms designed for disabled guests and 30 designated no-smoking; all rooms have exceptionally good amenities, including well-designed bathrooms with power showers as well as full baths, air conditioning, ISDN lines, teletext TV and many other features. The hotel also has conference facilities/ meeting rooms (70/20) with back-up business services available on request, and a restaurant, Francesca's. • Acc££££ •

Dublin 2 — Bruno's

30 East Essex Street Temple Bar Dublin
RESTAURANT   Tel: 01 670 6767   Fax: 01 677 5155

Open since 1997, Bruno's is starting to make quite an impact on the Dublin dining scene. It's stylish, with clean lined lightwood and plain white walls providing a pleasingly simple background for owner-chef Bruno Berta's contemporary cooking. • L£ & D££ Mon-Sat •

Dublin 2 — Burlington Hotel

Upper Leeson Street Dublin
HOTEL   Tel: 01 660 5222   Fax: 01 668 8086

Ireland's largest hotel, the Burlington has more experience of dealing with very large numbers efficiently and enjoyably than any other in the country. All bedrooms have been refurbished within the last two years and banquets for up to 2200 guests are not only catered for but can have a minimum choice of three main courses on all menus. The Burlington also offers particularly good facilities for business guests; all rooms have email sockets and 250 of the 520 bedrooms are designated executive, with fax machines (and air conditioning). Conference/banqueting facilities are available for up to 2000 and there are 20 meeting rooms with excellent facilities and backup business services. On-site entertainment is available at Annabel's night club and their bar, Buck Mulligan's, has won awards for the last three years. • Acc££££ • Open all year •

Dublin 4 — Butlers

44 Lansdowne Road Ballsbridge Dublin

ACCOMMODATION   Tel: 01 667 4022   Fax: 01 667 3960

email: cmo@indigo.ie

On a corner site in the "embassy belt" and close to the Lansdowne Road stadium, this large townhouse/guesthouse has been extensively refurbished and luxuriously decorated in a Victorian country house style. Public rooms include a comfortable drawing room and an attractive conservatory-style dining room where breakfast is served. Rooms are individually decorated and furnished to a high standard, some with four-poster beds. • Acc£££ •

Dublin 2 — Café en Seine

40 Dawson Street Dublin

CAFÉ/BAR   Tel: 01 677 4369   Fax: 01 671 7938

The first of the continental style café-bars to open in Dublin, in 1993, the large and lively Café en Seine is still just as fashionable now. It's a most attractive place, too, and offers sustenance as well as drinks at lunchtime (quiches, pasta dishes, smoked salmon salad and roast meats), snacks from late afternoon and coffee and pastries all day. Live jazz on Sundays, 1-4 pm, when a brunch menu is served. • All day £-££ •

Visit our web site - www.ireland-guide.com

Dublin 2 — Camden Court Hotel

Camden Street Dublin

HOTEL   Tel: 01 475 9666   Fax: 01 475 9677

A stylish new hotel (opened 1998) with two entrances – one next to the Bleeding Horse pub, the other via an arched passageway through a courtyard. The spacious reception area, with a partly tiled floor and lots of natural wood, leads to a smart restaurant, where an enticing breakfast buffet is laid out. But perhaps the hotel's finest asset is the atmospheric and rustic Piseogs pub, themed around Irish myths with differently decorated areas, the most intriguing being a fairytale forest! All of the bedrooms (some no-smoking) are practically and similarly furnished and decorated with co-ordinating fabrics and fitted furniture and the usual facilities (plus satellite TV which can show your room bill, speeding check-out). Some 45 rooms have their own fax machines. Bathrooms are neat, but quite small. Meeting rooms for up to 120; a leisure centre, including a swimming pool, is due to open towards the end of 1998. Staff are very friendly and the hotel seems to have 'lifted' this thriving locality, a mixture of big business and old shops. No hidden charges in the rates. • Acc££££ • Open all year •

Dublin 2 — Camden Hall Hotel

1 Upper Camden Street Dublin

HOTEL/RESTAURANT   Tel: 01 475 7906   Fax: 01 475 7905

email: onepico@iol.ie

Several connecting town houses make up this pleasant and well-run small hotel, where guests will feel comfortably at home. There's a lounge next to the reception (on the other side is the restaurant – see below – and next door a cellar bar, both with their own entrances), and behind the hotel, a converted church (the Abbey Room) that's used as an atmospheric meeting room. Also, at the rear of the hotel is a small car park, accessed under an arched building (where the quietest bedrooms are located) from the narrow street behind, and a patio terrace, popular with students. The well-furnished bedrooms offer everything you need, from multi-channel TV and tea/coffee tray to trouserpress and hairdryer. Bowls of fruit, mineral water and biscuits greet guests on arrival. Bathrooms are compact rather than grand but well equipped nonetheless.

141

Camden One Pico ⭐

Eamonn O'Reilly's elegant country house-style restaurant, sited in the Camden Hall Hotel, is a welcome addition to the Dublin eating-out scene. Perhaps surprisingly, given the smart surroundings, the cooking is much more modern than anticipated, with worldwide leanings – but none the worse for that. Indeed, the involved dishes are quite exemplary and great attention (almost too much at times!) is paid in their presentation. Though some of the menu descriptions could be simplified, it's the flavours of the ingredients that stand out and the precision of the cooking. For a main course you could choose fillet of beef with foie gras butter, spiced couscous and onion confit; best end of lamb with basil mash and crispy polenta; seared scallops with saffron mash, tomato salsa and sweet chili jam or seared monkfish with hot pepper marmalade and chive and tomato crème fraîche. Splendid desserts include warm chocolate tart with vanilla bean ice cream; praline parfait served with a confit of berries and champagne sabayon or a gratin of red fruits with red berry sorbet surrounded by spun sugar. Irish farmhouse cheeses, in tip-top condition, for those without a sweet tooth. Service is solicitous, the wine list agreeable. • L£ Mon-Fri, D££ Tues-Sat • Acc£££ •

Dublin 4   Canaletto's

71 Mespil Road Ballsbridge Dublin

RESTAURANT   Tel: 01 667 0699/01 667 5220   Fax: 01 628 1120

Since 1992 owner-chef Terry Sheehan has been delighting diners at this unpretentious canalside restaurant with his lively, wholesome cooking. In addition to good food – including a phone-in take-out service (no deliveries) – specialities of the house include Sunday brunch, from 10.30, which they also run on bank holiday Mondays. Most unusual however, is the in-house fortune teller every Monday night; advance bookings essential, fee £10! • Open all day L£, D££ •

Dublin 2   La Cave

28 South Anne Street Dublin

RESTAURANT   Tel: 01 679 4409   Fax: 01 670 5255

Margaret and Akim Beskri have run this well-known wine bar just off Grafton Street since 1989. With its classic French cooking and a wide range of wines by the glass (22), it makes a handy place to take a break from shopping. Marrakesh, an authentic Moroccan restaurant run by the Beskris and previously located in Ballsbridge, is now also in the South Anne Street premises, on the first floor. • Mon-Sat all day £, D££ daily • Closed 25-26 Dec & Good Fri •

Dublin 4   Cedar Lodge

98 Merrion Road Ballsbridge Dublin

ACCOMMODATION   Tel: 01 668 4410   Fax: 01 668 4533

Conveniently located near the RDS show grounds and conference centre, this recently refurbished guesthouse has spacious rooms, with a full range of amenities and good bathrooms (four shower only). Public rooms are comfortably furnished and there is one room suitable for disabled guests. • Acc££ •

Dublin 2   Central Hotel

1-5 Exchequer Street Dublin

HOTEL   Tel: 01 679 7302   Fax: 01 679 7303
email: reservations@centralhotel.ie www.centralhotel.ie

Very conveniently located, as its name implies, this hotel is over a hundred years old and currently in the midst of a major refurbishment programme. The reception and central staircase areas have been completed and there is a very congenial library bar which serves light snacks. A very handy place to stay and not unreasonably priced; it's worth asking about special offers, including weekends, when car parking used by a local office during the week becomes available for guests. • Acc££-£££ •

Dublin 1   Chapter One

18/19 Parnell Square Dublin

RESTAURANT   Tel: 01 873 2266/2281   Fax: 01 873 2330

Since 1993 chef-proprietor Ross Lewis and his partner, restaurant manager Martin Corbett, have been operating this successful restaurant in the basement beneath the Dublin Writers' Museum (where they also run a coffee shop, 10-5 pm daily). The restaurant has facilities for small conferences and secure parking – and they are most obliging about fitting in with the times of the nearby Gate Theatre. Ross has built up quite a following for cooking which is based on first class seasonal ingredients and he leans towards the New Irish Cuisine style, with world influences. (He prepared a much-praised lunch for the Irish Food Writers' Guild in 1998, when a portrait of the food writer Theodora Fitzgibbon, their first President, was presented to the museum.) • L£ Mon-Fri, D££ Mon-Sat • Closed 2 wks Xmas •

Dublin 2 — The Chili Club

1 Anne's Lane Dublin

RESTAURANT   Tel: 01 677 3721 Fax: 01 493 8284/677 3721

This cosy restaurant, in a laneway just off Grafton Street, was Dublin's first authentic Thai restaurant and is still as popular as ever, nearly ten years on. It is currently owned and managed by Patricia Kenna, who supervises a friendly and efficient staff. The head chef, Supot Boonchouy, prepares a fine range of genuine Thai dishes which are not "tamed" too much to suit Irish tastes. • L£ Mon-Sat, D££ daily •

Dublin 3 — Clontarf Castle Hotel

Clontarf Dublin

HOTEL   Tel: 01 833 2321   Fax: 01 833 2542

email: info@clontarfcastle.ie

This historic 17th century castle is convenient to both the airport and city centre. It has been family-owned and operated for 25 years (by the Houlihan family), who have recently completed a major refurbishment and extension programme. This has included banqueting, conference and business facilities (business centre and secretarial services, same day laundry and dry cleaning and exercise room for guests) as well as major changes to public areas and the addition of 100 deluxe rooms. Bedrooms, which include two executive suites and two junior suites, are furnished to a high standard and well-equipped for business guests with ISDN lines, voicemail and US electrical sockets in addition to the usual amenities; all south-facing rooms have air conditioning and bathrooms are well-designed and finished. The new building has been imaginatively incorporated into the old castle structure, retaining the historic atmosphere – some rooms, such as the restaurant and the original bar, have been left untouched and bedrooms have old-world details to remind guests of their castle surroundings. The "new" castle is very welcome in an area where extra facilities and accommodation were badly needed. • Acc££ • Open all year • Amex, Diners, MasterCard, Visa •

Dublin 2 — Clarence Hotel

6-8 Wellington Quay Dublin

HOTEL/RESTAURANT   Tel: 01 670 9000   Fax: 01 670 7800

email: clarence@indigo.ie www.theclarence.ie

The Clarence Hotel dates back to 1852 and – largely because of its convenience to Heuston Station – has long had a special place in the hearts of Irish people, especially the clergy and the many who regarded it as a home from home when "up from the country" for business or shopping in Dublin. Since the early '90s, however, it has achieved a different kind of fame through its owners, U2, The Edge and Harry Crosbie, who have completely refurbished the hotel, creating the coolest of jewels in the crown of Temple Bar. No expense has been spared to get the details right, reflecting the hotel's original arts and crafts style whenever possible and complementing it with specially commissioned furniture and artefacts in contemporary style. Luxurious accommodation includes The Penthouse, which has wonderful river views (and an outdoor hot tub as well as a terrace from which to enjoy them to the full). All of the individually designed, double glazed bedrooms have king size beds, white-tiled bathrooms reminiscent of an earlier era and excellent amenities including mini-bar, private safe, PC/fax connections, remote control satellite television and video and temperature control panels. Public areas include the oak panelled, clublike Octagon Bar, which is a popular Temple Bar meeting place, and The Study, which has an open fire and makes a quieter spot for reading and writing.

The Tea Room

Approached from its own entrance on Essex Street this high-ceilinged room is furnished in the light oak which is a feature throughout the hotel. Pristine white linen, designer cutlery and glasses, high windows softened only by the filtered damson tones of pavement awnings, all combine to create an impressive dining room. Under the direction of restaurant manager Niki Sullivan, discreet staff move quietly, quickly offering aperitifs, menus and excellent breads which come with a dip. Head chef Michael Martin presents fashionably international menus which offer plenty of choice, including vegetarian options, but which are not overlong or overpriced. Seasonal à la carte dinner menus offer around nine starters – carpaccio of wild salmon with a salad of warm potatoes and fried quail egg, perhaps, or salad of aubergine crisps, mesclun leaves, roast garlic and red onion oil. From a dozen or so main courses, typical dishes might be: grilled tuna with braised french onions and jus of herbs; or roast cannon of lamb with black olive and parmesan mash and oven roast garlic; and also a vegetarian wonton of baked goat's cheese and mozzarella with cucumber and ginger relish. The style is modern, bright and sassy, with strong but not overworked presentation. Desserts range from updated nursery classics like vanilla and coconut cream pot with rum raisin ice cream to an artistic assiette gourmandise, or there is farmhouse cheese, a nicely presented selection with tossed salad, grapes and toasted "brioche" and a choice of coffees or tea. Lunch menus (£13.50/£17.50) offer a more restricted but well-balanced choice and are good value. Although there is no specific "House" wine, an interesting, fairly priced wine list offers plenty of choice for under £20. • L££ Mon-Fri, D£££ daily • Acc ££££ •

Dublin 2   Clarion Stephen's Hall Hotel

The Earlsfort Centre Lower Leeson Street Dublin
HOTEL/RESTAURANT   Tel: 01 638 1111   Fax: 01 638 1122
email: stephens@premgroup.com   www.premgroup.com

Conveniently located just off St Stephen's Green, Dublin's only "all-suite" hotel has recently been refurbished and upgraded. Most suites now have wooden floors, all have ISDN lines, voice mail, modem access, fax machines and CD players – and computers are to be introduced to all rooms shortly.

Restaurant

Morels Bistro is in a semi-basement adjacent to the hotel and accessible directly from it or from offices at the back. Sister restaurant to the well-known southside restaurant Morels of Sandycove, the kitchen here is also under the direction of Morels proprietor Alain O'Reilly; sunny decor and a bright and colourful style of cooking both echo the parent restaurant's Mediterranean theme. • L£ Mon-Fri, D££+ daily • Acc£££ • Closed 25-26 Dec •

Dublin 2   The Commons Restaurant

Newman House 85-86 St Stephen's Green Dublin
RESTAURANT   Tel: 01 478 0530/475 2597   Fax: 01 478 0551

Sited in the basement of Newman House, considered one of Dublin's finest examples of Georgian splendour, the restaurant (formerly the college dining room of University College Dublin) still evokes literary memories, with several works of modern art dedicated to James Joyce, a scholar at the turn of the last century. Other luminaries associated with the Palladian building are John Henry Cardinal Newman, former rector, and Gerald Manley Hopkins, professor. The spacious restaurant, with a polished wood-block floor, French doors opening on to a secluded south-facing terrace (perfect for pre-meal drinks on a warm summer's day) and smartly laid tables, is surprisingly bright and suggests a serious dining-room, further confirmed by an array of unfailingly polite and professional staff. Little canapés on arrival (blue cheese and walnut), an amuse-gueule of lobster and sauerkraut – a marriage destined to end in divorce – and several breads continue this notion that something special is about to occur, but somehow there is insufficient spark, no crescendo. Dishes, though technically very sound and beautifully presented, lack inspiration; for instance a vegetable mosaic (terrine) with rabbit confit, foie gras, leaves and a balsamic vinaigrette left no discernible taste of the foie gras – rather a waste of an expensive ingredient, followed by a quite irrelevant mulled wine granité (palate cleanser? Mulled wine is best served hot on ski slopes!) Two chunks of a pan-fried red mullet were perfectly cooked and served with a mould of ratatouille, and layered beetroot potato Lyonnaise, but the almost turquoise basil dressing (in fact a tiny pool) had no taste at all, rendering the dish almost dull, to the point of being boring. Finally, a well-executed strawberry and mascarpone tart would have been greatly enhanced by a little chocolate sauce, rather than half a dozen artistic blobs, the whole constituting less than a dip of a teaspoon! You cannot fault the cooking, but with a little more attention to flavours it would be exceptional. The set four-course table d'hôte menu (£35) offers three choices in each section, or else choose from the à la carte, but this will add considerably to the final bill. Service, and very good it is too, is now discretionary (it used to be a whopping 15%). • L££ Mon-Fri, D£££ Mon-Sat • Closed Sun, Bank Hols & Xmas wk •

Dublin 2

HOTEL 🏛

Conrad International

Earlsfort Terrace Dublin
Tel: 01 676 5555   Fax: 01 676 5424
email: info@conrad-international.ie   www.conrad-international.ie

Just a stroll away from St Stephen's Green and right opposite the National Concert Hall, the hotel celebrates its tenth anniversary in 1999. Nothing stands still here, however, and apart from the ongoing refurbishment of the air-conditioned bedrooms, a new fitness centre has opened and individual fax machines (alongside three telephones) have been installed in every bedroom, confirming the hotel's attraction to business/corporate guests. Note, too, the fully-equipped and staffed business centre, complemented by an exceptional conference room (370 theatre-style), executive boardroom (12) and banqueting facilities (260). Many of the generously-sized bedrooms enjoy views of the piazza below and across the city, and offer plenty of workspace, at least one double bed, mini-bar, remote-control satellite TV with free in-house movie channel, clock/radio and safe. The well-equipped bathrooms have bathrobes and environmentally-friendly toiletries. A nightly turn-down service (hand-made Irish chocolates and bottles of mineral water are left beside the pillow) is provided, an example of the outstanding and professional service by committed staff, under the direction of long-serving general manager Michael Governey. Public areas include a raised lounge, two restaurants, the Alexandra and Plurabelle Brasserie (breakfast served here), and Alfie Byrne's Pub (serving splendid pub lunches) that opens on to an external terrace. • L£, D££-£££ • Acc££££ • Open all year •

Dublin 2

RESTAURANT

Cooke's Café & The Rhino Room

14 South William Street Dublin
Tel: 01 679 0536/7/8   Fax: 01 679 0546

John Cooke has always been ahead of fashions in the Dublin restaurant scene and his stylish café, Cooke's, was among the first of the current wave of trendy café-bistro style places doing Mediterranean and Cal-Ital food. The formula is still working well at Cooke's, where there is always a good buzz and you can be sure of stylish, well cooked food based on the best of ingredients. They even have a pavement area with an awning, which is "covered, heated and secure" – perfect for people-watching. More recently they have opened The Rhino Room, a first floor restaurant over the café but with its own entrance on South William Street. The food is much the same – pastas, salads, char-grilled meats and vegetables, all very competently prepared – but it is quieter and suits people who prefer a slightly more formal atmosphere and well-spaced tables. • L£-££ & D££ daily • Closed Bank Hols •

Dublin 4

RESTAURANT

Coopers Café, Ballsbridge

Sweepstake Centre Ballsbridge Dublin
Tel: 01 660 1525   Fax: 01 660 1537

The flagship of the Coopers chain of restaurants, Coopers Café Ballsbridge is in the dashing premises opposite the RDS originally occupied by the ill-fated Brubecks. Well-situated for the Ballsbridge hotels and exhibition crowds, the Café serves global cuisine – salsa, szechuan, rocket and chilli are the kinds of words that leap off the menu – but it is reassuring to know that, on request, they will also cook a plain steak perfectly and serve it with a simple green salad. • L£ & D££ daily except Sat L •
Other Coopers Restaurants are situated at Lower Leeson Street (01-6768615), Greystones (01-2873914) and Kilternan (01-2959349)

Dublin 4

RESTAURANT ★
Irish Pork Award Winner

Le Coq Hardi

35 Pembroke Road Ballsbridge Dublin
Tel: 01 668 9070   Fax: 01 668 9887

Granite steps lead up to the classic Georgian doorway of John and Catherine Howard's fine Ballsbridge restaurant – and there is always a warm welcome awaiting at the top. Sumptuously furnished in classical style, this beautiful restaurant provides a fine setting for some of the best food in the land – including, if you are lucky, John's wonderful roast loin of kassler with green cabbage, fresh herb mash and Calvados jus, winner of our Irish Pork Award. Famous down the years for his refusal to be a slave to food fashions, John's steadfast sureness of purpose has served the restaurant well in the long term. Over the years his background of classical French cooking has blended with a love of traditional

Irish themes to produce dishes that show New Irish Cuisine at its best and, paradoxically perhaps for a man so uninterested in fashion, are very much of our time. House specialities which have become permanent features on the menu over the years include "smokies," a Scottish-influenced appetizer of baked smoked haddock, marbled with tomato, double cream, and Irish cheese and also 'Coq Hardi', chicken breast filled with potatoes, mushrooms and herbs, wrapped in bacon, oven-baked, and finished with Irish whiskey – a substantial dish which is perhaps best suited to lunch. Upbeat Irish classics also appear in dishes like Clonakilty black pudding served with a traditional potato cake and apple sauce, and baked white fish served with bacon and cabbage with a whiskey cream sauce. Seasonally influenced table d'hôte menus include many of the best choices from the carte and the £21 set lunch possibly represents the best value in town. Seafood often includes lobster from Howth or the west coast and game in season is a particular strength, often including rare treats such as partridge (pot-roasted, perhaps, with wild mushrooms and winter berries). Desserts are equally good and there's always a fine choice of Irish farmhouse cheeses in good condition. An outstanding wine list is particularly strong in John's favourite areas – Bordeaux, Burgundy, Loire, and Champagne; while there is little choice under £20, house wines (c.£16) are chosen with care. • L££ Mon-Fri, D£££ Mon-Sat • Closed Bank Hols, 2 wks Aug & Xmas •

Dublin 2 — Da Pino

38-40 Parliament Street Dublin
RESTAURANT   Tel: 01 671 9308   Fax: 01 677 3409
email: m.jimenez@tinet.ie

Just across the road from Dublin Castle, this busy youthful Italian/Spanish restaurant is always full – and no wonder, as they serve cheerful, informal, well cooked food that does not make too many concessions to trendiness and is sold at very reasonable prices. The pizzas are especially good and are prepared in full view of customers. • L£ & D££ daily •

Dublin 2 — The Davenport Hotel

Merrion Square Dublin
HOTEL   Tel: 01 607 3500   Fax: 01 661 5663
email: davenporthotel@tinet.ie   www.davenporthotel.ie

On Merrion Square, close to the National Gallery, this striking hotel is fronted by the impressive 1863 facade of Merrion Hall, which was restored as part of the hotel building project in the early '90s. Inside, the hotel has been imaginatively designed to be both interesting and comfortable, with a pleasing mixture of old and new influences and bold, confident colours used in both public areas and bedrooms. A high proportion of the bedrooms are designated no-smoking and there is one suitable for disabled guests; all are furnished to a high standard and have excellent amenities. Conference/banqueting facilities are available for 300/400 respectively, with back-up business services as required. • Acc££££ • Open all year •

➤ Dublin 2 — Davy Byrnes

21 Duke Street Dublin
PUB   Tel: 01 677 5217   Fax: 01 671 7619
www.visit.ie/dublin

Just off Grafton Street, Davy Byrnes is one of Dublin's most famous pubs – having been mentioned in Joyce's *Ulysses* means it is very much on the tourist circuit. Despite all this fame it remains a genuine, well-run place and equally popular with Dubliners, who find it a handy meeting place and also enjoy the bar food. This is a particular point of pride and always includes a list of daily specials as well as the regular menu. • L£ & D£ Mon-Sun •

➤ Dublin 2 — Dish

2 Crow Street Dublin
RESTAURANT   Tel: 01 671 1248   Fax: 01 671 1249
email: dish@indigo.ie

Trevor Browne and Gerard Foote have made quite an impact with their stylishly spartan restaurant in the Temple Bar area. Again we find the global cuisine which seems to have engulfed kitchens everywhere recently, but it is in Gerard Foote's capable hands here so you can be sure of substance as well as style. From the à la carte dinner menu, starters such as crab and sweet potato cakes with orange braised fennel and rocket salad with basil essence would be typical, with main courses such as angel hair pomodoro with tomatoes, basil, garlic, extra virgin olive oil – available as a vegetarian dish or with added sautéed tiger prawns. Lunch menus are slightly simpler and offer less choice than dinner, but the style is essentially the same. • L£ & D££ Mon-Sun • Closed 25 Dec & Good Fri •

Dublin 2   Dobbins
15 Stephens Lane Dublin
RESTAURANT   Tel: 01 676 4670/9, 01 661 3321   Fax: 01 661 3331

Now something of an institution, this restaurant has operated in a "Nissen hut" near Merrion Square since 1978 under the close supervision of owner John O'Byrne and manager Patrick Walsh. It has a conservatory area at the far end, which is very popular in summer, and a dark intimate atmosphere in the main restaurant. Gary Flynn, head chef since 1985, has attracted a loyal following for consistently good cooking in a style which has not abandoned tradition but incorporates new ideas too. Good details include generous, plain wine glasses and lovely home-baked brown bread. • L£-££ Mon-Fri, D££-£££ Mon-Sat • Closed Bank Hols •

Dublin 22   Doyle Green Isle Hotel
Naas Road Dublin
HOTEL   Tel: 01 459 3406   Fax: 01 459 2178

Situated on the Naas Road, close to the major industrial estates, this is a popular hotel for conferences and business. Over half of the bedrooms are executive rooms and there are conference facilities for up to 250 delegates, four meeting rooms for a maximum of 50 each and some business back-up service if required. • Acc££ • Open all year • Amex, Diners, MasterCard, Visa •

Dublin 4   Doyle Montrose Hotel
Stillorgan Road Dublin
HOTEL   Tel: 01 269 3311   Fax: 01 269 1164

This south-city hotel near the University College campus has undergone extensive refurbishment. Removing balconies and rebuilding the whole front has updated the exterior, while interior improvements include the addition of more suites and rooms for the disabled. Rooms 180. • Acc£££ • Open all year • Access, Amex, Diners, Visa.

Dublin 9   Doyle Skylon Hotel
Upper Dtumcondra Road Dublin
HOTEL   Tel: 01 837 9121   Fax: 01 837 2778

Three miles north of the city centre, this 1960s hotel is conveniently situated for the airport, which is just four miles further out. • Acc£££ • Open all year •

Dublin 6   Dunville Place
25 Dunville Place Ranelagh Dublin
RESTAURANT   Tel: 01 496 8181   Fax: 01 491 0604

Michael Duignan and Sophie Ridley are operating a very stylish neighbourhood restaurant at Dunville Place, particularly in summer when the little courtyard at the back can also be used for drinks, or eating out in fine weather. The restaurant is informally well-appointed and Michael Duignan presents imaginative, contemporary seasonal menus which are carried through with style and include strong vegetarian choices. Asian influences come through quite strongly in the spicing, but Europe is represented too – in a vegetarian Greek plate with stuffed vine leaves, hummus, tabbouleh and various other little dishes, all served with warm pitta bread. Good desserts might include a classic crème brûlée. • L£ daily, D££ Tues-Sat • Closed Bank Hols •

Dublin 2   Eastern Tandoori
34/36 South William Street Dublin
RESTAURANT   Tel: 01 671 0428/0506   Fax: 01 677 9232

The flagship of a small chain of Indian restaurants, the Eastern Tandoori opened in 1984 and was one of Ireland's earliest good ethnic restaurants. It's a fine, well-appointed establishment with friendly staff and reliably enjoyable food. • L£ Sun-Fri, D££ daily • Closed 25-26 Dec •
Other branches are at: Deansgrange, Co Dublin (01 2892856), Malahide, Co Dublin (01 8454155), Emmet Place, Cork (021 272020); Spanish Parade, Galway (091 564819) and Steamboat Quay, Limerick (061-311575).

Dublin 2   L'Ecrivain

109a Lower Baggot Street Dublin

RESTAURANT   Tel: 01 661 1919   Fax: 01 661 0617

Derry and Sallyanne Clarke's city centre restaurant has a welcoming atmosphere: aperitifs and olives are served promptly in the ground floor bar/reception area where the writers theme – seen in portraits throughout the restaurant – is underlined by a disconcertingly lifelike statue of Brendan Behan having a pint. Menus are presented later, once guests are seated in the first floor restaurant above. This is a light and airy room, with a terrace for fine weather, cheery Mediterranean-toned walls. Owner-chef Derry Clarke, who is currently Ireland's Commissioner General for Euro-Toques, is not likely to disappoint. He presents a number of dinner menus: a 5-course table d'hôte (£29.50), an à la carte and a special weekday 3-course menu (6.30-7.30 Monday -Thursday only, £17.50 including service) – and a two/three course set lunch menu (good value at £12.50/£15.50). New Irish Cuisine-style cooking is a strength – a starter of oysters with chopped bacon & cabbage and a Guinness sabayon, for example, is an inspired example. There are also Mediterranean influences, as in a dashing dish of hot goat's cheese, layered in a modish "tower" with char-grilled Mediterranean vegetables and crisp potato curls. Well-balanced main courses are strong on seafood, lamb and beef, also game in season, but could also include neglected ingredients like rabbit – roasted, boned and appealingly served in slices, with black and white pudding, an onion relish and vegetable "chips". Wonderful puddings are presented with panache and might include a super crème brûlée with armagnac. Presentation generally is impressive but not ostentatious and attention to detail – garnishes designed individually to enhance each dish, careful selection of plates, delicious home-made breads and splendid farmhouse cheeses – all create the impression of a very caring approach. Service, under the direction of restaurant manager Ray Hingston, is professional although, as everything is cooked to order, not necessarily speedy. A thoughtfully selected wine list includes 15 wines available by bottle, half bottle or glass and the 10% service charge is added to the food only. • Mon-Fri L££, Mon-Sat D£££ • Closed 25 Dec & 1 Jan •

Dublin 2   Eden

Meeting House Square Dublin

RESTAURANT   Tel: 01 670 5373   Fax: 01 670 3330

In the heart of Temple Bar on Sycamore Street, next to the Irish Film Theatre and opposite Diceman's Corner (The Diceman, Thom McGinty, was a popular and well-known Dublin street performer, particularly famous for his costumes), lies this spacious and modern restaurant, with its own outdoor terrace on the square. It is on two floors, with lots of greenery and hanging baskets and an open kitchen that ground floor customers can observe. The lunch menu (two courses £13, three £15) changes weekly, perhaps salmon tartare with crème fraîche and paprika, spicy lamb meat balls with lemon rice and tomato sauce, sticky toffee pudding with caramel sauce, while the dinner menu is seasonal, with many of the dishes employing organic produce. A caramelised lemon tart (actually two slices) finishes off the meal nicely and comes with a scoop of blackcurrant sorbet. A well-balanced and not-too-expensive wine list offers several wines by the glass. Friendly staff are efficient and observant. • L & D£-££ daily • Closed Bank Hols •

Dublin 9   Egan's Guesthouse

7-9 Iona Park Glasnevin Dublin

ACCOMMODATION   Tel: 01 830 3611   Fax: 01 830 3312

email: eganshouse@tinet.ie   www.holiday-ireland.com

Within walking distance of the Botanic Gardens, this long-established, family-run guesthouse offers comfortable en-suite accommodation and warm hospitality at a reasonable price. • Acc££ • Closed 24-27 Dec •

Dublin 2   Elephant & Castle

18 Temple Bar Dublin

RESTAURANT   Tel: 01 679 3121   Fax: 01 679 1399

John Hayes and Elizabeth Mee do a consistently good job at this buzzy Temple Bar restaurant – it was one of the first new-wave restaurants in the area and is still one of the best. Ingredients are carefully sourced and served in a range of big, generous and wholesome salads (their special Caesar salad is legendary), pasta dishes, home made burgers and great big baskets of chicken wings. Service can sometimes be a problem –

waiting staff are usually foreign students (often with little English) and, although willing and friendly, it can take longer than anticipated to finish a meal here. • All day L&D£-££ • Closed 24-26 Dec •

Dublin 4   Ernie's

Mulberry Gardens Donnybrook Dublin

RESTAURANT   Tel: 01 269 3300   Fax: 01 269 3260

Unless you know Dublin, it is best to ask directions (and where to park) to this long-established restaurant, named after the late Ernie Evans and still owned by the family. The dining-room looks out on to a pretty courtyard garden, floodlit at night, though the abiding memory of the restaurant is the fantastic art collection, mostly Irish paintings, many of Kerry, that cover the walls entirely. Both the cooking and service are straightforward, almost old-fashioned, in the classical sense (real sauces!) and a welcome respite in this new era of retro and minimalist restaurants. However, there is a hint of modernism and a nod to foreign influences in some of the dishes: grilled bratwurst with wild mushrooms and onion jus, oven-baked parcel of brie served with fruit chutney and red pepper relish, home-made fish cakes on a bed of leaves with a pink peppercorn vinaigrette, and baked cod with fresh basil pesto and black olives. Alternatively, regular patrons can still enjoy dishes they have become accustomed to, such as roast rack of Wicklow lamb with a Madeira glaze, escalope of veal with a mushroom and Calvados cream sauce and pan-fried lambs liver with sage, avocado and red wine jus. For dessert, a gingered crème brûlée or poached pears and plums with Mascarpone cheese fit the bill perfectly. Good wine list, strong on clarets. • L££ Tues-Fri, D££+ Tues-Sat •

Dublin 4   Expresso Bar Café

47 Shelbourne Rd Ballsbridge Dublin

CAFÉ BAR   Tel/Fax: 01 660 8632

The flagship restaurant of a small but growing chain of cool, informal eating places in Dublin. It is notable for clean-lined minimalism, and colourful Cal-Ital food, well-prepared and carefully presented with good coffee. Saturday and Sunday brunch are a must. Other branches are at Westbury Mall, St Mary's Road (Ballsbridge), and Powerscourt Townhouse Centre. • Mon-Sun all day £-££ •

Dublin 4   Fitzers Ballsbridge Café

Royal Dublin Society Merrion Road Dublin

RESTAURANT   Tel: 01 667 1301/2   Fax: 01 667 1303

Flagship of the Fitzers Café group, this dashing neo-classical restaurant is in the members' annexe of the Regency style Royal Dublin Society building – sculptures and old paintings from the RDS archives look stunning against deep orange walls. New and old meet well, providing a high level of comfort with great style – a dramatic setting for Cal-Ital influenced cooking. Private function rooms are also available and there is ample secure parking available exclusively to the restaurant. • L£ Mon-Fri & Sun, D£££ Mon-Sat • Closed Bank Hols •

Other Fitzers Cafés are in Dublin at: Temple Bar Square (01-679 0440), Dawson Street (01-677 1155), National Gallery, Merrion Square (01-661 4496).

Dublin 2   Fitzwilliam Hotel

St Stephen's Green Dublin

HOTEL   Tel: 01 478 7000   Fax: 01 478 7878

email: eng@fitzwilliamh.com   www.fitzwilliamh.com

Newcomer of the Year

This stylish contemporary hotel enjoys a superb location overlooking St Stephen's Green and close to Dublin's most prestigious shopping area. Behind its deceptively low-key frontage lies an impressively sleek interior created by Sir Terence Conran's design group CD Partnership. Public areas combine elegant minimalism with luxury fabrics and finishes, notably leather upholstery and an unusual pewter bar counter – and, although only open a short time before we went to press, the bar was already becoming established as the chic place to meet in the Grafton Street area. Bedrooms, while quite compact for a luxury hotel, are finished to a high standard with fax/modem points, stereo CD players and minibars, and care has been lavished on the bathrooms too, down to details such as the choice of toiletries. As we went to press Conrad Gallagher's "Peacock Alley" restaurant was poised to move from its South William Street premises to become "Peacock Alley at The Fitzwilliam" (in an upper floor location, close to the roof garden) while the all-day brasserie-style mezzanine restaurant "Christopher's", which is also operated by Gallagher, was just opening. • Acc££££ • Meals£-££££ • Open all year •

Dublin 2 — The Fitzwilliam Park Hotel

 HOTEL

5 Fitzwilliam Square Dublin
Tel: 01 662 8280   Fax: 01 662 8281
www.fitzparkhotel.ie

Mary Madden has recently opened this elegant Georgian house after extensive renovation and refurbishment, yet retaining many of the original features. It's a big house – one of the largest and oldest buildings on the eastern side of the garden square (private, but residents have access) – with a fine back stone staircase, though guests will probably use the lift! The Grand Salon, a lofty and opulent room with fine antiques, paintings and objets d'art on the first floor, is where a hearty Irish breakfast is served in splendid surroundings. The bedrooms – the higher you go, the smaller they become – are well-appointed and furnished with black and white tiled bathrooms (all with shower attachment), satellite TV, radio and direct-dial telephone, as well as plenty of desk-writing space – important for business travellers, who can also make use of a boardroom on the ground floor. Secure free parking behind the building via Lad Lane. • Acc£££ • Closed 25 Dec •

Please note that price indications are intended only as a guideline - always check current prices (and special offers) when making reservations.

Dublin 2 — Les Frères Jacques

74 Dame Street Dublin
RESTAURANT   Tel: 01 679 4555   Fax: 01 679 4725

One of the few genuinely French restaurants in Dublin, Les Freres Jacques opened beside the Olympia Theatre in 1986, well before the development of Temple Bar made the area fashionable. The staff are all French, the atmosphere is French – and the cooking is definitely French. Seasonal menus are wide-ranging and well-balanced but – as expected when you notice the lobster tank just beside the door on entering – there is a definite bias towards fish and seafood, all of it from Irish waters; there is also game in season. Lunch at Les Freres Jacques is a treat (and good value at £13.50 for the set menu) but dinner is a feast. The 4-course set dinner offers soup (sea food minestrone perhaps) and three choices on the other courses – smoked chicken & pigeon salad with pine kernels and hazelnut dressings, for example, or roast Wicklow lamb and juices. Poached pear & Roquefort sauce and soup of summer red fruits with pistachio ice cream are all typical examples. Suggestions from the à la carte are also made on the dinner menu; thus west coast oysters (native and rock), grilled lobster, turbot with girolles & roasting juices, individually priced. There are cheeses or beautifully presented desserts, as in a dramatic crème caramel in a sugar cage, with cappuccino cream. Service is efficient and discreet. • L£ Mon-Fri, D££-£££ Mon-Sat • Closed Xmas wk •

Dublin 4 — Furama Chinese Restaurant

Anglesea House Donnybrook Road Donnybrook Dublin
RESTAURANT   Tel: 01 283 0522   Fax: 01 668 7623

In the sleek black interior of Rodney Mak's long-established restaurant Freddie Lee, who has been head chef since the restaurant opened in 1989, produces terrific food with an authenticity which is unusual in Ireland. Even the menu does not read like other Chinese restaurants – dishes aren't numbered, for a start, and they are also presented and described with great individuality. Thus, starters of soft shell crab in spicy salt and pepper or sweet and sour sauce; king size mussels in rich garlic sauce or spicy chilli sauce; lobster on shell (various ways), stir fried oyster with ginger and scallion, and much more. They do offer Set Dinners, which are more predictable – and many traditional Chinese dishes on the à la carte menu – but the option is there to try something different. Service, under the supervision of Rodney Mak and manager Stephen Lee, is friendly and efficient. • L£ Mon-Fri & Sun, D££ daily • Closed Bank Hols •

Dublin 4   Glenogra House

64 Merrion Road Dublin

ACCOMMODATION   Tel: 01 668 3661   Fax: 01 668 3698

A comfortable nine-room Ballsbridge guesthouse, run by Seamus and Cherry McNamee, conveniently located for the RDS and within 3 minutes walk of the Sandymount DART station. Personal service, very good breakfasts. • Acc££ •

Dublin 4   Glenveagh Townhouse

31 Northumberland Road Ballsbridge Dublin

ACCOMMODATION   Tel: 01 668 4612   Fax: 01 668 4559

A warm welcome and courteous service are the hallmarks of this fine period guesthouse, which has been renovated to a high standard and provides a comfortable base for both business guests and tourists. Although just off the centre of the city, on a fine day it's a pleasant 10-15 minute walk to Trinity College and the Grafton Street area. Bedrooms (which include three suitable for disabled guests) vary – they include singles, twins and family rooms, but all are well-furnished, with a high standard of amenities including complimentary mineral water and toiletries. There's a guest sitting room and facilities for small conferences (14). No dogs. • Acc££ • Closed 18-28 Dec •

Dublin 2   Good World Chinese Restaurant

18 South Great Georges Street Dublin

RESTAURANT   Tel/Fax: 01 677 5373

One of a cluster of interesting ethnic restaurants around Wicklow Street and South Great George's Street, the Good World opened in 1991 and is owner-managed by Thomas Choi. It has always been a favourite of the local Chinese community, because of its large selection of Dim Sum, which is served daily. The restaurant also prides itself on an especially full range of other Chinese dishes, suitable for both Chinese and European customers and Thomas Choi makes a welcoming and helpful host. • L£ & D££ daily • Closed 25-26 Dec •

Dublin 2   The Gotham Café

8 South Anne Street Dublin

RESTAURANT   Tel: 01 679 5266   Fax: 01 679 5280

A lively, youthful café-restaurant just off Grafton Street, the Gotham does good informal food: lovely starter salads – mozzarella, perhaps, with plum tomato, chargrilled zucchini, herbed olives and a basil dressing, hot sandwiches – BLT, chicken breast – a wide range of pasta, bigger dishes like char-grilled steaks and a great pizza menu. Sunday brunch is a speciality (12-4.30pm). • L£ & D£ daily • Closed 25 Dec & I Jan •

Dublin 2   Grafton Plaza Hotel

Johnsons Place Dublin

HOTEL   Tel: 01 475 0888   Fax: 01 475 0908

email: info@graftonplaza.ie www.graftonplaza.ie

In a prime city centre location just a couple of minutes walk from Grafton Street, this attractive hotel offers particularly well furnished rooms and good amenities (including fax/modem) at prices which are not unreasonable for the area. Rooms are also available for small conferences, meetings and interviews. The popular 'Break for the Border' nightclub next door is in common ownership with the hotel and offers guests live entertainment on Wednesday-Saturday nights. • Acc£££ • Closed 24-26 Dec •

Dublin 1   The Gresham

O'Connell Street Dublin

HOTEL   Tel: 01 874 6881   Fax: 01 878 7175

Ryan Hotels' flagship has seen a transformation in the past year with the addition of 100 new air-conditioned bedrooms, two lifts and multi-storey car parking. First opened in 1817, the hotel has always been at the centre of society in the centre of Dublin, and is now considered one of the city's finest business hotels – with a variety of meeting rooms (max 300) and a 24-hour business centre. However, at the same time it's still a favourite meeting place and the lobby lounge is renowned for its traditional afternoon tea, while the Gresham and Toddy's Bars are popular rendezvous for a pint. The Aberdeen Restaurant has been expanded to cope with the additional guests, and a small fitness room allows guests to work off those extra pounds. Obviously, the new (and spacious bedrooms) are the best, with smart furniture and colourful fabrics and the added benefit of separate walk-in shower in the well-equipped bathroom, but all the other bedrooms, including six penthouse suites, (one occupied for several months by Elizabeth Taylor and Richard Burton many years ago), offer the same facilities including voicemail and fax/modem points. The hotel prides itself on the quality of its staff, particularly the concierge. • Acc££££ • Open all year •

Dublin 2 — Grey Door Restaurant & Guesthouse

22/23 Upper Pembroke Street Dublin
RESTAURANT/ACCOMMODATION   Tel: 01 676 3286   Fax: 01 676 3287

P J Daly and Barry Wyse's Grey Door empire has grown so much of late that it is hard to know where to begin and end. (In addition to the premises described here, they also own the Hibernian Hotel in Ballsbridge and the new McCausland hotel in Belfast – see separate entries). The original Grey Door Restaurant changed its style quite dramatically a year or two ago; guests who remember it as a grand, classically elegant place featuring Russian specialities may be surprised to find a sleek, contemporary restaurant serving modern Irish food. The new fixed price lunch menu changes weekly and there is both a set dinner menu and an à la carte. The restaurant also has two private dining rooms, for parties of up to 70. Down in the basement, under the Grey Door, Pier 32 is quite different, with an Irish country atmosphere and traditional "home-made" food – soda breads, simple seafood, farmhouse cheeses and pints of stout convey the feeling, and it's all good fun as well as good eating. Above the Grey Door, accommodation is offered in seven rooms, furnished to a high standard with sitting areas and private bathrooms. • Acc££ • L£ Mon-Fri, D££ Mon-Sun •

> The best – independently assessed

Dublin 7 — Halfway House

Ashtown Dublin
PUB   Tel: 01 8383 3218

A well-supported local and handy meeting place just off the West-Link motorway, this well-known pub is very large, well-run and offers good quality popular bar food. • Closed 25 Dec & Good Fri •

Dublin 1 — The Harbourmaster

Custom House Docks Dublin
BAR/RESTAURANT   Tel: 01 670 1688   Fax: 01 670 1690

In a waterside setting at Dublin's financial services centre this old Dock Offices building has genuine character and makes a fine restaurant and bar. The bar is pleasant and very busy at times, but it's now more of a restaurant than a pub at meal times and most tables have an interesting (and increasingly attractive) view of the development outside. For fine weather there's also a decked outdoor area overlooking the inner harbour and fountain, with seating for 50. Eclectic menus offer everything from spinach roulade to seafood jambalaya and, while not exactly gourmet fare, it suits the surroundings. • Open weekdays from 7.30am, Sat & Sun 12pm £-££ • Closed 25 Dec & Good Fri •

Dublin 2 — Harcourt Hotel

60 Harcourt Street Dublin
HOTEL   Tel: 01 478 3677   Fax: 01 475 2013

This small, comfortable hotel lays claim to a unique distinction – it was, for several years, the home of George Bernard Shaw, writer, dramatist and wit. GBS would probably still be keen to stay, since the rooms are comfortable (though not large) and the atmosphere friendly. Being a strict teetotaller he might not approve of the two bars, but they are both very congenial, with the larger bar playing host to some of the best traditional Irish musicians and music, and the more intimate, panelled Barney Google's bar more suitable for quiet conversation or contemplation. GBS was also not known as an habitué of night clubs, but if he was he would be perfectly placed for visiting both the well-known POD (Place of Dance) and other clubs just a short walk away. The rooms have recently been refurbished and there is the recently opened GB Shaw Restaurant serving Irish and Mediterranean dishes. • Acc££-£££ • Closed 24-25 Dec •

Dublin 2   Harrington Hall

69/70 Harcourt Street Dublin

ACCOMMODATION   Tel: 01 475 3497   Fax: 01 475 4544

email: harringtonhall@tinet.ie   www.harringtonhall.com

Opened in March 1998 and conveniently located close to St Stephen's Green, this is a guesthouse (once the home of a former Lord Mayor of Dublin) of grand Georgian splendour. It has been sympathetically and elegantly refurbished, retaining many original features, especially the ornamental ceilings and fireplaces in the well-proportioned ground and first floor rooms (note the tranquil drawing room). At present the bedrooms are somewhat spartan, but nevertheless comfortable and practical with decent bathrooms. Given the need for some finishing touches – a few pictures here and there, and double-glazing installed in the rooms facing the busy street so that guests can enjoy an uninterrupted night's sleep – this is a welcome and considerably cheaper alternative to a city-centre hotel, with the huge advantage of free parking behind the building. • Acc££ • Open all year •

Dublin 2   Harvey's Coffee House

14-15 Trinity Street Dublin

CAFÉ/BAR   Tel: 01 677 1060

Just off Dame Street, this busy daytime café offers great coffee every-which-way and lots of lovely things to go with it – from toast, bagels and scones in the morning, through to lovely big open sandwiches and other more filling fare at lunchtime. There are also pastries and desserts to take your fancy later. Sunday brunch is a speciality. • Open all day £ •

Dublin 4   Herbert Park Hotel

Ballsbridge Dublin

HOTEL   Tel: 01 667 2200   Fax: 01 667 2595

This very large, striking hotel is near the RDS and the public park after which it is named. It is approached over a little bridge, which leads to an underground carpark and, ultimately, to a chic lower ground foyer and the lift up to the main lobby. Public areas on the ground floor are impressively light and spacious, with excellent light meals and drinks provided by efficient waiting staff. The bright and modern style is also repeated in the bedrooms – stylishly designed and well-finished with a high standard of amenities. • Acc££££ •

Visit our web site (www.ireland-guide.com) for new recommendations, news and other relevant travel and dining information.

Dublin 4   Hibernian Hotel

Eastmoreland Place Ballsbridge Dublin

HOTEL/RESTAURANT   Tel: 01 668 7666   Fax: 01 660 2655

email: info@hibernianhotel.com   www.slh.com/hibernia

The Hibernian Hotel feels as if it's in a peaceful backwater, yet this splendid Victorian building is only yards from one of Dublin's busiest city centre roads. It's a very friendly hotel, with a country house feeling in the size and proportions of its rooms and the elegant decorative style with warm country colours. The names of the rooms evoke a homely atmosphere too – the drawing room, the library and so on. Bedrooms are all individually decorated to a high standard with excellent bathrooms featuring a wide range of amenities. Service, under the direction of David Butt (who has been manager since the hotel opened in 1993), is outstanding.

Patrick Kavanagh Restaurant

In keeping with the rest of the hotel, the restaurant is well-appointed, with elegance and charm. David Foley, who has been head chef since 1994, presents lunch and dinner menus that change weekly, in addition to an evening à la carte and a separate vegetarian menu. Global influences are certainly at work here, but David takes great pride in using the best of Irish produce to advantage as, for example, in a dish of roast rack of Wicklow lamb with a tempura of vegetables and fondant potatoes. Desserts tend to be based more closely on classical dishes and Irish farmhouse cheeses are an option. Service is friendly and efficient. • L£ Mon-Fri & Sun, D£££ daily • Acc£££ • Closed 25 Dec •

Dublin 8 — Hole in the Wall

Blackhorse Lane Phoenix Park Dublin
PUB   **Tel: 01 838 9491**

PJ McCaffrey's remarkable pub beside the Phoenix Park is named in honour of a tradition which existed here for around a hundred years – the practice of serving drinks through a hole in the wall of Phoenix Park to members of the army garrison stationed nearby. Today the Hole in the Wall also claims to be the longest pub in Ireland – and it is certainly one of the most interesting, best-run and most hospitable. They do good food too – a buffet lunch every day, 12-3pm. • Normal pub hours • Closed 25 Dec & Good Fri •
In 1998 PJ McCaffrey also opened Nancy Hands pub, on the quays at 30-32 Parkgate Street, Dublin 8 – another pub definitely worth a visit.

Dublin 1 — Hotel St George

7 Parnell Square Dublin
HOTEL   **Tel: 01 874 5611   Fax: 01 874 5582**

Almost opposite the Gate Theatre at the top of O'Connell Street, this tall Georgian house has been a hotel since 1907. Both the ground floor lounge and bar are elegant, featuring lofty rooms with plasterwork ceilings, chandeliers, marble fireplaces and antique mirrors. The bedrooms (accessed by a period staircase) are more modest by comparison. They are nonetheless compact and comfortable, offering the usual facilities, and most have a shower. There's no lift at present, though one is planned. Own car park. Same ownership as Stauntons on the Green (see entry). Note: the basement 'Georgian' Brasserie is leased out. • Acc££ •

Dublin 2 — Il Primo

16 Montague Street Dublin
RESTAURANT   **Tel/Fax: 01 478 3373**

Dieter Bergman's cheery little first floor restaurant was way ahead of current fashions when it opened in 1991. It's simple (some would say spartan) but the essentials are right: warm hospitality and excellent, imaginative, freshly cooked modern Italian food. Then there's the wine, which is Dieter's special passion: all wines below £36 are available by the millilitre – customers drink as much as they want and that's the amount they pay for: brilliant. Dieter also organises regular wine tastings and dinners. This place is special. • L£ Mon-Fri, D££ Mon-Sat • Closed Xmas & Bank Hols •

► Dublin 2 — Imperial Chinese Restaurant

12A Wicklow Street Dublin
RESTAURANT   **Tel: 01 677 2580   Fax: 01 677 9851**

Oriental Restaurant of the Year

The rich variety and exoticism of the regional cuisines of China sometimes seem to be "lost in translation" when reproduced in Chinese restaurants in the West. Concessions to blandness are often made to increase the appeal of Chinese food to Western palates. Sadly, the compromises made can result in some dishes becoming uniformly dull, the more exotic ones not appearing at all, and Chinese cuisine in general acquiring a reputation for not being as innovative as, say, the food from Thailand. The Imperial has bucked this trend and presents a menu of both regular favourites done with a real concern for the authenticity of dishes (even with such modest dishes as spring rolls) along with an extensive special menu of more obscure dishes. Fixed price three-course lunches are very good value, as is Sunday dim sum. It should come as no surprise therefore that the restaurant, run by Mrs Cheung and her team, is strongly supported by perhaps that most demanding group of customers, the local Chinese community. • L£ & D££ daily • Closed 25-26 Dec •

Dublin 14 — Indian Brasserie

Rathfarnham Dublin
RESTAURANT   **Tel/Fax: 01 492 0260**

Although only open since summer 1998, Samir Sapru's Indian Brasserie has already made a remarkable impact – it prepared the Great Indian Banquet at Dublin Castle to celebrate the 50th anniversary of Indian Independence. The restaurant, which is run as a buffet, offers freshly prepared wholesome food, aiming to make it the nearest to home cooking that can be achieved in a restaurant. The usual selection includes around eight starters, five or six salads and seven or eight main courses, with each dish individually prepared from scratch and the selection worked out so that all the dishes complement each other. Breads – which are baked quickly at a very high temperature – are cooked to order. The hospitality is intended to make each guest feel as if they are visiting a private house – customers are encouraged to try a little of everything that has been prepared on the night. • Meals£-££ daily • Closed 25 Dec • Amex, Diners, MasterCard, Visa •

Dublin 6   Ivy Court Restaurant
88 Rathgar Road Dublin
RESTAURANT   Tel: 01 492 0633   Fax: 01 492 0634

Josef and Eileen Frei's Rathgar restaurant is a warm and welcoming place with friendly, efficient staff and good food at reasonable prices. A real neighbourhood restaurant, it has a great local following and is likely to be busy any day of the week. The decor of the first floor dining area is quite unusual, with huge Breughel-style murals the main feature – but there isn't too much time to dwell on them as service is swift. Josef Frei presents seasonal à la carte menus, mainly in a French country style, with a few other influences creeping in (pasta and spatzli for example) and it makes a refreshing change from the supercharged international menus which are currently almost universal. French onion soup, home made bisque with brandy, fillet of sea trout grand'mere, sirloin steak Café de Paris are all typical and very good. • D£-££ Mon-Sat • Closed 25-26 Dec & 1 Jan •

Dublin 2   Jacob's Ladder
4 Nassau Street Dublin
RESTAURANT   Tel: 01 670 3865   Fax: 01 670 3868

Adrian and Bernie Roche opened this smart restaurant overlooking the playing fields of Trinity College in 1997 and it was an immediate success. The modern decor provides an appropriate backdrop for Adrian's cooking which is in the New Irish style with international influences. He presents well-balanced seasonal menus, which always include some vegetarian dishes (marked on the menu), and there is a welcome heartiness about his food. Typical starters, for example, might include sauté of ducklivers & confit with parfait and a citrus salad and one of the half dozen main courses on the dinner menu could be roast cutlet of smoked pork with savoy cabbage, herbed mash, glazed turnip & grain mustard. To finish, Irish farmhouse cheeses feature alongside tempting desserts such as a lemon brûlée with orange ice. • L£ & D££ Mon-Sat • Closed 3 wks at Xmas •

Dublin 8   Jurys Christchurch Inn
Christchurch Place Dublin
HOTEL   Tel: 01 454 0000   Fax: 01 454 0012

The Jurys Inn chain provides competitively priced middle range accommodation throughout Ireland. Jurys Christchurch Inn is particularly well placed for both tourist and business travellers, with a location close to attractions such as Dublin Castle and Dublinia (the museum of medieval Dublin). Temple Bar and the central city are also close by. There is a large multi-storey car park at the rear with convenient access to the hotel. Rooms are confortable and spacious (though occasionally in need of greater attention to upgrading and maintenance), with large, well positioned work desks. • Acc££ • Closed 25-26 Dec •

Dublin 1   Jurys Custom House Inn
Custom House Quay Dublin
HOTEL   Tel: 01 607 5000   Fax: 01 829 0400
www.jurys.com

Right beside the financial services centre, overlooking the Liffey and close to train and bus stations, this hotel meets the requirements of business guests with better facilities than is usual in budget hotels. Large bedrooms can sleep up to four and have all the usual facilities, but also fax/modem lines and a higher standard of finish than earlier sister hotels; fabrics and fittings are better quality and neat bathrooms are more thoughtfully designed, with more generous shelf space – although bath tubs are still tiny. As well as a large bar, there is a full restaurant on site, plus conference facilities for up to 100 and a staffed business centre. No room service. No private parking but there is a 400-space multi-storey park with direct access to the hotel. • Acc££ • Closed 24-26 Dec • Amex, Diners, MasterCard, Visa •

Dublin 4 — Jurys Hotel Dublin and The Towers

Pembroke Road Ballsbridge Dublin

HOTEL 🏛

Tel: 01 660 5000   Fax: 01 667 5276

Business Hotel of the Year

Jury Hotel in Ballsbridge has long been something of a Dublin institution – centrally located in the Ballsbridge area, always full of life, it has achieved a rather unusual distinction – it somehow manages to pull off the trick of being both an international hotel providing high levels of service to business and leisure guests while remaining a genuinely popular local hotel in which Dubliners themselves feel welcome and at home. It is a formula that works to everyone's benefit. For leisure guests the hotel has a well-stocked newsagent and shop, a swimming pool, fitness centre and cabaret with highly popular and long-running show. Rooms are of a very high standard in both Jurys (the front section of the hotel which has undergone a major refurbishment) and The Towers (the quieter, more exclusive section of the hotel located to the rear). The Towers pays tribute to Dublin's strong literary heritage, with floors named after major Irish writers – busts and short biographies grace the lift areas of each floor, making waiting for a lift an unusually edifying experience. For businesses and business people both sections of the hotel together provide everything that could be required – a business centre, secretarial services, conference rooms (up to 850), banqueting (for up to 600), corporate meeting rooms, computing, presentation, internet and other facilities, along with the peace and quiet (in The Towers) needed to recover from the demands of business and travel. – in other words, all of the essential ingredients for any hotel hoping to compete in this highly competitive and specialised market. The hotel is, therefore, a worthy winner of our Business Hotel of the Year Award. There have been many new hotels built for the business market in Dublin in recent years, and Jurys has had to ensure that, while it has long been held in high regard as a Dublin institution, it also continued to upgrade its facilities and levels of service to match the increasingly tough competition. This has been done, and perhaps one reason for its continued success is the commitment on the part of all levels of staff to high quality service for its customers, delivered with a friendly and relaxed helpfulness. Added to this are the facilities provided for business (and non-business) guests to dine, entertain or relax – complimentary early evening drinks for Towers guests and a pub (appropriately named The Dubliner), a cocktail bar, coffee shop (The Coffee Dock, open virtually all day and night) and restaurant (Raglan's) offering high quality food and genuine Dublin hospitality, variety and local colour. • Acc£££-££££ • Open all year •

Dublin 9 — Kavanagh's

Prospect Square Glasnevin Dublin

PUB

John Kavanagh's is also known as "The Gravediggers" because of its location next to the Glasnevin cemetery (with its rich folk history). It lays claim to being the oldest family pub in Dublin – it was established in 1833 and the current family are the 6th generation in the business. This is a genuine Victorian bar, totally unspoilt – and it has a reputation for serving one of the best pints in Dublin. Theme pub owners eat your hearts out. • Closed 25 Dec & Good Fri •

Dublin 2 — Kilkenny Restaurant & Café

6 Nassau Street Dublin

CAFÉ/RESTAURANT

Tel: 01 677 7066   Fax: 01 677 3891

Situated on the first floor of the shop now known simply as Kilkenny, with a clear view into the grounds of Trinity College, the refurbished Kilkenny Restaurant is one of the pleasantest places in Dublin to have a bite to eat – and the food matches the view. It looks good and the experience matches the anticipation. Real home cooking has always been the strength of the Kilkenny kitchen. All their ingredients are fresh and additive-free (as are all the products on sale in the shop's Food Hall). Salads, quiches, casseroles, home-baked breads and cakes are the specialities of the Kilkenny Restaurant and they are very good. For quicker bites the shop has a second eating place, Kilkenny Café, where the same principles apply. A range of Kilkenny preserves and dressings – all made and labelled on the premises – is available in the shop. • Shopping hours daily meals£ • Closed 25 Dec & 1 Jan •

Dublin 22

Kingswood Country House

Old Kingswood Naas Road Clondalkin Dublin

RESTAURANT/ACCOMMODATION   Tel/Fax: 01 459 2428

Just off the Naas Road and very close to the industrial estates around Newlands Cross, the country house atmosphere of this guesthouse and restaurant comes as a very pleasant surprise. The restaurant has a lovely cosy atmosphere and a loyal following, for both the service and atmosphere as well as the food. This is an interesting combination of classic French and traditional and new Irish styles. Ingredients are top quality and the policy is to use as much local and free range produce as possible Private rooms are available for groups and small business meetings. Accommodation: There are seven guest rooms, all en-suite, and like the rest of the house they have an old-fashioned charm. • Acc££-£££ • L£ Mon-Fri & Sun, D££ daily • Closed 25-26 Dec & Good Fri •

Dublin 4

Langkawi

46 Upper Baggot Street Dublin

RESTAURANT   Tel: 01 668 2760

email: hosey@indigo.ie

Malaysian cuisine is a synthesis of three main distinct national cuisines – Malay, Chinese and Indian – and the result is a distinctive mix that offers something for everyone, from hot, fiery dishes through to more subtle flavours. The now very popular Langkawi sets out to do all styles justice, but there is an understandable emphasis on Malay dishes since this is the rarer cuisine in Ireland. Satays make a good start for the more timid. For the more adventurous diner there is plenty to choose from (with clear menu guidance on heat levels). Chef Alex Hosey uses genuine imported ingredients to achieve an authentic Malaysian taste. Well worth visiting for a lunch or dinner that is out of the ordinary. • L£ Mon-Fri & D££ Mon-Sat • Closed 25 Dec, Easter Sun & Good Fri •

Dublin 4

Lansdowne Manor

46-48 Lansdowne Road Ballsbridge Dublin

ACCOMMODATION   Tel: 01 668 8848   Fax: 01 668 8873

Situated in the heart of "embassyland", Lansdowne Manor comprises two early Victorian mansions which have been recently refurbished and decorated in period style. It now offers some of the most comfortable guesthouse accommodation in the city. • Acc££ • Closed 22-27 Dec •

Dublin 2

Little Caesar's Palace

Balfe Street Dublin

RESTAURANT   Tel: 01 671 8714

This genuine little pizza place is just a stone's throw from the door of the Westbury Hotel – fresh, tasty and inexpensive pizzas (with good crisp bases) cooked before your very eyes could be the perfect antidote to too much luxury, or too much shopping. Open 12noon-midnight. • Closed 25 Dec & Good Fri • Amex, Diners, MasterCard, Visa •

Dublin 2

Lloyds Brasserie

20 Merrion Street Upper Dublin

RESTAURANT   Tel: 01 662 7240/1/2   Fax: 01 662 7243

email: conradallagher@tinet.ie   gallaghergroup@tinet.ie

Conrad Gallagher is one of the city's best known chef/restaurateurs and this, his second eaterie, is much more casual than his serious Peacock Alley restaurant (which, at the time of going to press, is about to move to the Fitzwilliam Hotel)). Lloyds is open seven days a week for lunch (brunch at weekends) and dinner; additionally, bar food is served all day and there's usually a lively crowd in the piano bar on Thursday, Friday and Saturday evenings from 9pm- 2am. The basement restaurant is minimalist in the extreme, very chic, with red banquettes, marble-topped tables cheek by jowl, aluminium chairs, tiled floor and blue walls. It's a modern and trendy restaurant (incidentally, the eager young staff are quite in keeping), serving excellent modern food, with dishes influenced by cuisines from around the globe. There's a good and reasonably priced wine list with a decent showing from the New World. • Open all day (from 1pm Sat & Sun) • Meals from £ • Closed 25-26 Dec, 1 Jan & Good Fri •

➤ Dublin 4

RESTAURANT

The Lobster Pot

9 Ballsbridge Terrace Ballsbridge Dublin
Tel/Fax: 01 668 0025

Situated in a conspicuous position on the first floor of a redbrick Ballsbridge terrace, this long-established restaurant has lost none of its charm and quality over the years. How good it is to see old favourites like dressed Kilmore crab, home-made chicken liver pâté and fresh prawn bisque on the menu, along with fresh prawns Mornay and, would you believe, Coq au Vin. All this and wonderfully old-fashioned service too. Long may it last.
• L£ Mon-Fri, D££ Mon-Sat • Closed 25 Dec, 1 Jan & Good Fri •

Dublin 8

RESTAURANT

Locks

1 Windsor Terrace Portobello Dublin
Tel: 01 454 3391   Fax: 01 453 8352

Locks Restaurant is a very special place, in an old building with a lovely canalside setting. Inside it is furnished and decorated in a warm country house style and has a soothing atmosphere – soft lighting, open fires and a feeling that it has evolved rather than being designed by a decorator. Food and service echo that feeling – the short set menus for lunch and dinner offer the kind of food that might be served in a good country house; the seasonal à la carte menu is more ambitious in scale, but offers a similar combination of classic and country French and New Irish cooking; for example, a starter of Locks fish soup with aioli & croutons, and main courses such as roast loin of lamb with dauphinoise potatoes, caramelised onions, mushrooms & rosemary sauce. The cooking is sure, presentation very much in a house style and service professional. • L££ Mon-Fri, D£££ Mon-Sat • Closed last wk Jul, Xmas wk & Bank Hols •

Dublin 2

HOTEL/RESTAURANT

Longfields Hotel

9/10 Fitzwilliam Street Lower Dublin
Tel: 01 676 1367   Fax: 01 676 1542

Located in a Georgian terrace right in the heart of Georgian Dublin, this hotel is more like a well proportioned private house, furnished with antiques in period style. Public areas are elegant and comfortable and bedrooms individually furnished, all with en-suite bath/shower. They vary considerably in size as rooms are smaller on the upper floors. Staff are friendly and there is 24 hour room service. Morning coffee and afternoon tea are served in the drawing room.

No 10 Restaurant

In the basement, with direct access from the hotel or the street, this compact well-appointed restaurant makes a popular venue for both lunch and dinner. Head chef Tommy Donovan, who has been with the hotel since 1990, presents imaginative menus, based on seasonal local ingredients and cooks in a style combining French and Irish influences. French and Irish cheeses are offered, and a choice of coffee/speciality tea. • L£ Mon-Sat, D££ daily • Acc£££ • Closed 24-28 Dec •

Dublin 8

RESTAURANT

The Lord Edward

23 Christchurch Place Dublin
Tel/Fax: 01 454 2420

Dublin's oldest seafood restaurant is on three floors of a tall, narrow building overlooking Christchurch cathedral. Traditional in a decidedly old-fashioned way, The Lord Edward provides a complete contrast to the wave of trendy restaurants that has taken over Dublin recently, which is just the way a lot of people seem to like it. There are a few non-seafood options – traditional dishes like Irish stew, perhaps or corned beef and cabbage – and the seafood can be excellent. Simplest choices are usually best. • L£ Mon-Fri, D££ Mon-Sat • Closed Xmas wk & Good Fri •

Dublin 2

RESTAURANT

Café Mao

2 Chatham Row Dublin
Tel: 01 670 4899

In simple but stylish surroundings, Café Mao brings to the Grafton Street area the cuisines of Thailand, Malaysia, Indonesia, Japan and China – about as "Asian Fusion" as it gets. The atmosphere at Mao is bright and very buzzy – having a queue at the door, as has happened here from the start, probably zips up the atmosphere a notch or two. Interesting food is based on seasonal ingredients, the standard of cooking is consistently good and so is value for money, although the bill can mount up quickly if you don't watch the number of Asian beers ordered! The "no reservations" policy seems to be working well for the restaurant, although it puts off some potential customers. • L££, D££ daily •

Dublin 13   Marine Hotel
Sutton Cross Dublin

HOTEL   Tel: 01 839 0000   Fax: 01 839 0442

This attractive, well-maintained hotel is on the sea side of this busy junction, with ample car parking in front and a lawn reaching down to the foreshore at the rear. Public areas, which have all been recently renovated, give a good impression; they include a smart foyer and adjacent bar, an informal conservatory style seating area overlooking the garden and a well-appointed restaurant. First floor corridors and bedrooms, some of which have sea views, were much less impressive on a recent visit, but refurbishment is ongoing and 12 new executive rooms are due for completion by April 1999. A popular venue for conferences and social gatherings, especially weddings – capacity up to 200.
• Acc£££ • Open all year •

Dublin 4   McCormack's Merrion Inn
188 Merrion Road Dublin

PUB   Tel: 01 269 3816/2455   Fax: 01 269 766

The McCormacks are a great pub family (see separate entry for their Mounttown establishment) and this attractive contemporary pub on the main road between Dublin and Dun Laoghaire has always had a good name for food. At lunchtime chef John Teehan puts up an excellent buffet, with a choice of four hot main courses – a roast and a fish dish plus two others – as well as a wide range of salads; it's a well-organised operation and details (such as having chilled drinks to hand) are well-planned. In the evening the style moves up a notch or two, with a menu including the likes of warm crispy bacon & crouton salad, pastas, stir-fries and serious main courses such as medallions of fillet beef (chargrilled and served with a choice of sauces and salads). There are always a few good fish dishes and vegetarian options, and homely desserts always include homemade apple tart. • L£, Meals£, D£ daily • Closed 25 Dec & Good Fri •

Dublin 2   La Mère Zou
22 St Stephen's Green Dublin

RESTAURANT   Tel/Fax: 01 661 6669
email: merzou@indigo.ie

Situated in a Georgian basement not far from the Shelbourne Hotel, Eric Tydgadt's French/Belgian restaurant has been open since 1994 and just gets on with doing what it does best, without the fuss and flurry so many other restaurants are prone to at the moment. Although there are some concessions to current cuisine (especially on the lunch menu), this establishment's reputation is based on French country cooking, as in terrine of wild rabbit with pistachio nuts (albeit with a raspberry & onion compote), grilled chicken chasseur (with a mushroom, tomato & white sauce) and specialities such as steamed mussels (various ways) with French fries and even traditional Alsatian sauerkraut with four meats. Prices are reasonable, a policy carried through to the wine list too; well-chosen French house wines, for example, are £10. • L£ Mon-Fri, D££ daily • Closed 25 Dec & 1-6 Jan •

Dublin 2   Mermaid Café
69-70 Dame Street Dublin

RESTAURANT   Tel: 01 670 8236   Fax: 01 670 8205

Interesting decor and imaginative American-inpired cooking are to be found at this restaurant on the edge of Temple Bar. Small, but with every inch of space used with style, owner-chef Benedict Gorman's cooking is among the best in the area and his front-of-house partner, Mark Harrell, is a quietly solicitous host. Examples which indicate the style include starters like New England crab cakes with piquant mayonnaise and smoked mackerel rillette with scallion and tomato salad. Terrific vegetarian main courses such as pumpkin & red onion tart with cumin & parmesan are to be found beside the likes of hearty home-made venison & port sausage with celeriac & elderberry gravy and 'Giant Atlantic Seafood Casserole', a speciality which changes daily depending on availability. Irish cheeses are imaginatively served and in good condition. Espresso and cappuccino arrive with crystallised pecan nuts. Wines are imported privately and are exclusive to the restaurant. • L£ daily & D££ Mon-Sat • Closed Xmas wk •

Dublin 4 — Merrion Hall

ACCOMMODATION

54-56 Merriom Road Ballsbridge Dublin
Tel: 01 668 1426   Fax: 01 668 4280

Spacious, friendly guesthouse opposite the RDS, with small amount of off-street parking, bedrooms to a high standard, comfortable roomy sitting room and very good breakfasts.
• Acc£££ • Open all year •

Dublin 2 — The Merrion Hotel

HOTEL/RESTAURANT 🏛🏛

Upper Merrion Street Dublin
Tel: 01 603 0600   Fax: 01 603 0700
email: info@merrionhotel.ie www.merrionhotel.ie

Set in the heart of Georgian Dublin opposite the Government Buildings, the city's grandest and most luxurious hotel opened its doors in October 1997. The Main House of the hotel comprises four meticulously restored Grade I listed townhouses built in the 1760s, and a contemporary garden wing has been added, overlooking two private period and formal landscaped gardens. Inside, Irish fabrics and antiques reflect the architecture and original interiors, such as rococo plasterwork ceilings, varied woodwork and classically proportioned windows. The elegant and spacious Front Hall, with marble columns, features a series of murals for the neo-classical main stairwell by Martin Mooney, one of Ireland's foremost young artists (indeed, the hotel boasts one of the most important private collections of 20th-century art throughout), while the three interconnecting drawing rooms (one is the cocktail bar with a log fire), have French windows giving access to the gardens. The elegant and gracious bedrooms with individually controlled air-conditioning, have been beautifully designed by Alice Roden, and incorporate the very latest technology, ranging from three telephones, personalised voice-mail with remote access, fax/modem and ISDN lines and video conference facilities. In addition to the usual amenities there is a mini-bar and safe (VCRs and CD players are available on request). Sumptuous Italian marble bathrooms, with a separate walk-in shower, pamper guests to the extreme. The six meeting/private dining rooms combine state-of-the-art technology and Georgian splendour, contrasting with the arched and rough stone-walled Cellar Bar, originally the wine vaults. On the other hand, the splendid leisure complex, The Tethra Spa, with classical mosaics, is almost Romanesque. Staff, under the excellent direction of General Manager Peter MacCann, are quite exemplary and courteous, suggesting standards of hospitality from a bygone era. Complimentary underground valet parking. Restaurant Patrick Guilbaud (see separate entry) is also on site.

Mornington Restaurant

Executive chef Ed Cooney's dishes reflect the contemporary style of the elegant dining-room, combining fine Irish ingredients with Mediterranean cooking influences. An inexpensive table d'hôte lunch menu contrasts with more choices in the evening, but nonetheless shows off competent and precise cooking, backed up by excellent service. The wine list is grand, but prices are not over the top for such an illustrious establishment. • Meals££-£££ •Acc££££• Open all year •

Dublin 4 — Mespil Hotel

HOTEL

Mespil Road Dublin
Tel: 01 667 1222   Fax: 01 667 1244
email: mespil@leehotels.ie www.iol.ie/lee

This fine modern hotel enjoys an excellent location in the Georgian district of the city, overlooking the Grand canal and within easy walking distance of the city centre. Public areas are spacious and elegant in an easy contemporary style and generously-sized bedrooms (including eight suitable for disabled guests and 30 non-smoking rooms) are comfortably furnished with good amenities. Facilities are also available for meetings and small conferences (up to 50) and banquets (110). Special breaks offer good value. Sister hotel to Sligo Park Hotel (see entry). • Acc££ • Closed 24-26 Dec •

Dublin 2 — Milano

RESTAURANT

38 Dawson Street Dublin
Tel: 01 670 7744   Fax: 01 679 2717

This stylish modern restaurant at the top of Dawson Street is best known for its wide range of excellent pizzas (it's owned by the UK company PizzaExpress), but it's more of a restaurant than the description implies. They run a very popular crèche facility on Sunday afternoons (12-6) and live jazz on Monday evenings. A second branch opened in Temple Bar more recently and they have a jazz duo at Sunday lunchtime (2-4). • L£ & D£ daily • Closed 25 Dec & Good Fri •

Dublin 2   Mitchell's Cellars

21 Kildare Street Dublin

RESTAURANT   Tel: 01 662 4724   Fax: 01 661 1509

Run by Patricia Hogan and Anne McCartney since 1978, this lunchtime restaurant in the arched cellars underneath the old Mitchell's wine merchants has become something of an institution. The 'no reservations' policy ensures an early crowd and the food, as ever, revolves around wholesome classics – beef in Guinness, lamb provençal – and good fish dishes such as salmon with coriander & lime in filo pastry and seafood platters. Vegetarian dishes are always available. If there isn't a table ready when you arrive, there's a characterful wine bar at the far end where you can wait in comfort. • L£ Mon-Fri (& Sat off-season) • Closed 24-29 Dec, 1 Jan & Easter •

Dublin 2   Mont Clare Hotel

Merrion Square Dublin

HOTEL   Tel: 01 607 3800   Fax: 01 661 5663

email: montclare@tinet.ie   www.montclarehotel.ie

A few doors away from the National gallery, the Mont Clare is in common ownership with the nearby Davenport and Alexander Hotels. It has recently been totally renovated and refurbished and now has all the amenities expected of a good modern hotel. It is imaginatively decorated in contemporary style – except the old stained glass and mahogany Gallery Bar, which has retained its original pubby atmosphere. Compact bedrooms are well furnished and comfortable, with full marbled bathrooms and good amenities, including a personal safe. There are no on-site leisure facilities but guests have a complimentary arrangement with a nearby fitness centre. • Acc£££ •

Dublin 2   The Morgan

10 Fleet Street Temple Bar Dublin

HOTEL   Tel: 01 679 3939   Fax: 01 679 3946

email: morganht@iol.ie   www.iol.ie/~morganht

Situated in deepest Temple Bar, this unusual boutique hotel opened in 1997 and has already completed a major extension programme, including de-luxe bedrooms and junior suites. With the exception of a luxurious Odeon duplex suite in Art-Deco style, the overall design concept is of chic minimalism (with excellent amenities, including the latest technology in bedrooms), 'warmed' by the use of natural materials such as stone, timber and leather. Other special features of the Morgan include a roof-top garden with residents' cocktail bar, a private fitness centre and a "new age" hair salon. Although it may seem at odds with the Morgan's air of cool sophistication, The All Sports Café next door also belongs to the hotel. • Acc£££ •

Dublin 2   Muscat

64 South William Street Dublin

RESTAURANT   Tel: 01 679 7699

Brian Corish and Bernadette Doherty's tiny restaurant is in a very old building a couple of steps down from the street, and it's a little gem. The logistics of the operation are, theoretically, impossible (and it's fascinating to watch how they do actually work) but the hospitality is warm, Seamus Commons' Irish/Mediterranean cooking is excellent and the service is a miracle. They even have very nice little loos with extras normally associated with much grander places. • L£ Tues-Fri, D££ Tues-Sat • Close Xmas wk, New Year & 2 wks Sept •

Establishments recommended have all met our stringent entry requirements at the time of assessment. However, standards are sometimes not always as consistent as they should be. If you are disappointed by any aspect of a visit to a listed establishment, we suggest that you try to sort it out at the time if possible, as speedy, amicable solutions are by far the best. If you are still dissatisfied, put your complaints in writing to the proprietor or manager as soon as possible after the event - and send a copy to the guide if you wish.

Dublin 2

Number 31

31 Leeson Close Dublin

ACCOMMODATION   Tel: 01 676 5011   Fax: 01 676 2929

email: number31@iol.ie

The former home of Dublin architect Sam Stephenson, Brian and Mary Bennett's renowned guesthouse provides "an oasis of tranquility"; spacious, unusual accommodation of a very high standard and very fine hospitality – just off St Stephen's Green. Excellent breakfasts. Not suitable for children under 10. • Acc££ • Closed Xmas wk •

We aim to be as up to date as possible, but changes will inevitably occur after we go to press. We would request that listed establishments inform us as quickly as possible of major changes, eg sale of property or key staff changes, so that our records may be updated through the year. Readers will have access to important changes by visiting our website (www.ireland-guide.com).

Dublin 2

O Sushi

12 Fownes Street Dublin

RESTAURANT   Tel: 01 677 6111

Dublin's first sushi bar is one of the more interesting restaurants in Temple Bar. They also serve teriyaki, tempura, sashimi, norimaki rolls and other Japanese specialities. The tasting plate selection is a good choice for beginners. • L£ Mon-Sat, D Mon-Sun • Closed 25-26 Dec & Good Fri •

Dublin 2

O'Neill's Public House

2 Suffolk Street Dublin

PUB   Tel: 01 679 3656   Fax: 01 679 0689

email: mikeon@indigo.ie

A striking pub with its own fine clock over the door and an excellent corner location, it has been in the O'Neill family since 1920 and is equally popular with Dubliners and visitors alike. Students from Trinity and several other colleges nearby home into O'Neill's for its wide range of reasonably priced bar food, which includes a carvery with a choice of five roasts and an equal number of other dishes (including traditional favourites such as Irish Stew) each day. • Meals£ • Closed 25-26 Dec & Good Fri •

Dublin 8

The Old Dublin

90/91 Francis Street Dublin

RESTAURANT   Tel/Fax: 01 454 2028

Eamonn Walsh's oasis of civilised dining is one of Dublin's longest-established fine restaurants. The standard of cooking is high and the food is lively, with new dishes regularly taking their place alongside established favourites. The dining area is broken up into several domestic-sized rooms with special features – a marble fireplace, some very good pictures – creating a cosy old-world atmosphere. While most famous for its Russian and Scandinavian specialities like blini (buckwheat pancake with cured salmon, prawns and herrings), and planked sirloin Hussar, which still feature on the à la carte, recent menus have been noticeably modern, with starters such as seared duck liver crostini followed by main courses like baked fillet of monkfish wrapped in speck, tomato and coriander dressing. Desserts include good home-made ices and a trio of farmhouse cheeses, served plated. A vegetarian menu is offered, also a reasonable early-bird 2-course dinner. Hospitable, thoughtful service. • L£ Mon-Fri, D££ Mon-Sat •

Establishments recommended have all met our stringent entry requirements at the time of assessment. However, standards are sometimes not always as consistent as they should be. If you are disappointed by any aspect of a visit to a listed establishment, we suggest that you try to sort it out at the time if possible, as speedy, amicable solutions are by far the best. If you are still dissatisfied, put your complaints in writing to the proprietor or manager as soon as possible after the event - and send a copy to the guide if you wish.

Dublin 7

CAFÉ/BAR

The Old Jameson Distillery

Bow Street Dublin
Tel: 01 807 2355   Fax: 01 807 2369
email: rdempsey@iol.ie

While most visitors to Dublin will visit the recently restored Old Jameson Distillery to do the tour (which is fascinating), it's also a good spot for a bite to eat. There are special menus for groups (including evening functions, when the Distillery is not otherwise open) but The Still Room Restaurant is also open to individuals – light food served all day and lunch, featuring Irish specialities like bacon & cabbage soup and John Jameson casserole, from 12.30-2.30 daily. • L£ daily • Closed 25 Dec & Good Fri •

Dublin 2

PUB

The Old Stand

37 Exchequer Street Dublin
Tel: 01 677 7220   Fax: 01 677 5849

This fine traditional pub, which is a sister establishment to Davy Byrnes, off Grafton Street and equally well-run, occupies a prominent position on the corner of Exchequer Street and St Andrew Street. It has a loyal following amongst the local business community, notably from the "rag trade" area around South William Street. They do a good line in reliable no-nonsense bar food at reasonable prices. A blackboard at the door proclaims daily specials as well as a selection of regulars from the menu – steaks (with or without sauce), grilled salmon steak, omelettes and chips, Irish stew and a vegetarian pasta dish of the day are all typical. • Meals£ daily • Closed 25 Dec & Good Fri •

The guide aims to provide comprehensive recommendations of the best places to eat, drink and stay throughout Ireland. We welcome suggestions from readers. If you think an establishment merits assessment, please write or email us.

Dublin 2

HOTEL

Parliament Hotel

Lord Edward Street Dublin
Tel: 01 670 8777   Fax: 01 670 8787
email: parl@regencyhotels.com www.reghotels.com

Conveniently located near the entrance to Dublin Castle, and on the edge of Temple Bar, the Parliament Hotel will probably appeal most to tourist travellers. Rooms are well appointed and there is a large bar at street level which serves casual food. Breakfast is excellent and is served in a more private basement restaurant. • Acc££ • Closed 25 Dec •

Dublin 2

RESTAURANT

Pasta Fresca

2, 3 & 4 Chatham Street Dublin
Tel: 01 679 2402

This chic Italian wine bar-delicatessen is just off the Grafton Street shopping area. The popular all-day menu is based on good home-made pastas, interesting vegetarian options and a wide range of salads with well-made dressings. Evening menus offer more choice. • Open all day, L£ & D££ daily •

Dublin 2

RESTAURANT

Pizza Stop

6-10 Chatham Lane Dublin
Tel: 01 679 4769

This cheap and cheerful little restaurant has been doing good pizzas in style since the late '80s. Just the place to meet up with the family for a tasty meal that won't break the bank. Also good for nightbirds since it stays open until 2 am every day. • Meals£ daily •

Dublin 6W

RESTAURANT

Popjoys

4 Rathfarnham Road Terenure Dublin
Tel: 01 492 9346   Fax: 01 492 9293

Chef-proprietor Warren Massey opened this neighbourhood restaurant in partnership with restaurant manager John Coleman in August '96. With a comfortable and well-appointed dining room, Warren's progressive cooking – always based on the best of local and seasonal ingredients – and good service have attracted a loyal following. • L£ Tues-Fri & Sun, D££ Tues-Sat •

Dublin 2

PUB ⭐

Pub of the Year

The Porterhouse

16-18 Parliament Street Dublin
Tel: 01 679 8847   Fax: 01 670 9605
email: PorterH.indigo.ie

When this stunning pub opened in 1996, it changed Dubliners' perception of what a pub could be, opening up a whole new range of possibilities that simply hadn't been considered before. It was, for a start, Ireland's first micro-brewery and, although several others have since set up and are doing an excellent job, The Porterhouse started this admirable new trend in the brewing of real ale. Ten different beers are brewed on the premises, several of which have won international awards, and beer connoisseurs can sample a special "tasting tray" selection which gives information on the various brews. These include: plain porter (a classic light stout), oyster stout (brewed with fresh oysters, the logical development of a perfect partnership), Wrasslers 4X (based on a west Cork recipe from the early 1900s, and said to be Michael Collins' favourite tipple), Porter House Red (an Irish Red Ale with traditional flavour), An Brain Blasta (dangerous to know) and the wittily named Temple Brau. But you don't even have to like beer to love The Porterhouse. The whole concept is an innovative move away from the constraints of the traditional Irish pub and yet it stays in tune with its origins – it is emphatically not just another theme pub. The loving attention to detail which has gone into the decor and design is a constant source of pleasure to visitors – the bottles in glass cases that line the walls, the brewing-related displays in glass-topped tables – and the food, while definitely not gourmet, is a cut above the usual bar food and, like the pub itself, combines elements of tradition with innovation. This is a real Irish pub in the modern idiom and we applaud it. • L£ & D£ daily •

Dublin 4

ACCOMMODATION

Raglan Lodge

10 Raglan Road Ballsbridge Dublin
Tel: 01 660 6697   Fax: 01 660 6781

Helen Moran's elegant mid19th-century residence is peacefully situated and yet convenient to the city centre, which is only a 10-15 minute walk away. Well-proportioned, high-ceilinged reception rooms are reminiscent of more leisurely times and the en-suite bedrooms are exceptionally comfortable, with all the necessary amenities. Having been restored and converted to its present use in 1987, Raglan Lodge is now one of the city's most desirable guesthouses – not only for the high level of comfort and service provided, but most particularly, for outstanding breakfasts. Theatre reservations can be arranged. Private parking. • Acc£££ • Closed 23 Dec-7 Jan • Amex, Diners, MasterCard, Visa •

Dublin 2

RESTAURANT

Rajdoot Tandoori

26 Clarendon Street Dublin
Tel: 01 679 4724/4280   Fax: 01 679 4274

A member of a small UK chain of restaurants specialising in subtle, aromatic North Indian cuisine, this restaurant has had a fine reputation for its food and service since it opened in 1984. Tandoori dishes are the main speciality, based on a wide range of ingredients authentically cooked. Set price daily menus include a keenly priced 4-course lunch (£7.95). • L£ & D££ Mon-Sat • Closed Bank Hols, Xmas & New Year • All cards •

Dublin 6

HOTEL

Rathmines Plaza Hotel

Lower Rathmines Road Rathmines Dublin
Tel: 01 496 6966   Fax: 01 491 0603

Secure parking across the road is a distinct advantage for this modern hotel a few minutes' drive from the city centre in the characterful Rathmines district. Spacious bedrooms, each with a good tiled bathroom, offer the usual facilities including fax and computer points, and breakfast is taken in a rustic themed restaurant/bar (that can get very lively at night). Notably friendly staff. • Acc£££ • Closed 24-26 Dec •

The guide aims to provide comprehensive recommendations of the best places to eat, drink and stay throughout Ireland. We welcome suggestions from readers. If you know of an establishment which you think merits assessment for the guide, please write or email us.

Dublin 22 — Red Cow Moran's Hotel

Red Cow Complex Naas Road Dublin

HOTEL

Tel: 01 459 3650 Fax: 04 459 1588

Strategically located close to the motorway and known as a pub for many years, it may come as a surprise to discover that the Red Cow has now grown into an hotel. An impressive staircase sweeping up from the marble lobby gives an indication of the style to follow and, although it will also be of interest to private guests, this is definitely a location to check out if you are considering visiting the area on business or wish to organise conferences or meetings. Bedrooms are all of executive standard, with excellent amenities for business guests including voice mail and fax/modem lines. The purpose-built conference centre offers a wide range of facilities, backed up by full secretarial services and ample car parking. • Acc£££-££££ •

Dublin 2 — Restaurant Patrick Guilbaud

Upper Merrion Street Dublin

RESTAURANT ★

Tel: 01 676 4192 Fax: 01 661 0052

Dessert of the Year

Originally in St James's Place off Lower Baggot Street, Patrick Guilbaud has again utilised the services of designer Arthur Gibney & Partners to create this spectacular and elegant ground-floor restaurant in the Main House of The Merrion Hotel, opening on to a terrace and landscaped garden (with al fresco eating in fine weather). The entrance to the restaurant is the original entrance to the Georgian townhouse built in the 1760s by Lord Monck (access can also be gained via the hotel). Customers should particularly note some fine works by Irish artists (Roderic O'Connor, Mary Swanzy, Louise le Brocquy and William Scott, to name but a few – look out especially for Harry Kernoff's 'Jammet's Restaurant', probably Dublin's finest restaurant in the 'sixties). All in all, it's a very fine setting for one of Ireland's most renowned restaurants, and the cooking has lost nothing in the transfer; if anything it has moved up a gear. Patrick himself is much in evidence, as charming as ever, and head chef Guillaume Le Brun presides over a fine kitchen. The table d'hôte lunch is a snip at £20 inclusive for two courses (perhaps steamed fillets of wild sea trout with olives and a basil sauce and pan-fried fennel, followed by fillets of Irish beef with a red wine sauce and honey-glazed apricots), while the £65 menu surprise is just that – you are only told what the dishes are, as they are served. Unusually for a French restaurant, the à la carte menu is written in English – no fuss, with a short description, thus starters such as King Scallops, pan-fried Bantry Bay king scallops with rhubarb compote and citrus vinaigrette, Lobster Ravioli, poached and infused with coconut jus, served between two layers of home-made pasta, seasoned with curried olive oil, and (probably a first this) organic spelt, wheat grains perfectly cooked risotto-style with diced Perigord truffles. Main courses include Sea Bass, roasted and served with deep-fried squid and cockles; Brill, steamed and served with a basil purée and red pepper oil; Pigeon, boned, roast corn-fed squab pigeon with Bunratty mead and almond jus; Crubeens, pigs' trotters, boned and served with mushroom bread pudding and rosemary jus, and Veal Cutlets, milk-fed veal, pan-fried with a foie gras sauce. So, the best of Irish ingredients, combined with the precision and talents of a team of gifted chefs, produces dishes of dexterity, appeal and flavour. Desserts are particularly interesting – a Nougatine Millefeuille served with an amazing caramelised Fennel Confit is an unlikely-sounding but superbly successful dish and a worthy winner of our Dessert of the Year Award. Other less unusual but extremely good desserts could include fresh apricot tart with dried fruit and chartreuse ice cream or the assiette gourmand, assorted mini-chocolate desserts, including a melting chocolate fondant. Cheeses come from Philippe Olivier, breads are home-made, and the mostly French wine list includes some great classics, with some reasonably-priced offerings. Service is spot on. • L££ & D££££ Tues-Sat • Closed 25 Dec, first wk Jan & Good Fri •

Dublin 4 — Roly's Bistro

7 Ballsbridge Terrace Ballsbridge Dublin

RESTAURANT

Tel: 01 668 2611 Fax: 01 660 8535

A smash hit since the day it opened, a visit to this bustling Ballsbridge bistro invariably begins with a warm welcome – usually from Roly Saul or his partner John O'Sullivan (on duty at the desk). Aperitifs at the table are quickly followed by a selection of breads and the menu. Head chef Colin O'Daly is one of Ireland's most highly regarded chefs and has been part-owner of the restaurant since it opened in 1992. He presents imaginative, reasonably priced menus at lunch (£11.50 plus £2 supplement for the cheese plate) and an evening à la carte menu, all changed fortnightly. The style has its base in Colin's classical French experience but it also gives more than a passing nod to Irish traditions and world cuisines. Thus, starters of grainy Clonakilty Black Pudding wrapped in Brioche served on a well-reduced glaze and pleasingly runny, crisp-coated Deep-fried Brie served with a complementary Braised Red Cabbage & Apple Salad. Similarly, main course's of Roast Loin of Pork with Cajun Spices and Dublin Bay Prawns Newberg, which have become something of a speciality and come with a tian of mixed long grain and wild rice. Wholesomely delicious puddings are worth saving a space for: Pear & Apple Bake with Cinnamon Cream, perhaps, or dark chocolate and apricot slice. Service is efficient but discreet. • L£ & D££ Mon-Sun • Closed 25-27 Dec & Good Fri •

Dublin 2   Royal Garden
Westbury Centre Clarendon Street Dublin
RESTAURANT   Tel: 01 679 1397   Fax: 01 626 7643
Since the early 1980s this well-appointed Chinese restaurant at the back of the Westbury Hotel has been pleasing a loyal local clientele and visitors to the city with its authentic Cantonese cooking and excellent service. • L£ & D££ daily • Closed 25-26 Dec & Good Fri •

Dublin 8   Ryans of Parkgate Street
28 Parkgate Street Dublin
PUB   Tel: 01 671 9352   Fax: 01 671 3590
Ryans is one of Ireland's finest and best-loved original Victorian pubs. Its most distinguishing feature is its atmosphere, but there is also magnificent stained glass, original mahogany bar fixtures and an outstanding collection of antique mirrors. Good bar food is available at lunch time and in the evening, and there's a separate restaurant upstairs. • Meals£-££ • Closed first 2 wks Jan & Bank Hols •

Dublin 2   Saagar
16 Harcourt Street Dublin
RESTAURANT   Tel: 01 475 5060/5012   Fax: 01 475 5741
email: saagar@iol.ie www.bigsavings.ie/saagar
Saagar, Meera and Sunil Kumar's basement restaurant just off St Stephen's Green, is one of the most authentic and highly-respected ethnic restaurants in Ireland. The restaurant offers a wide range of speciality dishes, all prepared from fresh ingredients and thoughtfully coded with a range of one to four stars to indicate the heat level. Thus Malai Kabab (chicken marinated in traditional spices) is a safe one-star dish, while traditional Lamb Balti and Lamb Aayish (marinated with exotic spices and cooked in a cognac-flavoured sauce) is a three-star and therefore pretty hot. The vegetarian selection is good, as is to be expected of an Indian restaurant, and the side dishes, such as Naan breads which are made to order in the tandoori oven, are excellent. The Kumars also have a tandoori and take-way restaurant, Little India, at Dublin Bridge, Mullingar (044-40911). • L£ Mon-Fri, D££ Mon-Sun •

Dublin 4   The Schoolhouse Hotel
2-8 Northumberland Road Ballsbridge Dublin
HOTEL   Tel: 01 667 5014   Fax: 01 667 5015
Dating back to its opening in 1896 as a school, this building beside Mount Street Bridge has seen many changes lately, culminating in its opening in 1998 as one of Dublin's trendiest small hotels. The Inkwell Bar is always a-buzz with young business people of the area. Rooms are finished to a high standard, with air conditioning, power showers and the usual amenities expected of a quality hotel. A private room is available for small conferences and meetings of up to 25 delegates. • Acc£££-££££ • Closed 25 Dec •

Dublin 2   Shalimar
17 South Great Georges Street Dublin
RESTAURANT   Tel: 01 671 0738   Fax: 01 677 3478
Just across the road from the Central Hotel this welcoming, well-appointed basement restaurant serves generous portions of a wide-range of Indian dishes. Balti dishes are a speciality – diners are invited to mix and match items on the menu to suit individual tastes – and there's also a wide choice of Tandoori and Biryani basmati rice dishes. This is a friendly, relaxing restaurant and prices are reasonable. • L£ & D££ Mon-Sun • Closed 25-26 Dec & Good Fri •

Dublin 2   Shelbourne Hotel

HOTEL/RESTAURANT 🏛 🏛

27 St Stephen's Green Dublin
Tel: 01 676 6471   Fax: 01 661 6006
email: jricoux@shelbourne.ie   www.shelbourne.ie

One of Ireland's most historic buildings – the Irish constitution was drafted here – this opulent 18th-century hotel is still central to Dublin life today, and the many improvements which have recently taken place ensure its ranking among the world's great hotels. Overlooking Europe's largest garden square, St Stephen's Green, the hotel has retained all its grandeur, and the entrance creates a strong impression with its magnificent faux-marble entrance hall and Lord Mayor's Lounge, a popular meeting place for afternoon tea. Pressure on bar space was reduced by the opening of the Shelbourne Bar on Kildare Street, which allowed the famous Horseshoe Bar, renowned as a meeting place for local politicians and theatrical society, to be completely refurbished recently. This is regarded as a huge success, largely because everybody loved it as it was and the improvements are hardly noticeable. Under the direction of general manager Jean Ricoux, who joined the hotel in 1997, much renovation work is in progress – and a real change of direction came about in 1998 with the opening of the Health, Fitness & Relaxation Centre, which has an 18 metre swimming pool, sauna, jacuzzi, steam room, aerobics and state-of-the-art workout equipment, with individual tv screens and headphones. As is to be expected in an old building, accommodation varies somewhat, but new rooms have recently been added and all rooms are well-appointed, with good bathrooms, bathrobes, mini-bars and three telephones as standard. The best rooms are very luxurious, including 24 suites with private sitting rooms; these, and the spacious, elegantly furnished superior and de-luxe rooms, have traditional polished wood furniture and impressive drapes. The hotel has two restaurants, No 27 The Green (see below) and The Side Door At The Shelbourne which has a separate entrance from Kildare Street and, with its striking minimalist decor and Cal-Ital menus, provides a complete contrast to the ultra-traditional atmosphere of the hotel. The Side Door, which serves breakfast, lunch and dinner, can also be reached via The Shelbourne Bar, where bar food is served from 11am to 9 pm. Valet parking. A 15% service charge is added to all bills.

Restaurant: No 27 The Green

Recently refurbished in yellow and blue, this is an elegant and lofty dining-room in which to enjoy some very good cooking, combining the best of Irish produce with some traditional/continental flair and expertise. Alongside the daily-changing table d'hôte menus (four choices of starter and main course with dinner providing an additional soup course), there's a substantial à la carte offering the likes of a giant ravioli (two open slices) of wild mushrooms and asparagus with sage and port cream, or sautéed langoustines with deep-fried egg noodles, chicory and ginger butter. Main courses include grilled chateaubriand with béarnaise sauce and rack of herb and nut-crusted Kildare lamb. A wonderful cappuccino dessert consists of coffee crème brûlée topped with white chocolate mousse and covered with a dark chocolate sauce accompanied by a perfect crisp tuile. An example of a table d'hôte menu (lunch: £18.50 for 3 courses, dinner £28.50 for 4 courses) is a warm salad of duck livers with smoked bacon and croutons, curried vegetable soup, pan-fried Gressingham duck with an orange glaze, a fresh strawberry meringue, coffee and chocolates. All in all, this is a slick operation – several breads are offered with butter or (novel this) a dish of raw diced vegetables, and service is ultra-professional. • L££ & D£££ daily • Acc££££ • Open all year •

Dublin 1   The Stag's Head

1 Dame Court Dublin
PUB   Tel: 01 679 3701

In Dame Court, just behind the Adams Trinity Hotel, this impressive establishment has retained its original late-Victorian decor and is one of the city's finest pubs. In recent years it has also had a reputation for good food, although changes were being made in this area as we went to press – well worth investigation however. • Meals££ (daytime) • Closed 25 Dec & Good Fri •

Establishments recommended in the guide are entitled to display the current year's plaque or certificate. However, we strongly recommend that you also read the guide's entry as some establishments may be praised for certain aspects of their operation and criticised for others.

Dublin 2

HOTEL/RESTAURANT

Stakis Dublin

Charlemont Place Dublin
Tel: 01 402 9988   Fax: 01 402 9852
www.stakis.co.uk

Overlooking the Grand Canal, this recently-opened hotel, a few minutes walk from the city centre, caters for all needs of the modern day guest. However, the somewhat institutional atmosphere of the lobby (and television sets in the nearby Champions' Bar) do little to prepare guests for the quality of accommodation. Each double-glazed bedroom provides a worktop with modem point, swivel satellite TV, individual heater, tea/coffee-making facilities, trouser press, hairdryer and compact bathroom (club rooms also offer a bathrobe, additional toiletries and chocolates). Every floor has a vending machine operated and billed by the room key card. The perfect venue for meetings, the ground floor air-conditioned Charlemont Suite (with its own private bar and reception area) can accommodate up to 400 theatre-style, and benefits from natural daylight. It can also be subdivided into separate rooms. There are additional meeting/syndicate rooms on the first floor. A large underground car park has direct access to the hotel. The well-appointed Waterfront Restaurant offers a buffet-style breakfast and, since the arrival of Gavin McDonagh as head chef in June 1998, the restaurant rates as a serious choice among Dublin dining destinations. The glass-walled kitchen provides entertainment for guests who are not overlooking the canal and food – in the modern Irish idiom – is imaginative, well cooked and well presented. • Acc£££ated • L£ & D£ daily • Open all year •

Visit our web site (www.ireland-guide.com) for new recommendations, news and other relevant travel and dining information.

Dublin 2

RESTAURANT

La Stampa

35 Dawson Street Dublin
Tel: 01 677 8611   Fax: 01 677 3336

Reminiscent of a grand French belle epoque brasserie, this is one of Ireland's finest dining rooms – high-ceiling, large mirrors, wooden floor, Roman urns, statues, busts, candelabra, Victorian lamps, plants, flowers and various bits of bric-a-brac, the whole noisily complemented by a constant bustle, the staff's bright waistcoats, and, most importantly, admirable food. On entering, there's a small bar with a variety of different styles of pictures on display and a few comfortable seats. Here you can sip a drink while studying a menu that encompass dishes from around the world. The set lunch menu (a steal at £12.95) offers plenty of choices in each section, as well as several dishes that can either be eaten as starters or main courses. Choosing from the à la carte, fresh oysters with shallot vinegar, Caesar salad with spiced chicken or French onion soup with Gruyere croutons might fit the bill, with main courses such as fillet of turbot with champ, green pea and herb sauce, fillet of beef Rossini with spinach and Dauphinoise potatoes, and open ravioli of monkfish and scallops served with a rocket salad and parmesan. Equally tasty are the desserts – a tarte tatin, here served with yoghurt ice cream, or a duo of strawberry and coconut mousse with a lemon sorbet. Alternatively, a £2 supplement enables you to sample some prime Irish cheeses. The breads are good (but why charge 50p?), as is the coffee, and there are some excellent wines on an inexpensive list, including several by the glass. This is a fun and lively place, offering good food in delightful surroundings. At the time of going to press we were informed that La Stampa was due to expand next door (with some twenty bedrooms above). • L£ Mon-Fri, D££ daily • Closed Xmas wk, Easter & Bank Hols •

Dublin 2

ACCOMMODATION

Stauntons on the Green

83 St Stephen's Green Dublin
Tel: 01 478 2300   Fax: 01 487 2263
email: hotels@indigo.ie   www.indigo.ie/~hotels

Stauntons on the Green is an exceptionally well-located guesthouse, offering moderately priced accommodation. It has views over St Stephen's Green at the front and its own private gardens at the back. Accommodation is all en-suite and of a good standard, with all the usual amenities. The house – which is in an elegant Georgian terrace and has fine period reception rooms – is in the heart of the business and banking district and the Grafton Street shopping area is just a stroll across the Green. Meeting rooms are available, with secretarial facilities on request. • Acc£££ • Closed 24-26 Dec •

Dublin 7

Ta Se Mahogani Gaspipes

17 Manor Street Stoneybatter Dublin

RESTAURANT   Tel: 01 679 8138   Fax: 01 670 5353

A small American-style restaurant in Stoneybatter, a very pleasant neighbourhood of the city near Phoenix Park, away from the bustle of Temple Bar (in the "undiscovered" Dublin). Drina Kinsley prepares an eclectic menu strong on spicy fare like Thai spring rolls with hot dipping sauce or bruschetta with spicy marinara and regato cheese. There's a fresh fish special daily and a late night jazz menu. • L£ Tues-Fri, D££ Tues-Sun • Closed 24-25 Dec, Good Fri & Bank Hols •

Dublin 2

Temple Bar Hotel

Fleet Street Temple Bar Dublin

HOTEL   Tel: 01 677 3333   Fax: 01 677 3088

This pleasant hotel is well-located for reaching locations on both sides of the river. Spacious reception and lounge areas create a good impression and bedrooms are generally larger than average, almost all with a double and single bed and above average amenities Neat, well-lit bathrooms have over-bath showers and marble wash basin units. A room is available for up to 100 people for private parties and small conferences, and there are also several smaller meeting rooms. No parking, but the hotel has an arrangement with a nearby car park. • Acc£££ • Closed 25 Dec •

Dublin 2

Thomas Read

Parliament Street Dublin

CAFÉ/BAR   Tel: 01 677 1487

This bustling café-bar was one of the first of its type and it is still one of the best. Attracting a wide variety of customers – including literary types from Trinity College and nearby newspapers – it serves a good cup of coffee, with (or without) light food. Its corner position and large windows looking down to Dame Street make this a fine place to sit and watch the world go by. • Closed 25 Dec & Good Fri •

Please note that price indications are intended only as a guideline - always check current prices (and special offers) when making reservations.

Dublin 8

Thornton's

1 Portobello Road Dublin

RESTAURANT ★★   Tel: 01 454 9067   Fax: 01 453 2947

Chef of the Year – Kevin Thornton

This large, square street corner restaurant stands out against the surrounding two-up, two-down dwellings and overlooks a section of the Grand Canal where optimistic anglers try their luck late into the summer evenings. Here one finds seriously good cooking in a seriously good restaurant. Muriel Thornton and her team of French waiting staff set the tone from the outset, providing a highly professional service to complement Kevin Thornton's superb cooking. There is a small reception bar downstairs (from which guests can see into the kitchen) and a private dining-room, with the main dining areas (candle-lit at night) upstairs in two rooms. Decor is modern and understated with muslin drapes, "distressed" painted tiles and a tall vase of flowers catching the eye. Service is impeccable, from the moment a basket of breads (fennel rolls, tomato and basil, walnut etc) arrive to the final presentation of assorted petits fours accompanying coffees and teas. In between, one could be offered an amuse-gueule of two plump sautéed prawns in a bisque and truffle sabayon, a trio of fillets of monkfish with tortellini arranged around the plate in a Jurancon jus, splendidly flavoured with herbs and seaweed, followed by perfectly cooked squab pigeon, roasted whole but served boned; breast, livers, webbed legs, the lot, with a small tartlet of shallots, artichoke mousseline topped with baby artichoke, a little mound of wild mushrooms and buttered baby new potatoes. Next, a pre-dessert of red fruits and passionfruit sorbet, followed by the real thing: a masterful bitter lemon tart, crystalised lemon rinds, blackcurrant sorbet and spun sugar. Other starters include foie gras with scallops, celeriac and cep jus or pressed terrine of goat's cheese and tomato with basil oil; main courses, tournedos of veal with tarragon rosti, lemon and ginger confit or fillet of turbot with toasted brioche, puréed potatoes, grapefruit and beetroot sauce. Alternatively, an entire table can choose the six-course 'surprise' menu at £49 per person (perhaps sautéed foie gras and scallops, ragout of wild mushrooms, fillet of sea bass, passionfruit sorbet, poularde de Bresse with fresh morels, pre-dessert, finishing with a pyramid of nougat with glazed fruits). This is creative cooking of the highest class, utilising first-rate seasonal ingredients, perfectly seasoned and beautifully presented – chef-patron Kevin Thornton certainly has a perfectionist's eye for detail and a palate to match. The wine list, though concise, provides a good selection, including several New World wines. A 12.5% service charge is added to the final bill. • D£££ Tues-Sat, L££ Fri only • Closed 2 wks Xmas •

Dublin 2 — Toners

139 Lower Baggot Street Dublin
PUB   **Tel: 01 676 3090   Fax: 01 676 2617**

One of the few authentic old pubs left in Dublin, Toners is definitely worth a visit (or two). Among many other claims to fame, it is said to be the only pub ever frequented by the poet W.B. Yeats. • Closed 25 Dec & Good Fri •

►Dublin 2 — Tosca

20 Suffolk Street Dublin
RESTAURANT   **Tel: 01 679 6744   Fax: 01 677 4310**

Owned by Norman Hewson, Tosca is one of the most stylish of the smaller café-bars in Dublin and serves excellent "global" food. Strongly recommended are the minestrone soup, served with large chunks of warm home-made bread, and Mick's Salad, a vibrantly coloured concoction which is a meal in itself. The front window seats provide an excellent view of passing Dublin street life. Next door n i n i is in the same ownership and specialises in sandwiches – over 45 varieties. (Orders can be taken by fax; a delivery service is also available). • Daytime Mon-Sun until late, meals£-££ • Closed Xmas & Good Fri •

Dublin 2 — Trinity Lodge

12 South Frederick Street Dublin
ACCOMMODATION   **Tel: 01 679 5044   Fax: 01 679 5223**
email: trinitylodge@tinet.ie

As centrally located as it is possible to get, Trinity Lodge offers a very high standard of accommodation just yards away from Trinity College. • Acc££ • Open all year •

►Dublin 2 — Unicorn Café & Restaurant

12B Merrion Court Merrion Row Dublin
CAFÉ/RESTAURANT   **Tel/Fax: 01 668 8552**

Lovely, secluded location just off a busy street near the Shelbourne Hotel. The doors open out onto a terrace which is used for guest seating in fine weather. A informal and fashionable restaurant, famous for its buffet hors d'oeuvres selection and "No 5" piano bar. (Weds-Sat 9pm-3 am) Café and Restaurant open Mon- Sat from 9 am. Closed Sundays and lunch on bank holidays. • Open all day Mon-Sat, L£ & D££ • Closed Bank Hols •

Dublin 2 — Westbury Hotel

Grafton Street Dublin
HOTEL/RESTAURANT   🏛 🏛   **Tel: 01 679 1122   Fax: 01 679 7078**

Possibly the most conveniently situated of all the central Dublin hotels, the Westbury is a very small stone's throw from the main shopping street in the city. Under the management of Billy Kingston since opening in 1984, the Westbury has all the benefits of luxury hotels – notably valet parking – to offset any practical disadvantages of the location. Unashamedly sumptuous, the hotel's public areas drip with chandeliers and have accessories to match – like the grand piano on The Terrace, a popular first floor meeting place for afternoon tea and frequently used for fashion shows. Accommodation is similarly luxurious, with bedrooms that include penthouse suites and a high proportion of suites, junior suites and executive rooms as well as four suitable for disabled guests and 41 non-smoking rooms. With conference facilities to match its quality of accommodation and service, the hotel is understandably popular with business guests; four meeting rooms are available (up to 170 delegates) with full back-up services and private dining.

Russell Room

After a drink in one of the hotel's two bars – the first floor Terrace bar and the Sandbank Bistro, an informal seafood restaurant and bar accessible from the back of the building – fine dining is available in the Russell Room. Executive Chef Paddy Brady offers a choice of set menus and à la carte dining at both lunch and dinner, plus a separate vegetarian menu. The style is classic French, with some global cuisine and New Irish influences. Each autumn the Westbury hosts an International Gourmet Food Season; the event runs for a number of weeks and features guest appearances by executive chefs of well-known hotels around the world. They present menus typical of their own establishments, with the Russell Room as their venue.

Dublin   Zen

89 Upper Rathmines Road Dublin

RESTAURANT   Tel: **01 497 9428**

Denis O'Connor's unusual Chinese restaurant in a converted church has a well-earned reputation for authenticity. Staff are sourced in Beijing and, although there are plenty of popular dishes on their menus, this is one of the relatively small number of oriental restaurants in Dublin where more adventurous diners are rewarded with food that is more highly spiced than normal. • D££ daily, L£ Thurs, Fri & Sun • Amex Diners, MasterCard, Visa •

COUNTY DUBLIN

The Greater Dublin area has been developing so rapidly in recent years that, not surprisingly, the citizens of what used to be County Dublin occasionally suffer from a minor identity crisis. For they are now in theory living in three new counties – Fingal in the north, South Dublin in the southwest, and Dun Laoghaire-Rathdown in the southeast. But although Dubliners of town and county alike will happily accept that they're part of a thrusting modern city, equally they'll cheerfully adhere to the old Irish saying that when God made time, He made a lot of it. So most folk are allowing themselves all the time in the world to get used to the fact that they are now either Fingallions, or South Dubliners, or – Heaven forbid – Hyphenators out in Dun Laoghaire-Rathdown. In this approach, they seem to be supported by the An Post, the Irish Post Office, which still – on the threshold of the 21st century – appears to have a sublime disregard for the creation some years ago of these new counties. All of which is good news for the visitor, for it means that if you feel that the frenetic pace of Dublin city is a mite overpowering, you will very quickly find that nearby, in what used to be and for most folk still is County Dublin, many oases of a much more easy-going way of life can be discovered. Admittedly the fact that the handsome Dublin mountains overlook the city in spectacular style means that even up in the nearby hills, you can sometimes be aware of the city's buzz. But if you want to find a vigorous contrast between modern style and classical elegance, you can find it in an unusual form at Dun Laoghaire's remarkable harbour, where one of the world's most modern ferryports is in interesting synergy with one of the world's largest Victorian artificial harbours. And should you head northward into Fingal, you'll quickly discover an away from-it-all sort of place of estuary towns, fishing ports, offshore islands alive with seabirds, and an environment of leisurely pace in which it's thought very bad form to hasten over meals in restaurants (where portion control is in its infancy).

Local Attractions and Information

Balbriggan	Ardgillan Castle 01 849 2212
Donabate	Newbridge House, Park & Traditional Farm 01 843 6534
Dun Laoghaire	American Week (early July) 01 284 1864
Dun Laoghaire	National Maritime Museum Haigh Terrace 01 280 0969
Dun Laoghaire	Tourist Information 01 280 6984/5/6
Lucan	Primrose Hill Garden (house attrib James Gandon) 01 628 0373
Malahide	The Talbot Botanic Gardens, Malahide Castle 01 872 7530
Malahide	Fry Model Railway, Malahide Castle Demesne 01 846 3779
Malahide	Malahide Castle & Demesne 01 846 2184
Sandycove	James Joyce Museum (Martello Tower) 01 280 9265
Sandyford	Fernhill Gardens (Himalayan species; walled garden) 01 295 6000

Blackrock   Ayumi Ya

Newpark Centre Newtown Park Avenue Co Dublin

RESTAURANT   Tel: 01 283 1767   Fax: 01 288 0428

email: info@ayumiya.ie   www.ayumiya.ie

Established in 1983, Ayumi-Ya was the first authentic traditional Japanese restaurant in Dublin and, together with its informal sister restaurant in Baggot Street (Ayumi-Ya Steakhouse), that position remains unchallenged. Sadly, the restaurant's founder Akiko Hoashi died recently, shortly after handing the business on to her son Yoichi, but it is still operated by the Hoashi family and thriving in their care. Ayumi-Ya is an exceptionally customer-friendly restaurant: their floral logo is a fusion of the Irish shamrock and Japanese chrysanthemum, encircled by a ring of friendship, symbolising a genuine desire to bring the two cultures together. In practical terms, this is demonstrated by exceptional helpfulness and encouragement in the restaurant, enabling Irish customers to get the best possible experience of Japanese food, and through the food, the caring service and the restaurant's restorative calm, an insight into the culture. Yoishi and his team ask customers to approach the menu with an open mind, perhaps making a traditional Japanese choice and selecting a variety of starters from a traditional tasting menu, thus experiencing as many tastes, textures and flavours as possible. At the other end of the scale they can choose from the set menus which have been carefully compiled to include the most popular dishes including yakitori (grilled skewered chicken with teriyaki sauce), tempura (vegetables or fish deep-fried in light batter), sushi (raw fish in vinegared rice), norimaki (vinegared rice wrapped in nori seaweed with fish or vegetable filling). An exceptional choice is available for vegetarians. • D£-££ only Mon-Sat •

Blackrock

Radisson SAS St Helen's Hotel Dublin

Stillorgan Road Co Dublin

HOTEL   Tel: 01 218 600   Fax: 01 260 2295

www.radisson.com

Set in four acres of formal gardens just south of Dublin's city centre, with views across Dublin Bay to Howth Head, the fine house at the heart of this impressive new hotel dates back to the 18th century, when it was built as a private residence. It has been carefully restored and imaginatively modernised to create some exceptionally interesting public areas, including a conservatory bar, the Orangerie (newly added but in the spirit of the old house), a pillared ballroom complete with minstrels' gallery and grand piano and a fine formal dining room with views over the garden. Bedrooms, in a new four-storey block adjoining the main building, include ten suites and 16 junior suites; all have garden views (some of the best rooms also have balconies) and air conditioning and are well-equipped for business guests (with desks and fax machines). Rooms are comfortably furnished to a high standard in contemporary style, although less spacious than might be expected in a new development; bathrooms, especially, fail to live up to the opulence that the old house promises: while all the essentials are there, they are small and far from luxurious, with economy baths and a level of design and finish expected of more budget-conscious establishments. It should be pointed out that the present owners were not involved in the original design – they took over the hotel shortly before it opened in the summer of 1998. • Acc£££££ •

Booterstown

La Tavola

114 Rock Road Booterstown Co Dublin

RESTAURANT   Tel: 01 283 5101

Easy to find at the lower corner of Booterstown Avenue, Kevin Hart's friendly, informal restaurant has been providing good popular food at very customer-friendly prices since 1992. Value-conscious menus include a 3-course early-bird (5-6.30) at only £10.95 (children £6.95); pasta and pizza predominate, but they are well-made and there are vegetarian options. Although the mainstays are similar on later menus, there is a wider choice including a range of more expensive poultry and meat dishes plus daily blackboard specials. • D£-££ Tues-Sat • Amex̄, Diners, MasterCard, Visa •

Dalkey

Daniel Finnegan

2 Sorrento Road Dalkey Co Dublin

PUB   Tel: 01 285 8505

An immaculately maintained pub of great character, much-loved by locals and visitors alike. Food served at lunchtime only. • Closed 25 Dec & New Year •

Dalkey

Moytura

Saval Park Road Dalkey Co Dublin

ACCOMMODATION   Tel: 01 285 2371   Fax: 01 235 0633

email: giacomet@indigo.ie

Surrounded by a lovely old garden and mature trees, Corinne Giacometti's delightful family home, designed by John Loftus Robinson, was built in 1881. Handily situated near the Dun Laoghaire car ferry (2 miles) and within a short walk of Dalkey village (great pubs, restaurants and the DART – a 20 minute train ride to Dublin city centre), Moytura has country house qualities with city convenience. The three guest bedrooms are quite different, but all have their own private bathrooms. Gracious, well-proportioned reception rooms include a dining room overlooking the garden where breakfasts are served. • Acc££ • Closed Nov-Apr •

Dalkey

The Queen's

12 Castle Street Dalkey Co Dublin

PUB   Tel: 01 285 4569   Fax: 01 285 8345

email: queens@club.ie

The oldest pub in Dalkey, and also one of the oldest in Ireland, The Queen's was originally licensed to "dispense liquor" as far back as 1745. Recent renovations and improvements have been done with due respect for the age and character of the premises – a new restaurant is due to be built upstairs and will no doubt be completed in the same spirit. Good bar food – chowders, casseroles, salads, quiches – is available every afternoon and there's an informal restaurant serving evening meals. Outdoor bar food in patio areas at the back and front in fine weather. • L&D daily £-££ •

Dalkey   Thai House

21 Railway Road Dalkey Co Dublin
RESTAURANT   Tel: 01 284 7304   Fax: 01 284 7304

Anthony Ecock's restaurant provided a major boost to the Dalkey dining scene when it opened in 1997 and standards have, if anything, improved since then. Although quite pricey, a welcoming atmosphere and authentic, interesting food have built up a loyal following – and a reputation for including dishes that are genuinely spicy and do not pander to blander tastes. Starters are always especially good and dishes which came in for special praise on a recent visit include the Thai House Special Starter Pack – a tasty sampling plate of six starters: crisp deep-fried dishes like spring rolls, prawns with Thai sauce, marinated skewered pork or chicken satay with sweet and spicy sauce – all well-known dishes but spiced and cooked without compromise. From a choice of soups that include the famous Tom Yam gung (spicy prawn soup with lemon grass and chilli) Tom Yam Rumit – a spicy soup with prawns, squid, crab and mussels – is perhaps the most interesting. Main courses include a range of curries, fried rice dishes and pan-fried dishes such as Bu Paht Pung Galee – delicious crab fried with spring onions, garlic and sugar in special Thai sauce – although, at £11, it's an expensive course when rice is charged as an extra. Vegetarian dishes are listed separately and there are several set menus for two to six people. • D££ Tues-Sat •

Dublin Airport   Great Southern Hotel

Dublin Airport Co Dublin
HOTEL   Tel: 01 844 6000   Fax: 01 844 6001
                              email: res@dubairport.ie   www.gsh.ie

This large modern hotel opened in the airport complex in 1998 and is just two minutes drive from the main terminal building (with a coach service available). Rooms, which are all double-glazed, are en-suite with proper bathrooms. There are four designed for disabled guests and a high proportion of executive rooms (12 of which are designated lady executive) and 24 are non-smoking. Large bar/bistro on the ground floor. • Acc££-£££ •

Dun Laoghaire   Bistro Vino

56 Glasthule Road Dun Laoghaire Co Dublin
RESTAURANT   Tel/Fax: 01 280 6097

This small first floor evening restaurant (up steep stairs) is near the seafront at Sandycove. It pre-dates surrounding establishments in this now fashionable area by a long chalk. But it's still a hit with the locals, who appreciate the moderate prices, unpretentious, good food and informal atmosphere. A la carte except for an inexpensive early set menu (5-7 pm). • D£-££ daily • Amex, Diners, MasterCard, Visa •

Dun Laoghaire   Brasserie Na Mara

1 Harbour Road Dun Laoghaire Co Dublin
RESTAURANT   Tel: 01 280 6767 Fax: 01 284 4649

The old Kingstown terminal building beside the Dun Laoghaire DART station makes a fine location for a harbourside restaurant. A recent overhaul transformed the old restaurant into a modern brasserie, but while it is certainly attractive in its way, it is no replacement for the elegance of the former classical interior, which enhanced the architecture of this grand old building so well. Comfort has also been sacrificed to the god of fashion, now that small tables and mean chairs have replaced the generously comfortable furniture remembered so fondly. The food, of a bright, modern style to suit the decor, includes plenty of seafood as one would expect and is more than competently cooked, although service can leave a lot to be desired. • L££ Mon-Fri, D££ Mon-Sat • Closed Bank Hols • Access, Amex, Diners, Visa •

Dun Laoghaire   Caviston's Seafood Restaurant

59 Glasthule Road Dun Laoghaire Co Dublin
RESTAURANT   Tel: 01 280 9120/2715   Fax: 01 284 4054
              email: caviston@indigo.ie   www.indigo.ie/~caviston

Seafood Dish of the Year

Caviston's of Sandycove has long been a mecca for lovers of good food. Here you will find everything that is good, from organic vegetables to farmhouse cheeses, cooked meats to specialist oils and other exotic items. But it was always for fish and shellfish that

Caviston's were especially renowned – even providing a collection of well-thumbed recipe books for on-the-spot reference. So what could be more natural than to cook their fish on the spot and open a little restaurant next door – which is just what they did in 1996. Here they do two sittings in their tiny restaurant at lunchtime, serving an imaginative range of seafood dishes influenced by various traditions and all washed down by a glass or two from a very tempting little wine list. You might even try our Seafood Dish of the Year: Roast Monkfish Fillets, Roast Red Pepper and Olive Oil Dressing. This lovely dish is not too complicated: a trio of golden brown, crisp monkfish pieces arranged bonfire style, along with strips of juicy, meltingly soft red roast pepper, all surrounded by a very lightly spiced dressing of olive oil and fresh herbs. Simple, colourful, perfectly cooked, it speaks volumes for how good seafood can be.• L£-££ Tues-Sat •

Dun Laoghaire   P McCormack & Sons

67 Lr Mounttown Dun Laoghaire Co Dublin
PUB   Tel: 01 280 5519   Fax: 01 280 0145
email: cormak@iol.ie

This fine pub (and "emporium") has been run by the McCormack family since 1960. It's one of the neatest pubs around, with a landscaped carpark (no less). The garden corner creates a very pleasant outlook for an imaginative conservatory extension at the back of the pub. The main part of the pub is full of traditional character and the whole place has a well-run hum about it. Good bar food includes fresh fish available on the day as well as classics such as beef hot pot, chicken a la king and loads of salads. Evening menus offer tasty light dishes: moules marinières, warm crispy bacon and crouton salad and steak sandwiches. Main dishes include a fish special, a 10 oz sirloin steak (with mushroom and Irish whiskey sauce perhaps) or pasta dishes with fresh parmesan. • L£ & D££ daily •

Dun Laoghaire   Morels

18 Glasthule Road Dun Laoghaire Co Dublin
RESTAURANT   Tel: 01 230 0210/0068   Fax: 01 230 0466

On the first floor of the Eagle House pub (a fine traditional establishment that is full of interest and serves excellent bar meals), the bistro is vividly decorated. Recently expanded into a third room and with a new seafood tank at the entrance (patrolled by blue lobsters awaiting their fate), Morels has a sister restaurant at Stephens Hall Hotel in Dublin city. At present open only in the evenings (apart from an all-day Sunday menu at £13.50, served from noon-8pm), early diners can choose from the reduced fixed-price menu or the à la carte (with choices ranging from crab and sesame croquette or warm confit of duck on a bed of salad leaves). Good-value wines with interesting £11 and £15 sections, in addition to the regular list. Irish-French service is endearing and swift. • D£-££ daily, L£ Sun only •

Dun Laoghaire   Royal Marine Hotel

Marine Road Dun Laoghaire Co Dublin
HOTEL   Tel: 01 280 1911   Fax: 01 280 1089

Overlooking Dublin Bay and the ferry port, this grand old Victorian hotel has ample parking and extensive landscaped gardens (perfect for weddings), and yet is only a twenty minute DART ride to the centre of Dublin. On entering the marble floored foyer a few steps take you up and through arched columns into the Bay Lounge (popular for afternoon teas) and the Powerscourt Restaurant. Most of the bedrooms, offering the usual facilities, have recently been refurbished with smart co-ordinating fabrics, fitted furniture, and decent bathrooms, including those on the executive floor that provide extras for the business traveller. Additionally, there are eight bay-windowed suites featuring four-poster beds and freestanding antique furniture. Substantial conference facilities: the ballroom can accommodate 500 theatre-style or 300 for a banquet. Good, professional staff. • Acc££-£££ • Open all year •

Glencullen   Johnnie Fox's Pub

The Dublin Mountains Glencullen Co Dublin
PUB   ★   Tel: 01 295 5647   Fax: 01 295 8911

Nestling in an attractive wooded hamlet in the Dublin Mountains, south of Dublin city, Johnnie Fox's has numerous claims to fame. Undoubtedly one of County Dublin's best-loved pubs in present times, it can also claim to be one of the oldest, with a history going back to the eighteenth century. Daniel O'Connell, who lived in Glencullen at one time, was a regular apparently, and it's "undoubtedly" the highest pub in the land. More to the point, however, is the fact that it's a warm, friendly and very well run place just about equally famous for its food – the "Famous Seafood Kitchen" – and its music – "Famous Hooley Nights" (booking advisable). Unlike so many superficially similar pubs that have popped up all over the world recently, it's also real – the rickety old furniture is real, the dust is real and you certainly won't find a gas fire here – there's a lovely turf or log fire at every turn. It's a lovely place to drop into at quieter times too, if you're walking in the hills or just loafing around. • Meals£-££, L Mon-Sat, D daily •

Howth   Abbey Tavern

Abbey Street Howth Co Dublin

PUB   Tel: 01 839 0307/01 832 2006   Fax: 01 839 0284

This famous pub is only 50 yards from the harbour. Part of it dates back to the 15th century, when it was built as a seminary for the local monks (as an addition to the 12th century Chapter House next door). Currently owned by James and Eithne Scott-Lennon – James' grandfather bought it in 1945 – the entire establishment was refurbished in 1998. The locals see changes worthy of discussion, but what the average visitor will find is a well-run and immaculately maintained pub with all the authentic features that have always made the Abbey special – open turf fires, original stone walls, flagged floors and gas lights. Bar food – Howth seafood chowder, smoked salmon with home-made brown bread, a hot traditional dish such as corned beef and cabbage, a ploughman's salad – is available at lunchtime. In 1956 a restaurant was opened, quite a novel move in a pub at the time; since the recent redevelopment this evening restaurant has been named The Abbot and has its own separate entrance. Attractively and comfortably refurbished in keeping with the building, with open turf fires at both ends of the room, it makes a fine setting for well-cooked and not over-complicated food. In 1960 the Abbey started to lay on entertainment and this, more than anything else, has brought the tavern its fame: it can cater for groups of anything between two and 200 and the format, which now runs like clockwork, is a traditional 5-course dinner followed by traditional Irish music. It's on every night but booking is essential, especially in high season. • L & D daily, meals£-££ •

Howth   Casa Pasta

12 Harbour Road Howth Co Dublin

RESTAURANT   Tel: 01 839 3823

Atmosphere in spades is what sets this first floor restaurant overlooking Howth harbour apart, and although this was partly due to its tiny size, doubling it in 1998 doesn't seem to have diminished its appeal – it's still notoriously hard to get into, especially at weekends. The secret is entertainment – paper tablecloths and crayons provided for budding artists, great jazz and other live music most nights (usually from 9 pm); interesting modern pictures; swift young servers; and blackboard menus featuring youthful international food (lots of pastas and salads) that is neither over-ambitious nor over-priced. Regulars that locals happily order without even consulting the menu include runny deep-fried brie with spicy chutney, big Caesar salads (possibly with slivers of chicken breast), home-made tagliatelle with mixed seafood in a creamy wine sauce – and desserts like gooey, boozy tiramisu and sticky banoffi pie. Wines are not quite as cheap and cheerful as might be hoped given the style of food and surroundings. • D daily, L Fri-Sun, meals£-££ •

* There is a sister restaurant in Clontarf: 55 Clontarf Road, Dublin 3.
Tel/Fax: 01 833 1402. A southside restaurant is also planned for 1999.

Howth   Citrus

1 Island View House, Harbour Road Howth Co Dublin

RESTAURANT   Tel: 01 832 0200

Along the front a little from Casa Pasta, and in the same ownership, Citrus is Howth's only really contemporary café/restaurant – and it's been a hit since the day it opened in March 1998. Very stylish, with a little chrome-seated outdoor eating area at the front, a buzzy ground-floor café/bar where live jazz attracts a regular crowd and a slightly more formal first-floor restaurant, John Aungier has once again achieved atmosphere in spades. The food is good too – joint head chefs Mark Feavnon and Jose Porfirio de Carvalho, who have been with the restaurant since it opened – offer zappy global cuisine with the emphasis on Thai influences. They do it well and without pretension. Appetisers like fishcakes with chilli sauce/lime and coriander mayonnaise, seafood wontons, rumaki (monkfish and chestnuts rapped in bacon) and vegetable tempura all come in at £3-4, and main courses like chicken and hot garlic sauce with rice, sole with coriander and chilli sauce and Thai Green and Red curries are mostly well under £10 – these prices plus service and friendliness make the atmosphere all the more enjoyable. A shortish list of world wines is well-pitched for the style of the place, although more informative tasting notes would be helpful. • L£ & D££ daily •

Howth   Deer Park Hotel & Golf Courses

Howth Co Dublin

HOTEL/RESTAURANT   Tel: 01 832 2624   Fax: 01 839 2405

email: sales@deerpark.iol.ie

Set high up on the Hill of Howth, in the midst of its own four parkland golf courses, the Deerpark Hotel enjoys wonderful views across Howth demesne (of which it is part) to the islands of Ireland's Eye and Lambay and, on a clear day, right up the coast to the distant Mournes. Although golf breaks are a particular attraction, especially in summer, the hotel makes a comfortable base for anyone visiting the area and rooms have extra large beds, a sofa or armchairs and, in some cases, not just a kettle and tray for making drinks, but a kitchenette with fridge and toaster too. Bathrooms in some of the older rooms are somewhat basic in design and finish (although all have full bath and shower) and general maintenance has sometimes been less than perfect too – but everything works and the overall standard of comfort is good. New rooms (27) and a large indoor swimming pool, sauna and steam room were recently added. A quarter of a century after opening, with 15 rooms and a nine hole golf course, Deer Park is now an 87 room hotel and is Ireland's largest golf complex.

Restaurant

The restaurant is situated at the front of the hotel, with sea views, and is well-appointed with comfortable chairs and white linen. Set 3-course lunch and dinner menus are not adventurous but are based on good ingredients, competently cooked and offer good value – in short, menus read as traditional hotel food, but the food on the plate is above average. • L£ & D££ • Acc££ •

Establishment reports for Dublin City and Greater Dublin can be found on the Dublin Live section of The Irish Times On Line site (www.irish-times.com).

Howth   Howth Lodge Hotel

Howth Co Dublin

HOTEL/RESTAURANT   Tel: 01 832 1010   Fax: 01 832 2268

email: howlodge@iol.ie

On the sea side of the DART tracks, this seaside hotel gives a good impression with its crisp black and white paintwork and neatly organised car parking. Although much extended since, the original building goes back 175 years and has been owner-run since 1975. They have made a number of improvements, including a leisure centre in the grounds and the addition of some spacious rooms at the back, which have been cleverly designed to maximise the sea views. The reception makes the most of an attractive staircase in a central position and public areas include a comfortably furnished lounge bar that leads through to a more characterful beamed bar at the back of the hotel. Rooms do vary widely in size, position and standard, so it is wise to discuss requirements when booking.

Restaurant

This well-appointed restaurant has a sea view from window tables and a prompt welcome ensures meals get off to a good start. Well-balanced dinner and à la carte menus offer a wide selection with (given the location) an understandable bias towards fish but also some more unusual options, such as kassler (smoked loin of pork) which might be served with an apple and cider sauce. Special value "Dine Early" menus are available Monday-Friday.

The Lodge Bistro

On the left of the lobby, the Bistro has a choice of two areas, one with a sea view and proper dining chairs as well as banquettes, the other more predictably bistro with bentwood chairs. A written menu is augmented by daily blackboard specials (especially fish), and although the tone throughout – menu, ambience, service – is informal, the same high standard of cooking prevails. Prices are reasonable and the Bistro successfully provides a contrast to the main restaurant. • L£ & D££ daily • Acc£££ •

Howth

King Sitric Fish Restaurant

East Pier Howth Co Dublin.

RESTAURANT Tel: 01 832 5235/6729 Fax: 01 839 2442

Named after an 11th century Norse King of Dublin who had close links with Howth and was a cousin of the legendary Brian Boru, The King Sitric is one of Dublin's longest established fine restaurants. Perfectly situated at the end of the East Pier, owner-chef Aidan MacManus can keep an eye on his lobster pots in Balscadden Bay on one side and the fishing boats coming into harbour on the other. Each day's menu depends completely on the availability of fresh seafood landed that day, which is one of the many good reasons for adding game to the repertoire in winter (when gales can keep the boats in harbour for days at a time). House specialities include shellfish of all kinds, notably crab and lobster, a particularly good Irish farmhouse cheese trolley, the dessert 'Meringue Sitric' (which was invented to make use of all the egg whites left over after making yolk-rich sauces for fish) and one of the best brown bread recipes in the country, handed down through generations of Aidan's family and made personally by his mother until quite recently. Courteous, efficient service from long-serving staff, under the direction of Joan McManus, adds greatly to the enjoyment of Aidan's fine food. Exceptional wine list At the time of going to press plans are afoot to make major changes to the restaurant and add accommodation for 1999. • D££-£££ Mon-Sat, light L££ in summer •

Killiney

Fitzpatrick Castle Dublin

Killiney Co Dublin

COUNTRY HOUSE Tel: 01 284 0700 Fax: 01 285 0207

Half an hour's drive from the city centre, this imposing castellated mansion overlooking Dublin Bay dates back to 1741. It is surrounded by landscaped gardens and, despite its size and grand style, has a surprisingly relaxed atmosphere. Bedrooms combine old-world charm with modern facilities. Spacious bedrooms include four junior suites and the 40 executive rooms have e-mail sockets. Extensive facilities include two large lounges, two restaurants, a basement disco, a conference suite for up to 400 delegates and a new Library Bar, opened in 1998. Five championship golf courses, including Druid's Glen, are nearby. • Acc£££ • Open all year • Amex, Diners, MasterCard, Visa •

Leixlip

Becketts

Cooldrinagh House Leixlip Co Dublin

HOTEL Tel: 01 624 7040 Fax: 01 624 7072

A handsome house on the Co Dublin side of the river that divides Leixlip, Becketts is a recently opened country house offering a special kind of service that business guests in particular will no doubt appreciate: from the moment you arrive a butler looks after all your needs, whether it be dining, laundry, limousine facilities or specific requirements for meetings or conferences. The house has been imaginatively converted to its present use and accommodation includes four boardroom suites and six executive suites, all furnished to a high standard in a lively contemporary style. All have a workstation equipped for computers, including modem/internet connection. Audio visual equipment, private fax machines etc are also available on request. Public areas, including a bar and a stylish modern restaurant, have a far less business-like atmosphere and would make an interesting outing for non-residents with no special business in mind, especially those who appreciate wine – this unusual establishment is, after all, the brainchild of John O'Byrne, proprietor of the distinctive Dublin restaurant Dobbins. Cooldrinagh House overlooks the Eddie Hackett-designed Leixlip golf course, for which golf tee off times may be booked in advance. • Acc££ • L£ Tues-Fri, D£-££ Tues-Sat •

Lucan

Finnstown Country House Hotel

Newcastle Road Lucan Co Dublin

COUNTRY HOUSE Tel: 01 628 0644 Fax: 01 628 1088

Very much the hub of local activities, this fine old manor house set in 45 acres of woodland is impressive, but also full of charm. A welcoming open fire in the foyer sets the right tone. All of the large, well-proportioned reception rooms – drawing room, restaurant, bar – are elegantly furnished in a traditional style well-suited to the house. Although quite grand, there is a comfortable lived-in feeling throughout. Bedrooms include studio suites, with a small fridge and toaster in addition to the standard tea/coffee making facilities, and all rooms have good facilities including full bathrooms (with bath and shower). Well set up for business meetings and conferences, the hotel has six rooms to suit meetings of various sizes (up to 60) and The Library, a large new room on the ground floor, for conferences/banqueting for up to 100/110 respectively. In addition to indoor leisure facilities within the grounds, the hotel has its own nine hole golf course and residential golf breaks are a speciality. • Acc£££ • Meals £-£££ • Open all year •

Malahide   Bon Appetit
9 St James Terrace Malahide Co Dublin
RESTAURANT   Tel/Fax: 01 845 0314

Patsy McGuirk's well-established basement restaurant is in a Georgian terrace near the marina. Attractive decor is enhanced by a collection of local watercolours and there's a welcome emphasis on comfort. Patsy's shortish, well-balanced lunch menu (£15) is deservedly popular and there's a 5-course dinner menu (£27.50), daily specials and "chef's recommendations" in addition to a full à la carte. The style tends to be classic French, sometimes tempered by Mediterranean and modern Irish influences. Seafood, mostly from nearby Howth, predominates but steaks, Wicklow lamb, farmyard duckling and ostrich, which is farmed nearby, also feature. Fresh prawn bisque with cognac is a regular and a long-established house speciality is Sole Creation McGuirk (a whole boned black sole, filled with turbot and prawns, in a beurre blanc sauce – a style so old-fashioned it must be due for revival) while simple sole on the bone is presented whole at the table, then re-presented bone-free and neatly reassembled. Pretty desserts: fresh strawberries in a crisp filo basket, sliced and sprinkled with Grand Marnier is typical, or there's an Irish cheese platter. A fine wine list has its heart in France; there are helpful tasting notes and a special selection, as well as six house wines (£11-£18.50). • L£ Mon-Fri, D£££ Mon-Sat • Closed Bank Hols •

Malahide   Grand Hotel
Malahide Co Dublin
HOTEL   Tel: 01 845 000   Fax: 01 845 0987

Just 8 miles from Dublin airport, and set in six acres of gardens, this seaside hotel is well-situated for business and pleasure. Many of the bedrooms have sea views, the beach (tidal estuary) is just across the road and there are numerous golf courses nearby. Indoor leisure facilities include a new leisure centre with 21 metre swimming pool. Excellent banqueting, conference and business facilities. • Acc£££ • Amex, Diners, MasterCard, Visa •

Malahide   Siam Thai Restaurant
Gas Lane Malahide Co Dublin
RESTAURANT   Tel: 01 845 4698   Fax: 01 478 4798
siames@tinet.ie

Handily located in a laneway close to the marina (although parking can be tricky), this large, well-appointed restaurant was opened in 1994, ahead of the wave of global and Pacific Rim restaurants that has hit the Dublin area recently. It is pleasing to note that it is holding its own in the face of growing competition. Suracheto Yoodsang, head chef since 1996, presents menus that offer many of the Thai classics on an extensive à la carte as well as the set menus. The balance of ingredients is "true Thai" and dishes not only have variety – in textures as well as flavours – but there's a willingness to vary the spiciness according to personal preference. Dishes attracting praise on a recent visit include Siam Combination Appetizers (a selection for two, including chicken satay, spring rolls, special coated prawns, marinated pork ribs, prawns wrapped in ham and bags of golden wonton with plum sauce) and main courses of Ghung Phad Phong Garee (a generous quantity of Tiger prawns with scallions, mushrooms and basil leaves and a good kick to the sauce) and Ped Makham (succulent boneless crisp-skinned duck with crispy noodles and plum sauce). Incidentally, no monosodium glutamate is used in the food (something we applaud). A sister restaurant, Siam Thai Restaurant, Monkstown, Co Dublin (Tel: 01 284 3308) is run on identical lines. • D££ daily •

Malahide   Silks Restaurant
5 The Mall Malahide Co Dublin
RESTAURANT   Tel: 01 845 3331

Coming into Malahide by the coast road, this attractive Chinese restaurant is on the left just after the Grand Hotel. A floodlit miniature garden feature, with stream and bridge, give it atmosphere, but it is the quality of the cooking (transforming inscrutable menus into fine meals) teamed with seamless service from charming staff that explains its strong local following. • D££ daily • Amex, Diners, MasterCard, Visa •

Monkstown

Chestnut Lodge

2 Vesey Place Monkstown Co Dublin
Tel: 01 280 7860

ACCOMMODATION

Nancy Malone's delightful Regency residence overlooks a wooded park above Monkstown village. While it now has all the amenities required to make a modern traveller comfortable, it has also retained its mid-19th century charm and character. A lovely warm house, spacious, homely and elegantly furnished, it has that special atmosphere unique to places where there is a genuinely caring owner running the operation. Chestnut Lodge makes a good base for touring south Dublin and Wicklow and is only six miles from Dublin city centre, easily reached by DART (rapid rail) or bus. It's also very handy to the Dun Laoghaire car ferry. Be sure to allow time to enjoy one of Nancy's special breakfasts. • Acc££ • Closed Xmas wk •

Monkstown

Empress Restaurant

Clifton Avenue Monkstown Co Dublin
Tel: 01 284 3200 Fax: 01 284 3188

RESTAURANT

Since opening in 1992 owner-chef Burt Tsang has built up a strong local following for this first-floor restaurant just off Monkstown Crescent. He offers regional Chinese dishes – Sichuan, Shandong and Beijing – plus Thai and Vietnamese cuisine, in set dinners for varying numbers in addition to an à la carte. Specialities include Beijing duck, carved at the table and served with fresh vegetables and hoi sin sauce on pancakes, which requires 24 hours notice. A good choice of vegetarian options is always available; typically Thai vegetable curries. Charming service. • D££ daily •

Monkstown

The Purty Kitchen

Old Dunleary Road Monkstown Co Dublin
Tel: 01 284 3576

PUB

Established in 1728 – making it the second oldest pub in Dublin (after The Brazen Head) and the oldest in Dun Laoghaire – this attractive old pub has seen some changes recently, but its essential character remains. It has retained the dim atmosphere that seems to be a constant feature of the best old Irish pubs and is well set up for enjoyment of the bar food, for which it has earned a good reputation. • Meals£-££ •

Portmarnock

Portmarnock Hotel & Golf Links

Strand Road Portmarnock Co Dublin

HOTEL/RESTAURANT

Tel: 01 846 0611   Fax: 01 846 2442
email: reservatins@portmarnak.com portmarnock.com

Originally owned by the Jameson family, of Irish whiskey fame, Portmarnock Hotel and Golf Links enjoys a wonderful beachside position overlooking the islands of Lambay and Ireland's Eye. Very close to the airport, and only eleven miles from Dublin city centre, the hotel seems to offer the best of every world – the peace and convenience of the location and a magnificent 18 hole Bernhard Langer-designed links course. Public areas, including an impressive foyer, are bright and spacious, with elegant modern decor and a relaxed atmosphere. The Jameson Bar, in the old house, has great character and there's also an informal Links Bar and Restaurant next to the golf shop. Accommodation is particularly imaginative, designed so that all rooms have sea or golf course views. Although there are several types of room – including some in the original house which are furnished with antiques, two suites with four-posters and private sitting rooms and executive rooms with balconies or bay windows – all are furnished to a very high standard of comfort and have excellent bathrooms.

The Osborne Restaurant

Named after the artist Walter Osborne, who painted many of his most famous pictures in the area including the view from the Jameson house, the restaurant has been a major addition to the north Dublin dining scene since the hotel opened in 1996. Eric Faussurier, who has been executive chef from the outset, makes full use of local ingredients – especially seafood from the nearby fishing port of Howth – in a classic style with New Irish Cuisine influences. • L£-££ & D£££ • Acc££££ •

The guide aims to provide comprehensive recommendations of the best places to eat, drink and stay throughout Ireland. We welcome suggestions from readers. If you think an establishment merits assessment , please write or email us.

Rathcoole

An Poitin Stil

Rathcoole (off Naas Rd dual carriageway) Co Dublin

PUB **Tel: 01 458 9205/9339**

An imposing thatched pub on the Naas dual carriageway, the Poitin Stil looks like a contemporary superpub from the road, but although it has changed a lot in recent years, it was actually established in 1643. Once inside this famous sporting pub, its daunting first impression is quickly forgotten as it is broken up into several quite different bars, all likely to be packed with punters from the nearby racecourses. A sense of history is a genuine part of its charm: there is a fine old copper still, from which the pub takes its name, and a lot of fascinating original 'Arkle' memorabilia. Good traditional bar food is available from the carvery at lunchtime and there's limited food throughout opening hours. Traditional music also draws the crowds on some evenings. • Meals£-££ daily, L carvery • Amex, Diners, MasterCard, Visa •

Skerries   The Red Bank Restaurant & Lodge

7 Church Street Skerries Co Dublin

RESTAURANT/ACCOMMODATION   **Tel: 01 849 1005/0439   Fax: 01 849 1598**

The Red Bank Restaurant was founded by Terry and Margaret McCoy in 1983, when the local bank moved into new premises and they converted the old premises into a restaurant of character and practicality (even the old vault had its uses – as a wine cellar). The name comes from a nearby coastal feature. Margaret provides a warm welcome, serving aperitifs and crudites in an elegantly furnished bar/reception area and overseeing service in the comfortable, traditional restaurant (where smoking is only allowed if a private party takes over a room). One of the great characters of contemporary Irish cooking – and currently President of the Restaurants Association of Ireland – Terry is an avid supporter of local produce and suppliers and is always experimenting to make the most of them. Fresh seafood from Skerries harbour provides the backbone of his menus, but without limiting the vision – this is a man who goes out at dawn with a bucket to gather young nettles for soup. Dishes conceived and cooked with generosity are often named after key points on the local land- and sea-scape, or are related to history – thus grilled goats cheese St Patrick is a reminder that the saint once lived on Church Island off Skerries. The dessert trolley is legendary (perhaps the traditional adjective "groaning" should apply to the diners – a large space should be left if pudding is to be part of your meal). Should the sauces and accompaniments prove too much, plainly cooked food is gladly provided and dishes suitable for vegetarians are marked on the menu.

Accommodation

Just across the road from the restaurant, the McCoys have recently acquired a large house and converted it to make a comfortable guesthouse with 12 en-suite bedrooms and facilities for meetings and small conferences (two rooms, with a capacity for up to 10 and 35 respectively). • D££-£££ Tues-Sat & L£-££ Sun only • Acc££ •

Stillorgan   China-Sichuan Restaurant

4 Lower Kilmacud Road Stillorgan Co Dublin

RESTAURANT   **Tel: 01 288 4817   Fax: 01 288 0882**

Five miles south of Dublin city centre, David and Julie Hui's China-Sichuan Restaurant is rather unique – it has been run in co-operation with the cultural exchange programme of the state-run China Sichuan Catering Service Company since opening in 1986. While it looks much the same as any other Chinese restaurant, its chefs and special spices are supplied direct from Sichuan province, and it quickly gained recognition for its authentic oriental food and refusal to "bland-down" the style to suit local tastes (although spicy and chilli-hot dishes are clearly identified on menus). "Bon Bon Chicken" for example, is a dish of cold chicken shreds in a hot and spicy sauce – but the kitchen is flexible enough to alter the spicing to suit individual tastes. While set menus are relatively limited (especially at lunch time), the à la carte offers plenty to tempt the most jaded palate. Poultry is a strength – smoked duckling in Sichuan style, for example, which is smoked over bay leaves, black Chinese tea leaves and camphor wood then deep-fried, producing a crisp-skinned and succulent dish with a delicate, subtle smoky flavour. Beef, lamb and especially pork marry well with traditional flavourings, and seafood dishes offer much more than the usual king prawns – black sole, monkfish, scallops and squid all feature – and there's a hot seafood combination in garlic. A separate vegetarian menu also includes plenty of hot and spicy dishes, and interesting vegetable side dishes include a choice of stir-fried vegetables (one choice from a list – the Chinese don't mix them all up as Westerners do) and fried long beans, flavoured with chopped Chinese radish. • L£ Mon-Fri & Sun, D££ daily •

Stillorgan

HOTEL

Stillorgan Park Hotel

Stillorgan Co Dublin

Tel: 01 288 1621   Fax: 01 283 1610

email: sales@stillorganpark.com

Since coming under new management in 1994 this hotel on the Stillorgan dual carriageway has had a complete makeover. Having cast off its previously dull, concrete block persona, it is now remarkable for a dashing modern style throughout. Public areas include a large new restaurant, Purple Sage, and the stylish reception and lounge areas are visible from the road. Bedrooms, which have been increased in number to 120, include four rooms designed for disabled guests, four suites and four junior suites. Some bedrooms have views of Dublin Bay. The hotel has good facilities for business guests, who have work space and fax/modem lines in rooms, and there are conference/banqueting facilities for up to 450. • Acc£££ •

Swords

RESTAURANT

Lukas

River Mall Main Street Swords Co Dublin

Tel/Fax: 01 840 9080

Kate Gibbons' informal first-floor restaurant – on the river side of the main street in Swords – is an atmospheric little place serving modern food at reasonable prices. Home-made pastas take pride of place on head chef Denis Murnane's eclectic menus, typically offering a choice of spaghetti, penne or tagliatelle served with accompaniments and sauces, such as chicken and blue cheese or tomato, basil and garlic. There are also the more traditional pesto and carbonara sauces. Spicier cuisines influence some of the starter choices – quesadillas, for instance, or chicken wings Tex-Mex style, and there are several Mexican/Cajun main courses plus a list of daily blackboard specials. Live music on Thursday and Friday nights. • D£-££ daily •

Swords

RESTAURANT

The Old Schoolhouse

Coolbanagher Church Road Swords Co Dublin

Tel: 01 840 2846/4160   Fax: 01 840 5060

email: sincater@indigo.ie

In a quiet riverside site close to the Northern Cross motorway, and only 5 minutes from the airport, this 18th century stone school building has been restored by the Sinclair family to make a attractive country-style restaurant. Personal service and good home cooking are the aims; all ingredients are locally sourced and fresh every day, which allows for a seasonal à la carte and table d'hôte menus that change about twice a week (plus daily blackboard specials which include a lot of seafood). à la carte menus offer starters such as Westport mussels with garlic, shallots and white wine and an unusual Old Schoolhouse-style chowder, with big chunks of fish, whole crab claws and generous juices rather than soup – filling and excellent. Main courses include classics such as black sole on the bone meunière (faithfully rendered) and woodpigeon breasts served juicy, pink and tender, possibly with a luscious Madeira and balsamic sauce. • L£-££ Mon-Fri, D££ Mon-Sat • Closed Bank Hols •

Accommodation

At the time of going to press planning permission had been granted for 13 bedrooms, which should be open in time for the 1999 season.

CARLOW

Carlow punches way above its weight, for although it is Ireland's second smallest county, it confidently incorporates such wonderful varieties of scenery that it has been memorably commented that the Creator was in fine form when He m0ade this enchanting place. Whether you're lingering along the gentle meanderings of the waterway of the River Barrow, or savouring the soaring lines of the Blackstairs Mountains as they sweep upwards to the 793 m peak of Mount Leinster, this big-hearted little area will have you in thrall. There's history a-plenty if you wish to seek it out. But for those who prefer to live in the present, the county town of Carlow itself buzzes with student life and the energetic trade of a market centre, while a more leisurely pace can be enjoyed at riverside villages such as Leighlinbridge and Bagnelstown. The tidy town of Borris is a charmer, one of Ireland's better kept secrets, typical in fact of Carlow county, a place cherished by those who know it well.

Local Attractions and Information

Carlow Town,
Tullow

Tourist Information 0503 31554
Altamont Gardens 0503 59128

Bagnelstown

Lorum Old Rectory
Kilgreaney Co Carlow

COUNTRY HOUSE　　　　　　　　Tel: 0503 75282　　Fax: 0503 75455
email: lorum@indigo.ie　www.indigo.ie/hiddenireland/24.html

Lorum Old Rectory is close to many places of interest, including medieval Kilkenny, New Ross (where river cruises are available), Kildare's National Stud and Japanese Gardens. Close by is Gowran Park racecourse and activities such as golf and a riding school (offering both outdoor and indoor tuition). Elegant, spacious and very comfortable accommodation includes a lovely drawing room for guests and a bedroom with a four-poster (at a small supplement). But it is Don and Bobbie Smith's hospitality that keeps bringing guests back. Euro-Toques member Bobbie prepares good home cooking based mainly on organic ingredients. Dinner for residents is served at a long mahogany table (book by 3 pm). This is a family-friendly place – children enjoy swings in the orchard and there are many interesting animals. Private parties and small conferences for up to ten delegates can also be catered for. Dogs are welcome by arrangement. • Acc££ • Closed 22-30 Dec •

Carlow

Barrowville Townhouse
Kilkenny Road Carlow Co Carlow

ACCOMMODATION　　　　　　　　Tel: 0503 43324　　Fax: 0503 41953

Ex-hoteliers Marie and Randal Dempsey have built up a great reputation for this exceptionally comfortable and well-run guesthouse just a few minutes walk from the town centre. Although immaculately maintained the house is old, so bedrooms vary in size and character, but all are comfortable and attractively furnished with a mixture of antiques and fitted furniture. Good housekeeping and generous, thoughtfully designed and well-finished bathrooms contribute greatly to a generally high standard of comfort. Marie Dempsey is renowned for excellent breakfasts served in a lovely conservatory (complete with a large vine) overlooking the lovely back garden. There is also a particularly pleasant and comfortable residents' drawing room, with an open fire, grand piano and plenty to read. • Acc£ • Open all year • Amex, MasterCard, Visa •

Carlow

The Beams Restaurant
59 Dublin Street Carlow Co Carlow

RESTAURANT　　　　　　　　　　Tel: 0503 31824

Originally a coaching inn, this characterful building has been lovingly restored by the owners, Betty and Peter O'Gorman, who have run it as a restaurant since 1986. They also operate The Wine Tavern off-licence and specialist food shop next door. Massive wooden beams create a warm atmosphere and are a reminder of the building's long history (it has actually held a full licence since 1760). Classic French cuisine is the speciality of French chef Romain Chall, who has been at The Beams since it opened. He has established a reputation for fine fare, including game (such as wild duck and pheasant in season) and seafood such as scallops and sole, which are often on the dinner menu (at a very small supplement). Vegetarian dishes regularly feature on the menu and any special dietary requirements can be met at a day's notice. • Mon-Sat D££ • Closed 1 wk Xmas • MasterCard, Visa •

Carlow

Danette's Feast

Urglin Glebe Carlow Co Carlow

RESTAURANT   Tel: 0503 40817   Fax: 0503 40817

Danette O'Connell and David Milne opened their relaxed country house restaurant in 1994 and have built up a considerable reputation, particularly for the regular musical evenings which have become a special feature. Except when the weather is fine enough for aperitifs in the garden, David welcomes guests with drinks and nibbles in a little drawing room where there is an open fire in winter. Having taken orders from one of chef Danette's imaginative menus, diners are escorted through to one of two well-proportioned dining rooms furnished with antiques. Seasonal menus always include some interesting vegetarian options and feature specialist Irish products including bio-dynamically grown produce from west Wicklow and a fine range of farmhouse cheeses. The famous musical evenings take place once a month – a soirée followed by an 8-course Tasting Menu. As both David and Danette are musicians, the background music for each meal is also treated as an important element of the dining experience. • Weds-Sat D£££ Sun L££• Closed 1 wk Xmas and Bank Hols • MasterCard, Visa •

Leighlinbridge

The Lord Bagenal Inn

Leighlinbridge Co Carlow

PUB   Tel: 0503 21668   Fax: 0503 22639

Whether to break a journey or as a destination in its own right, The Lord Bagenal has much to offer, including a very pleasant walk along the river. A great deal of development was taking place at the time of going to press and yet more is planned. The proprietor, James Kehoe, has taken care to retain some of the best features of the old building – notably the old end bar, with its open fire and comfortably old-fashioned air and the restaurant section beside it – while incorporating many interesting new ideas. The grandest is around the harbour area (which was not complete at the time of our visit) but the most novel is undoubtedly the supervised indoor playroom, which is in the bar but behind glass so that, in time-honoured fashion, offspring can be seen and not heard. The new bar arrangement includes a fine buffet that shows every sign of maintaining the high standards for which The Lord Bagenal is famous. Seasonal restaurant meals offer a fairly robust modern Irish style, based on French country cooking; speciality seasonal dishes could include cod with roasted red peppers and new potatoes & spinach in summer, for example, or noisettes of lamb with fresh rosemary and minted pea purée, plus vegetarian options like spinach & mushroom tortelloni. Local farmhouse cheeses and a strong wine list add to the pleasure of dining at The Lord Bagenal. • Open all day daily meals £, D££ • Closed Good Fri & 25 Dec • Diners, MasterCard, Visa •

CAVAN

Because its main roads naturally follow the easiest routes through the least resistant territory, most visitors have an abiding impression of Cavan as a watery place of low-lying rounded little hills, intertwined with many lakes and rivers. And certainly much of Cavan is classic drumlin country, almost with more water than they know what to do with. But if you take your time wandering through this green and silver land – particularly if travelling at the leisurely pace of the deservedly renowned Shannon-Erne Waterway which has joined Ireland's two greatest lake and river systems – then you'll become aware that this is a place of rewardingly gentle pleasures. And you'll have time to discover that it does have its own mountain, or at least it shares the 667 m peak of Cuilcagh with neighbouring Fermanagh. In fact, Cavan is much more extensive than is popularly imagined, for in the northeast it has Shercock with its own miniature lake district, while in its southeast it takes in all of Lough Ramor at the charming lakeside village of Virginia. It also shares Lough Sheelin, that place of legend for the angler, with Westmeath and Meath, and always throughout its drumlin heartlands you can find many little Cavan lakes which, should the fancy take you, can be called your own at least for the day that's in it.

Local Attractions and Information

Belturbet	Tourist Office 049 22044
Cavan	Tourist Information 049 31942
Co Cavan Ballyjamesduff International Pork Festival (June)	049 44242

Ballyconnell   Slieve Russell Hotel & Country Club

Ballyconnell Co Cavan

HOTEL   **Tel: 049 26444**   **Fax: 049 26474**

email: slieve-russell@sqgroup.com

The Slieve Russell is close to the attractive town of Ballyconnell, on the recently re-opened canal linking the Shannon and Lough Erne. This is a particularly unspoilt area well known for its myriad lakes and fine fishing. Named after a nearby mountain, this striking flagship of the Sean Quinn Group is set amongst 300 acres of landscaped gardens and grounds, including 50 acres of lakes, and is now firmly established as the social and business centre of the area. In the foyer, generous seating areas are arranged around the marble colonnades and a grand central staircase, flanked by a large bar on one side and two restaurants at the other. Everything at the Slieve Russell is on a generous scale and the accommodation, which includes 10 suites, is no exception: all rooms have extra large beds and spacious marble bathrooms and all have pleasant country views. Excellent leisure facilities in the Golf and Country Club adjoining the hotel include a 20 metre pool while the championship golf course, which opened in 1992, has become one of the top golfing venues in Ireland. It is complemented by a putting green, practice area and nine hole, par 3 course. • Acc£££-££££ • Open all year • Amex, Diners, MasterCard, Visa •

Belturbet   International Fishing Centre

Loughdooley Belturbet Co Cavan

RESTAURANT   Tel: 049 22616

Michel and Yvette Neuville's International Fishing Centre offers residential fishing holidays, mainly for continental guests, and they also run a restaurant which is open to non-residents. As well as attracting local diners, the restaurant provides an excellent facility for holidaymakers on river cruises, as there are pontoons at the bottom of the garden – where, with typical French practicality, the menu is clearly displayed. The centre is like a little corner of France, with all signage in French and a very French menu that includes specialities from Alsace and is accompanied by a sensible wine selection – and a refreshingly reasonable bill. When the weather allows, tables are set out on the terrace. Accommodation, which can be self-catering or B&B, is sometimes available. • D£ daily • Closed mid Nov-early April • Visa •

Blacklion   MacNean House & Bistro

Blacklion Co Cavan

RESTAURANT/ACCOMMODATION   🍴   Tel: 072 53022 Fax: 072 53404/43004

Maguire's pub across the road is a very pleasant local to relax in over a drink before the serious business of addressing Neven Maguire's ambitious cooking. Since winning the Euro-Toques Young Chef competition in 1994 – with a prize giving him experience in a Luxembourg restaurant – Neven has attracted a sizeable following and put this little border town firmly on the culinary map. Here, in a small and distinctly low-key family restaurant run with his parents Joe and Vera Maguire, Neven sources the best local produce and prepares menus that reflect international trends rather than local preferences. Lamb, beef, guinea fowl, quail, scallops, langoustine ("Dublin Bay Prawns"), cod, halibut and organic produce from nearby Eden Plants are now more typical than the exotic kangaroo and ostrich of previous years. There is a lot of choice for a small establishment and, on our most recent visit, we felt that less might be more – not only in choice but also style, which is perhaps becoming over complicated. Desserts have always been a particular passion for Neven and it is a must to leave a little room for one of his carefully crafted confections – the grand finale is just that in this case. Sunday lunch is an interesting occasion at MacNean, somehow combining the elements of the traditional meal with more adventurous choices – and very good value at £12. Service, under Joe Maguire's direction, is friendly. No children under 10 in the restaurant after 7 pm.

Rooms

Accommodation is available in 5 en-suite bedrooms (2 shower only). Children are welcome. Nearby attractions include golf, fishing and hill walking, Marble Arch Caves and Florence Court. • D£-££ Tues-Sun, L£ Sun • Acc£ • Closed 25 Dec & Good Fri • MasterCard, Visa •

Butlersbridge   Derragarra Inn
Butlersbridge Co Cavan

PUB   **Tel: 049 31003**

Heading north on the N3, a few miles along from Cavan town, this well-known thatched inn makes a useful place to break a journey. It's easily spotted by the famous collection of agricultural memorabilia around the door – and there's more of the same inside. Renovations were in progress during the guide's recent visit, but there's no reason to expect very major changes. Food has always been reliable – popular bar staples, plus some more ambitious dishes with the emphasis on seafood. • Meals£ all day • Closed 25 Dec & Good Fri • MasterCard, Visa •

Cavan   Hotel Kilmore
Dublin Road Cavan Co Cavan

HOTEL   **Tel: 049 32288   Fax: 049 32458**

The leading hotel of the area, the Kilmore has an impressive foyer and spacious public rooms. The focal point of local business and social activities, it has good conference and banqueting facilities. Bedrooms, which include a bridal suite, are comfortable and well-equipped with direct dial phones, TV and tea/coffee trays. Leisure activities nearby include golf, fishing and horseriding. • Acc££ • Open all year • Amex, Diners, MasterCard, Visa •

Cavan   Lifeforce Mill
Mill Rock Cavan Co Cavan

CAFÉ/RESTAURANT/VISITOR CENTRE   Tel: 049 62722   Fax: 049 62923

The Lifeforce Mill, in the centre of Cavan town, dates back to 1846. Although the commercial milling operation closed down in the 1950s, it is now enjoying a new lease of life welcoming visitors and producing Lifeforce Stoneground Wholemeal Flour. All of the original machinery has been restored to working order, including what is believed to be the only working McAdam Water Turbine – designed by Belfast engineer Robert McAdam, the turbine was used to harness the power of the Kennypottle River and drive the great stone wheels instead of the usual, but slower and less efficient, water wheel. The mill tour is distinctly innovative as visitors experience the end result as well as learning about the workings of the mill itself: each visitor begins the tour by making a loaf of traditional soda bread with the stoneground flour produced by the mill and collects it, hot from the ovens of the coffee shop, on leaving. Wholesome fare is served in the coffee shop/restaurant – and even that has a tale to tell. Although also Victorian, it is not part of the original mill site – it was transported from Drogheda to avoid demolition during road improvements, then re-erected beside the mill. The mill is normally open Tuesday-Sunday from 9-5, May to September and for groups by arrangement at other times. • Tues-Sun daytime meals £ •

Kingscourt

Cabra Castle Hotel

Kingscourt Co Cavan

HOTEL   Tel: 042 67030   Fax: 042 67039

email: cabrach@iol.ie

Formerly known as Cormey Castle and renamed Cabra Castle in the early 19th century, this impressive hotel is set amidst 100 acres of garden and parkland, with lovely views over the Cavan countryside, famous for its lakes and fine fishing. (The nearby Dun A Ri Forest has many walks and nature trails on land once part of the Cabra estate.) Although initially imposing, with its large public rooms and antique furnishings, the atmosphere at Cabra Castle is relaxing. Due to the age of the building, the bedrooms vary in size and outlook, but all are comfortable and individually decorated. Accommodation includes some ground floor rooms suitable for less able guests, four suites and, in addition to rooms in the main building, the newer rooms in an extension are particularly suitable for families. There are also some romantic ones complete with old beams, in a courtyard which has been converted to provide modern comforts without sacrificing character. A special combination of formal background and easy ambience make this a good venue for private and business functions; it is popular for both weddings and conferences but special interest breaks such as golf, fishing and horseriding are also a great attraction. • Acc££ • Closed 25 Dec & 2nd wk Jan • Amex, MasterCard, Visa •

Kingscourt

Gartlans Pub

Main Street Kingscourt Co Cavan

PUB   Tel: 042 67003

This pretty thatched pub is a delightfully unspoilt example of the kind of grocery/pub that used to be so typical of Ireland, especially in country areas. Few enough of them remain, now that the theme pub has moved in, but this one is real, with plenty of local news items around the walls, a serving hatch where simple groceries can be bought, all served with genuine warmth and hospitality. The Gartlans have been here since 1911 and they have achieved the remarkable feat of appearing to make time stand still.

Mountnugent

Ross House & Castle

Mountnugent Co Cavan

COUNTRY HOUSE   Tel/Fax: 049 40218

email: rosshouse@tinet.ie   www.indigo.ie/~BehitaLH/fishing/ireland.htm

In mature grounds on the shores of Lough Sheelin, Peter and Ulla Harkort's old manor house enjoys a very lovely location and offers a good standard of accommodation at a modest price. Bedrooms, which are distinctly continental in style, have telephone, TV and tea/coffee trays and some unusual features: three have their own conservatories, four have fireplaces (help yourself to logs from the shed) and all have an unfamiliar type of shower not likely to be seen elsewhere in Ireland. Peace and relaxation are the great attraction, and there's a fine choice of activities at hand: a pier offers boats (and engines) for fishermen to explore the lake, there's safe bathing from a sandy beach, tennis and a sauna. At the castle nearby, Peter and Ulla's daughter Viola Harkort provides most unusual accommodation (it is a very real castle) and organises pony trekking and horseriding. Ulla cooks for everyone, making packed lunches, sandwiches and High Tea (£3-£10) and a 4-course dinner (£14/£18). • Acc£-££ • Open all year • MasterCard, Visa •

CLARE

There's a heroic quality to Clare which other places deny at their peril. This, after all, is "The Banner County" of Gaelic sporting legend. This is the homeland of some of the finest traditional music in the land. This is a larger-than life county which is bounded by the Atlantic to the west, Galway Bay to the north, the Shannon and Lough Derg to the east, and the Shannon Estuary to the south. And it's typical of Clare that, even with its boundaries marked on such a grand scale, there is always something extra added. Thus the Atlantic coasts include not only the astonishing and majestic Cliffs of Moher, but also one of Ireland's greatest surfing beaches at Lahinch on Liscannor Bay. As for that Galway Bay coastline, it is where The Burren, the fantastical North Clare moonscape of limestone which is home to so much unexpectedly exotic flora, comes plunging spectacularly towards the sea around the attractive village of Ballyvaughan. To the eastward, Lough Derg is one of Ireland's most handsome lakes, but even amidst its generous beauty, we find that Clare has claimed one of the most scenic lake coastlines of all. As for the Shannon Estuary, well, Ireland may have many estuaries, but needless to say the lordly Shannon has far and away the biggest estuary of all. Yet despite the heroic scale of its geography, the urban centres of Clare such as the county town of Ennis and the increasingly busy recreational port of Kilrush, together with smaller places like Ennistimon, Milltown Malbay, Corofin and Mountshannon – they all have a very human and friendly dimension. For this is a county where the human spirit defines itself as being very human indeed in the midst of scenic effects which at times seem to border on the supernatural.

Local Attractions and Information

Ballyvaughan	Aillwee Cave, 065 81171
Bunratty	Bunratty Castle & Folk Park 061 361020
Cliffs of Moher	(Tourist Information) 065 81171
Ennis	World Irish Dancing Championships (March) 01 4752220
Kinvara	Dunguaire Castle (medieval banquets etc) 061 360788
Quin	Craggaunowen Project (Celts &Living Past) 061 360788
Shannon Airport	Tourist Information 061 61664 / 61565

Ballyvaughan   Aillwee Cave

Ballyvaughan Co Clare

CAFÉ/RESTAURANT/VISITOR CENTRE   **Tel: 065 77036**

About 2 miles south-west of Ballyvaughan; well-signposted throughout the area. Visitors to this 2-million-year-old cave will see more than the amazing illuminated tunnels and waterfalls, for there is much of interest to foodlovers as well. Driving up to the entrance, look out for the sign to the cheese-making demonstrations – for it is here that the local Burren Gold cheese is made. Even if the process is in a quiet phase at the time of a visit, there is still plenty to see – and buy – as the cheesemaking takes place alongside a well-stocked food shop. Just inside the entrance to the cave there is a souvenir shop with a good book section (including travel and cookery books of Irish interest) and a café/restaurant serving inexpensive, wholesome fare. • Meals£ all day Mon-Sun •

Ballyvaughan   An Fear Gorta (Tea & Garden Rooms)

Ballyvaughan Co Clare

RESTAURANT   **Tel: 065 77023   065 77127**

Approached from the harbourfront through a lovely front garden, Katherine O'Donoghue's delightful old stone restaurant dates back to 1790, when it was built as a residence for 'coast security officers'. Having been rebuilt by the present owners in 1981, it is now just the spot for a light bite to eat. In fine weather the beautiful back garden or the conservatory can be idyllic; otherwise the homely indoor room offers comfort and shelter, with its informal arrangement of old furniture and a tempting display of home-baked fare. This is the speciality of the house – all laid out on an old cast-iron range and very reasonably priced – beginning at only 70p for scone, butter & home-made jam. Speciality teas are available as well as savoury choices including farmhouse cheeses, home-baked ham and Tea Room Specials including Open Smoked Salmon Sandwich on Brown Bread. 2-3 course lunch specials are available at £6/£7 and there's even home-made jam and marmalade to take away. • Open all day Mon-Sat meals£ • Closed Oct-May • No credit cards •

Ballyvaughan

COUNTRY HOUSE

Gregans Castle

Ballyvaughan Co Clare

Tel: 065 77005 Fax: 065 77111

email: res@gregans.ie www.gregans.ie

Gregans Castle has a long and interesting history, going back to a tower house, or small castle which was built by the O'Loughlen clan (the region's principal tribe) between the 10th and 17th centuries and which is still intact. The present house dates from the late 18th century and has been continuously added to, up to the present day. The present owners, Peter and Moira Haden, opened Gregans Castle as a country house hotel in 1976 and (true to the traditions of the house) have continued to develop and improve it (recently with their son Simon-Peter who is now Manager). The exterior is grey and stark, in keeping with the lunar landscape of the surrounding Burren, serving only to heighten the contrast between first impressions and the warmth, comfort and hospitality to be found within. Spacious accommodation, which includes four suites and two mini-suites, is furnished to a very high standard and rooms all have excellent bathrooms and lovely countryside views. Peace and quiet are the dominant themes – the otherwise luxurious rooms are deliberately left without the worldly interference of television. Yet this luxurious hotel is not too formal or at all intimidating; non-residents are welcome to drop in for lunch or afternoon tea in the Corkscrew Room bar – named after a nearby hill which, incidentally, provides the most scenic approach to Ballyvaughan. In fine weather guests can sit out beside the Celtic Cross rose garden and watch patches of sun and shade chasing across the hills.

Restaurant

The dining room is elegantly furnished in keeping with the rest of the house, overlooking the Burren (which on fine summer evenings enjoys very special light effects as the sun sets over Galway Bay). Dinner is often gently accompanied by a pianist or harpist and offers a wide choice of dishes based on the best of local produce, including organic vegetables. There is always a selection of local cheeses, with homemade biscuits. • D££-£££ daily, Bar L£-££ • Acc£££ • Closed late Oct-Easter • Amex, MasterCard, Visa •

Establishment reports for Dublin City and Greater Dublin can be found on the Dublin Live section of The Irish Times On Line site (www.irish-times.com).

Ballyvaughan

HOTEL

Hyland's Hotel

The Square Ballyvaughan Co Clare

Tel: 065 77037 Fax: 065 77131

email: hylands@tinet.ie

In the centre of Ballyvaughan, beside the harbour, this delightful family-run hotel dates back to the 18th century. Ownership is currently in the capable hands of 7th and 8th generation family members Marie & Deirdre Hyland. Open fires, comfortable well-crafted furniture and sympathetic lighting create a welcoming atmosphere that is carried through into all areas of the hotel. Food served is based on excellent local produce – locally caught seafood, Burren lamb, farmhouse cheeses, organic vegetables and herbs. New bedrooms have recently been added and all are very comfortable, with good amenities. • Meals £-££ • Acc££ • Closed late Dec and all Jan • Amex, Diners, MasterCard, Visa •

Ballyvaughan

PUB

Monks Pub

The Quay Ballyvaughan Co Clare

Tel: 065 77059

Michael and Bernadette Monks' famous pub has been drawing people along the pier at Ballyvaughan since 1981. It's an informal, cottagey kind of a place with several small bars well set up for the comfortable consumption of Bernadette's delicious seafood. They do their own special version of seafood chowder. There is also real prawn cocktail or mussels steamed in garlic, or open prawn or salmon sandwiches. The fishcakes are a speciality. If you want to splash out a bit and spend more than a fiver, there's a seafood platter (or, for the faint-hearted, a half platter), baked crab and, after 6 pm, poached fresh salmon served with hot vegetables. There's always a vegetarian dish of the day and a nice choice of wines to wash it all down with. Just lovely. • Meals£ • Closed 25 Dec, Good Fri • Amex, MasterCard, Visa •

Ballyvaughan

ACCOMMODATION

Rusheen Lodge

Knocknagrough Ballyvaughan Co Clare
Tel: 065 77092   Fax: 065 77152
email: jmcgann@iol.ie

Just on the edge of Ballyvaughan, Rusheen Lodge is well-signed from the Aillwee Cave direction. Since they first welcomed guests to Rusheen Lodge in 1991, Rita and John McGann have built up an enviable reputation for hospitality. Generously proportioned, well-appointed bedrooms, good bathrooms and spacious public rooms make this a very comfortable place to stay. Breakfast – whether traditional Irish or continental- is a major feature of a stay. Evening meals are not provided, but the pubs and restaurants of Ballyvaughan are only a few minutes walk. It was John McGann's father, Jacko McGann, who discovered the Aillwee Cave, an immense network of caverns and waterfalls under the Burren which is now a major attraction in the area. • Acc££ • Closed Dec & Jan • Amex, MasterCard, Visa •

Ballyvaughan

RESTAURANT

Whitethorn Restaurant

Ballyvaughan Co Clare
Tel: 065 77044   Fax: 065 77155
email: whitethorne@tinet.ie

A quarter of a mile from Ballyvaughan village, on the sea side of the Galway road, is Sarah and John McDonnell's fine craft shop and restaurant. John also runs a wine business and they've recently added a visitor centre, "Burren eXposure". Here visitors learn about the formation of the Burren rockscape, its history and the amazing diversity of flora which brings so many visitors to the region in early summer. The restaurant has magnificent sea views and offers excellent home-made fare throughout the day (which visitors can take indoors or out depending on the weather and inclination). Evening brings a more formal dining arrangement, but offers the same good cooking and excellent value in imaginative menus based on local produce. Tempting vegetarian dishes, nice homely desserts – and, of course, an especially interesting wine list. • L£ daily & D££ Mon-Sat • Closed Nov-Apr • MasterCard, Visa •

Bunratty

PUB

Durty Nelly's

Bunratty Co Clare
Tel: 061 364861

Although often seriously over-crowded with tourists in summer, this famous and genuinely characterful old pub in the shadow of Bunratty Castle somehow manages to provide cheerful service and above-average food to the great numbers who pass through its doors. All-day fare is served downstairs in The Oyster restaurant; upstairs there is a more exclusive restaurant, The Loft, open in the evening only. Both areas offer à la carte menus. •Closed 25 Dec, Good Fri • Amex, Diners, MasterCard, Visa •

Bunratty

HOTEL

Fitzpatrick Bunratty Hotel

Bunratty Co Clare
Tel: 061 361177   Fax: 061 471252
email: info@fitzpatrick.com

Conveniently located just ten minutes from both Shannon International Airport and Limerick city, Fitzpatrick Bunratty is in wooded grounds beside Bunratty Castle and Folk Park and offers good facilities for both business and leisure guests. The style of the building is typical of many hotels established in the 1960s, but the Fitzpatrick Hotel Group have been energetic in their efforts to update facilities. Public areas, including the foyer area which is large and decorated to a distinctive Irish theme, are quite impressive, as are recent additions. These include a fine fitness centre with 20 metre swimming pool and an excellent conference & banqueting centre (that offers a state-of-the-art range of conference facilities and can cater for up to 1,500 people). Bedrooms are well-equipped, with the facilities expected of a hotel of this calibre, although on a recent visit we felt that the decor in some (including a suite) was somewhat dated. However, refurbishments are due to take place before the 1999 season, including redecoration of 30 bedrooms and changes to the lounge area and the restaurant (which is to become a bistro). It may be advisable in the meantime to inquire about the decorative state of bedrooms when booking. • Acc£££ • Closed 25 Dec • Amex, Diners, MasterCard, Visa •

Clarecastle

COUNTRY HOUSE

Carnelly House

Clarecastle Co Clare

Tel: 065 28442   Fax: 065 29222

email: rgleeson@iol.ie   www.carnelly-house.com

Dermott and Rosemarie Gleeson's fine redbrick Georgian house is easily found (just back a little from the N18) and is set on 100 acres of farm and woodland. Conveniently located for Shannon airport and for touring the west of Ireland, this beautifully proportioned house is in excellent order and offers discerning guests very special accommodation. Reception rooms include an impressive drawing room with Corinthian pillars, Francini ceiling, grand piano and a striking panelled dining room where communal dinners are taken at 8 pm. (Residents only, except groups for lunch or dinner by arrangement.) Bedrooms are large and furnished to a very high standard, with antiques, canopied king size or twin beds and luxurious private bathrooms. Yet the grandeur is not at all daunting and Carnelly – which is also well-placed for a wide range of country pursuits, including many of the country's most famous hunts – has been described as "one of the warmest, friendliest and most entertaining houses in Ireland". Not normally suitable for children under 10. There is also a gate lodge, which is available by the night, week or month. • Acc£££• Closed Dec-Mar • Amex, MasterCard, Visa •

Cratloe

ACCOMMODATION

Bunratty View

Bunratty Co Clare

Tel: 061 357352   Fax: 061 357491

A modern house, providing comfortable, spacious accommodation conveniently close to Bunratty Castle and Shannon Airport. Rooms have double and single beds, phone, tea/coffee facilities, satellite TV, hairdryers and en-suite bathrooms which vary somewhat (some shower only). There's a comfortable residents' lounge with an open fire and bright dining room, where good breakfasts are served. Signed off the dual carriageway. • Acc£ • Open all year • MasterCard, Visa •

Doolin

HOTEL

Aran View House Hotel

Doolin Coast Road Co Clare

Tel: 065 74061   Fax: 065 74540

Just outside Doolin, and commanding dramatic sea views across to the islands, the Linnane's family-run hotel makes a good base for a family holiday – it is only a mile to a good beach, there is sea-angling and golf nearby and, of course, there is the traditional music for which Doolin is world famous. Public rooms include a comfortable bar for all weathers – it has a sea view and an open fire. Bedrooms vary considerably in size and outlook due to the age and nature of the building: rooms at the front are most desirable – several at the back have no view, but are otherwise pleasant. A high proportion – six rooms – are suitable for disabled guests and there are two extra large ones and two singles; six are non-smoking. All are en-suite with over-bath showers, tea/coffee trays and TV (local stations) Children are welcome – outdoor play area and children's menu provided. There is a restaurant (open to non-residents) with very reasonably priced set menus (£10 at lunch and dinner) available as well as an à la carte offering local produce, including lobster. • Acc££ • Closed Nov-Apr •

Doolin

PUB

O'Connor's Pub

Doolin Co Clare

Tel: 065 74168   Fax: 065 74668

Famous world-wide for its nightly traditional music, song and dance, O'Connor's pub has brought many people to Doolin. But, although the music may be the initial incentive to travel to this small fishing village, once they get there people find that the food and hospitality is every bit as good as the sessions. Although the pub changed hands just as the guide was going to press, cooking is still being done by the same team, so we anticipate that standards should be maintained. Everything is sourced locally and made freshly every day. Seafood is a speciality – their own version of chowder (served with home-baked bread), open crab sandwiches, Lisdoonvarna smoked salmon, smoked mackerel salad and a hot Catch of the Day – but red meats are also well-represented (beef stew in Guinness is a complete meal, served with potatoes) and vegetarians won't go hungry either. Prices are very reasonable and it is anticipated that credit cards (probably MasterCard and Visa) will be accepted for food in 1999. • L£ daily & D£ daily • Closed 25 Dec & Good Fri •

Ennis   Auburn Lodge Hotel

Galway Road Ennis Co Clare

HOTEL   Tel: 065 21247   Fax: 065 21202

This pleasant modern hotel just 20 minutes from Shannon airport is built around a central courtyard containing a soothing garden, creating a peaceful atmosphere throughout the building. Quite spacious rooms have good facilities and include some larger executive suites and a pretty bridal suite. • Acc££ • Amex, Diners, MasterCard, Visa •

Ennis   The Cloister

Club Bridge Abbey Street Ennis Co Clare

PUB   Tel: 065 29521   Fax: 065 28352

This remarkable pub and restaurant has been run by Jim and Annette Brindly since 1991, and although improvements have been made – including the addition of a conservatory a couple of years ago – they have been careful to retain the character of the building, which is actually built into the walls and garden of the adjacent 13th-century abbey. The food style tends towards traditional dishes such as Irish stew and fish pie on the bar menu with more classical dishes in the restaurant. The character of the place – stone walls and floors, open fires – and nightly traditional music sessions are a great attraction. • L£ & D££ daily • Closed 25 Dec, New Year, & 1-2 weeks Jan •

Ennis   Cruise's Pub

Abbey Street Ennis Co Clare

PUB   Tel: 065 28628

There is a real sense of history about this pub, which is beside the ruins of the Ennis Friary and dates from 1658. Although quite recently renovated it has retained original features and avoided the "theme pub" atmosphere. Nightly traditional music sessions are a major feature and there's a medieval room, "The Sanctuary", available for folklore evenings and private functions for up to 200 guests. • Closed 25 Dec & Good Fri • Amex, Diners, MasterCard, Visa •

Ennis   Garvello's

Clareabbey Limerick Road Ennis Co Clare

RESTAURANT   Tel: 065 40011   Fax: 065 40022

'More than just good food' is an appropriate motto for Gay O'Hara's well-appointed restaurant on the outskirts of Ennis. It is unusual for the area, not least for its very striking modern style – incorporating a bright bar/reception area, wooden floors and very special individual carpets throughout. Unlike most of the local competition, which tends towards traditional Irish themes, head chef Michael Foley's style is modern Irish, with the international influences that this implies. Wording on the menu could benefit from simplification but the cooking is good and employs the finest local produce in contemporary dishes. A vegetarian menu is also available. Interesting wine list and well-trained service under the management of Derek Halpin. Open for lunch on Sunday (and, although not obviously a family kind of place, genuinely welcoming to children) although the sophisticated atmosphere is really best suited to the primary evening business. • D££ Mon-Sat, L£ Sun only • Closed Bank Hols, 25 Dec & 1 Jan • Amex, Diners, MasterCard, Visa •

Ennis   Old Ground Hotel

O'Connell Street Ennis Co Clare

HOTEL   Tel: 065 28127   Fax: 065 28112

This ivy-clad former manor house dates back to the 18th century and, set in its own gardens, creates an oasis of calm in the centre of Ennis. One of the country's best-loved hotels, the Old Ground was bought by the Flynn family in 1995 and has been imaginatively extended and renovated by them in a way that is commendably sensitive to the age and importance of the building. Despite the difficulties of dealing with very thick walls in an old building, major improvements were made to existing banqueting/conference facilities in 1996/97, then an extra storey was added to provide new rooms. Again, this has been a sensitive development and, as the famous ivy-clad frontage continues to thrive, the external changes are barely noticeable to the casual observer. Major refurbishment has also taken place throughout the interior of the hotel, including all bedrooms, the O'Brien Room restaurant and a traditional style bar, Poet's Corner, which features equally traditional music on Wednesday, Thursday and Friday nights. • Meals£ • Acc£££ • Closed 25-26 Dec • Amex, Diners, MasterCard, Visa •

Ennis   Temple Gate Hotel
The Square Ennis Co Clare
HOTEL   Tel: 065 23300   Fax: 065 23322
email: templegh@iol.ie

Built in the centre of Ennis town, to a clever design that makes the best possible use of the site, this family-owned hotel opened to some acclaim in 1996. While retaining the older features (including a church which was first used as a pub and is now the Great Hall Banqueting/Conference room, seating up to 200) existing gothic themes have also been successfully blended into the new, creating a striking modern building which has relevance to its surroundings in the heart of a medieval town. Since then it has succeeded in providing the comfort and convenience expected by today's travellers at a reasonable price. In 1998 the hotel was extended to add 40 new deluxe rooms, two new state-of-the-art syndicate/conference rooms for up to 100 people, and a new bar to replace the old one in the church and the Great Hall. • Acc££ • Closed 25 Dec • Amex, Diners, MasterCard, Visa •

Ennis   West County Inn
Clare Road Ennis Co Clare
HOTEL   Tel: 065 28421   Fax: 065 28801
email: cro@lynchotels.com   www.lynchotels.com

Recently extended and refurbished, this modern hotel 5 minutes walk from the centre of Ennis town is not only a well-located and comfortable base for holidaymakers but also renowned for its exceptional conference facilities. The hotel's Island Convention Centre can seat 1,750 delegates in a range of four conference rooms and five meeting rooms that appear almost infinitely variable. There are also full business/office support services and a new Health and Leisure Club in which to wind down or shape up. Bedrooms include interconnecting rooms, mini-suites, family rooms and 43 recently added Premier standard rooms with fax/modem points. • Acc££-£££ • Open all year • Amex, Diners, MasterCard, Visa •

Kilbaha   Anvil Farm Guesthouse & Restaurant
Kilbaha Loop Head Co Clare
FARM STAY   Tel: 065 58018   Fax: 065 58133

On the family's clifftop farm at the end of the Loop Head peninsula, Maura Keating has five guest rooms providing comfortable en-suite accommodation (one with bath, the rest shower-only) in one of the country's most remote and unspoilt areas. Rugged cliff scenery, angling, diving, bird watching and walking are some of the attractions that bring visitors to this wild and windblown beauty spot – the perfect antidote to city life. There is plenty to visit in the area too -Maura has all the details for her guests – and good local food for dinner, including Aberdeen Angus beef from their own farm, locally caught Atlantic salmon and local Inagh and Cratloe cheeses. Visitors may also visit the farm, which has a variety of animals and a special interest in Irish sport horse breeding. • D£ • Acc£ • Closed Nov-Feb •

Kilfenora   Vaughan's Pub
Kilfenora Co Clare
PUB   Tel: 065 88004/59   Fax: 065 71750

One of the most famous music centres in the west of Ireland, traditional Irish music and set dancing at Vaughan's pub and thatched barn attract visitors from all over the world. In the family since about 1800, the present owners of this attractive old pub, John and Kay Vaughan, work hard to make sure that visitors have the best possible time. The pub is warm and homely, with an open fire in the front bar and a garden set up with tables at the back. Kay personally supervises the food, which has become an important part of the operation over the years: traditional Irish menus are based on good local ingredients, including organic meats, seafood and North Clare cheese. • Closed 25 Dec & Good Fri • MasterCard, Visa •

Lahinch
Aberdeen Arms Hotel

Lahinch Co Clare

HOTEL Tel: 065 81100 Fax: 065 81228

email: aberdeenarms@websters.ie

The Aberdeen Arms is the oldest golf links hotel in Ireland, with a history going back to 1850. Since Gerry Norton, the current owner, took over in 1995 a major refurbishment and extension programme has been completed, including the construction of a health centre, renovation of public areas and the addition of banqueting and conference facilities. Public areas are spacious and comfortably furnished, with a choice of bars – the lively Klondyke Bar (named after Lahinch's famous 5th hole) or the quieter residents' lounge – and an all-day grill room. Bedrooms are generously sized with good bathrooms and quality furniture (including queen-size orthopaedic beds). Most have views of the golf links and the long sandy beach which brings large numbers of keen surfers to ride the waves. • Acc££ • Closed Xmas wk, Jan & Feb • Amex, Diners, MasterCard, Visa •

Lahinch
Barrtra Seafood Restaurant

Lahinch Co Clare

RESTAURANT Tel: 065 81280

In 1998 Paul and Theresa O'Brien celebrated a decade of fine food and hospitality at their traditional, whitewashed restaurant on the cliffs just outside Lahinch. During that time they have built up a loyal following. Guests enjoy Theresa's good, unfussy cooking in dishes which, predictably, highlight seafood but also offer a wide choice (including a vegetarian menu). Paul provides warm and easy hospitality (and maintains good service). The decor is appealingly simple and the views of Liscannor Bay can be magic from window tables on a fine evening. Main courses include lobster, when available, and a wide range of other local seafood as well as alternatives such as steak and vegetarian dishes. An interesting and keenly priced wine list, good cheeseboard, home-baked breads and good cafetiere coffee show an attention to detail in tune with the overall high standard. • D££ Mon-Sat • Closed Jan & Feb • Amex, Diners, MasterCard, Visa •

Lahinch
Mr Eamon's Restaurant

Kettle Street Lahinch Co Clare

RESTAURANT Tel: 065 81050 Fax: 065 81810

Mr Eamon's is the longest established fine dining restaurant in the area and is very easy to find in the centre of the town. The ambience is cosy and welcoming, with excellent home-baked breads presented along with a menu that promises tasty starters and vegetarian dishes (such as grilled St Tola cheese with tapenade, local Bonina black pudding or courgettes stuffed with stir-fried vegetables) and a wide range of main courses including steaks (and, on winter menus, spiced beef) and rack of lamb. It is especially strong on local seafood. Hot buttered lobster is a speciality, also fresh crab, monkfish and turbot, which might be served with a classic sauce soubise. Good vegetables, farmhouse cheeses, simple well-made desserts and freshly brewed coffee to finish. • D££ • Closed mid Jan- mid Mar • Amex, Diners, MasterCard, Visa •

Visit our web site - www.ireland-guide.com

Lisdoonvarna
Ballinalacken Castle Hotel

Lisdoonvarna Co Clare

HOTEL Tel/Fax: 065 74025

Well away from the bustle of Lisdoonvarna, and with wonderful views of the Atlantic, Aran Islands, Cliffs of Moher and the distant hills of Connemara, Ballinalacken is easily identified by the 15th century castle still standing beside the hotel. In the O'Callaghan family ownership since its establishment in 1940, and currently managed by Marian O'Callaghan, Ballinalacken has retained a Victorian country house atmosphere with its welcoming fire in the hall and well-proportioned public rooms comfortably furnished with antiques. The drawing room and recently extended dining room both enjoy magnificent views. Additions and renovations are undertaken on an on-going basis at Ballinalacken and improvements are always noticeable on each visit. Bedrooms are all en-suite, varying according to age and location in the building – some have double and single beds, some are shower only; however, they are all comfortable and some have seating areas with sea views. • Acc££ • Closed mid Oct-Easter • MasterCard, Visa •

Lisdoonvarna

Sheedy's Spa Hotel

Lisdoonvarna Co Clare

HOTEL   Tel: 065 74026   Fax: 065 74555

Sheedy's has been in the Sheedy family for generations – after being in the capable hands of Frank and Patsy Sheedy since 1971 it moved into a new generation in 1998 when John and Martina Sheedy took the reins. Characterised by a high standard of maintenance indoors and out, attractive furnishings, warm ambience (in every sense – the sunny foyer has a comfortable seating area and an open fire for chillier days) and friendly hands-on management, it is not surprising that Sheedy's is one of the west of Ireland's best loved small hotels. Bedrooms vary in size, but are all en-suite, neatly decorated and well-equipped.

Orchid Restaurant

Frankie Sheedy, as previous head chef, had already established a national reputation for The Orchid Restaurant and, now that it has been taken over by John – who had been working at Ashford Castle as Chef de Cuisine since 1989 – it will be interesting to see what changes will be made. The guide's visit was made just at the time of the changeover, but menus do not indicate any dramatic changes as yet so a sense of continuity is likely to be retained. Whatever may develop, guests can have confidence that it will be good – and that hospitality will still be of paramount importance at Sheedy's.
* John and Martina have developed the cosy bar beside the foyer (previously open only at night) as an informal Seafood Bar, serving the likes of seafood platters, crab claws in garlic butter and crab salad from 12-9 daily. • Bar Meals£, D££ daily • Acc££ • Closed Nov-Mar • Amex, Diners, MasterCard, Visa •

Miltown Malbay

Berry Lodge

Annagh Miltown Malbay Co Clare

COUNTRY HOUSE   Tel/Fax: 065 87022

Near the coast of west Clare, between Kilkee and Lahinch, Berry Lodge is a pleasant Victorian country house and the family home of Rita Meade, who has run it as a guesthouse and restaurant since 1994. Comfortable accommodation is provided in five en-suite bedrooms (1 suitable for disabled guests, all shower only) furnished with an attractive mixture of old and new, including Irish craft items. A conservatory is planned for 1999. Cookery classes – given by Rita in her own kitchen – are a special feature of Berry Lodge. Information, including a short breaks brochure, is available on request. • MasterCard, Visa •

Restaurant

Rita cooks evening meals for guests and non-residents (booking advised). Quite ambitious menus are based on local and home-grown ingredients, many of them organic. Service was very slow on a recent visit, possibly because the menu is rather complicated for the size of the operation. • D££, SunL£ • Acc£ • Closed mid Jan-mid Feb • MasterCard, Visa •

New Quay

Linnane's

New Quay The Burren Co Clare

PUB   Tel: 065 78120

Right on the rocks – with a sliding door opening up in summer, the better to enjoy views clear across Galway Bay – the Linnane family's unpretentious pub has a great reputation for good pints of stout and seafood, especially lobster. In winter there's a cosy turf fire and a more limited selection of food – chowder and homebaked bread perhaps, or crab salad. A phone call is advised to check times of opening and whether food is available off-season. • MasterCard, Visa •

Newmarket-on-Fergus

Carrygerry Country House

Newmarket-on-Fergus Co Clare

COUNTRY HOUSE   Tel: 061 363739   Fax: 061 363823

Only 10 minutes from Shannon airport and in a beautiful rural setting, Carrygerry is a lovely residence dating back to 1793. It overlooks the Shannon and Fergus estuaries and, peacefully surrounded by woodlands, gardens and pastures, seems very distant from an international airport. After sensitive restoration in the late 1980s (which retained the farm cottages, stables, barns and a coach house that is ideal for weddings and private parties) Carrygerry has been run by the present owners, Marinus and Angela van Kooyk, as a country house hotel since 1996. Public rooms are large, elegantly furnished with antiques and very comfortable, with plenty of seating and open fires. Bedrooms are all non-smoking and include three suitable for disabled guests. Those viewed for the guide (in the main house) are spacious and furnished to a high standard in period style, with all the amenities. As well as catering for private guests, the hotel caters for small conferences, corporate and private dinners, including Christmas and New Year. • Acc££ • Closed Jan & Feb • Amex, Diners, MasterCard, Visa •

Newmarket-on-Fergus   Clare Inn

Dromoland Newmarket-on-Fergus Co Clare
HOTEL   Tel: 061 368161   Fax: 061 368622
email: cro@lynchotels.com   www.lynchotels.com
Built in the grounds of Dromoland Castle, this 1960s hotel overlooks the Shannon estuary and shares the Castle's golf course. Spacious, well-maintained public areas include a well-equipped leisure centre with 17-metre pool, gymnasium and sauna and well-run banqueting/conference facilities (for up to 350/400). Rooms are generally quite large and well-appointed, including some extra features including free movies and an in-room safe; some family rooms sleep up to four, although bathrooms may seem disproportionately small. • Acc££ • Open all year • Amex, Diners, MasterCard, Visa •

Newmarket-on-Fergus   Dromoland Castle Hotel

Newmarket-on-Fergus Co Clare
HOTEL/RESTAURANT 🏛 🏛   Tel: 061 368144   Fax: 061 363355
Dromoland is one of Ireland's grandest hotels, and also one of the best-loved . The ancestral home of the O'Briens, barons of Inchiquin and direct descendants of Brian Boru, High King of Ireland, it is one of the few Irish estates tracing its history back to Gaelic royal families. Today, the visitor is keenly aware of this sense of history, but will not find it daunting. Under the warm and thoughtful management of Mark Nolan, who has been General Manager since 1989, Dromoland is a very relaxing hotel, where the grandeur of the surroundings – the castle itself, its lakes and parkland and magnificent furnishings – does not overpower but rather enhances the pleasure for guests. It is an enchanting place, where wide corridors lined with oak panelling are hung with ancient portraits and scented with the haunting aroma of woodsmoke. Public areas are very grand, with all the crystal chandeliers and massive antiques to be expected in a real Irish Castle, but the atmosphere suggests that a lot of fun is to be had here. Bedrooms are all furnished to a very high standard and have luxurious bathrooms. The Brian Boru International Centre brought a new dimension to the Castle's activities a few years ago and can accommodate almost any type of business gathering, including exhibitions, conferences and banquets. Most recently, the Dromoland Golf and Country Club was opened on the estate last year; this incorporates not only an 18-hole parkland course but also a gym, a Health Clinic offering specialist treatments, and the Green Room Bar and Fig Tree Restaurant, which provide informal alternatives to facilities in the castle.

Earl of Thomond Room ⭐

The most beautiful room in the castle, the Earl of Thomond Dining Room is magnificent, with crystal, gilding and rich fabrics – and has a lovely view over the lake and golf course. Guests ease into the experience of dinner with an aperitif in the Library Bar, overlooking the eighth green, before moving through to beautifully presented tables and gentle background music provided by a traditional Irish harpist. In the evening a wide choice includes a table d'hôte menu (£38), vegetarian menu (£29.50) and an à la carte beginning with Head Chef David McCann's Dromoland signature dish, a "New Irish Cuisine" spectacular of traditional black pudding and buttermilk pancake topped with pan-fried foie gras and glazed apple; a superb dish and well worth trying. The à la carte continues in similar vein, offering a wonderful selection of luxurious dishes. The table d'hôte is more down-to-earth in tone, with a selection of four dishes in the starter and main course sections – a little less glamorous than the carte but with the same quality of ingredients and cooking. David McCann bases his menus on the best of local produce, all the little niceties of a very special meal are observed and service, under restaurant manager Tony Frisby, is excellent. Briefer lunch menus offer a shortened à la carte and a Chef's Suggested Lunch (£17.50) with a choice of three on each course. The wine list – about 250 wines, predominantly French – was under review at the time of going to press (House wines, £16.50). A 15% service charge is added to all prices. • L££, D£££-££££ • Acc£££ • Open all year • Amex, Diners, MasterCard, Visa •

Shannon

HOTEL

Oakwood Arms Hotel

Shannon Airport Shannon Co Clare
Tel: 061 361500   Fax: 061 361414
email: oakwoarm@iol.ie

John and Josephine O'Sullivan opened this mock-Tudor red brick hotel in 1991 and it created a good impression from the start, with its high standard of maintenance and neatly laid-out flower beds. The lounge bar and function room both have aviation themes: the bar honours the memory of the pioneer female pilot Sophie Pearse, who came from the area, and the restaurant is named after The Spruce Goose, Howard Hughes' famous flying boat. Public areas are quite spacious and comfortably furnished and there is ample evidence of a well-run establishment. Although not individually decorated, rooms have all the necessary comforts and are double-glazed; they include one room suitable for disabled guests, two suites, four executive rooms and 12 non-smoking rooms. 25 rooms were added a couple of years ago and it is hoped there will be a further 20 and a fitness centre for the 1999 season. Food in The Spruce Goose restaurant is moderately priced, fresh and homely. • Meals£ • Acc££ • Closed 25 Dec • Amex, Diners, MasterCard, Visa •

Shannon

HOTEL

Shannon Great Southern Hotel

Shannon Airport Shannon Co Clare
Tel: 061 471122   Fax: 061 471982
email: res@shannon.gsh.ie   www.gsh.ie

Just two minutes walk from the main terminal building at Shannon Airport, the Shannon Great Southern offers unbeatable convenience for travellers recovering from or preparing for international flights. The hotel is fully sound-proofed and bedrooms, all of which have been recently refurbished and upgraded, are spacious and comfortable, with all the amenities expected of a good modern hotel. Activities available include snooker and a recently completed mini-gym for residents, and there is golf and horseriding nearby. Day trips can be arranged to local sites, such as the Cliffs of Moher or the Aillwee Caves, including admission and full day transport. The hotel also has good conference facilities for groups of 12 to 170, backed up by a private business centre with full secretarial services. • Acc££-£££ • Closed 24-26 Dec • Amex, Diners, MasterCard, Visa •

Tulla

RESTAURANT

Flappers Restaurant

Main Street Tulla Co Clare
Tel: 065 35711

Run by Patricia and Jim McInerney – Patricia is the chef and Jim manages the restaurant – this simple little split-level restaurant (the lower part is non-smoking) has little decoration except for a pair of striking pictures and fresh flowers on the tables. Lunchtime sees the emphasis on fairly hearty food and good value, although you could easily work up to a rather smart 3-course meal too. In the evening the mood changes dramatically and, in addition to a set 2 or 3-course menu, there's an ambitious à la carte offering the likes of roast quail with raisin and pinenut couscous and deep fried calamari with spicy marinara sauce, followed by main courses like roast rack of lamb with basil pesto mash and port sauce or grilled salmon with vodka cream sauce and green peppercorns. Desserts are equally impressive and there's a fine and very fairly priced wine list. What's more, the locals even have a take-away service – a boon for holidaymakers self-catering in the area. In winter the restaurant opens later (from 7 pm) and is closed on Tuesdays. • L£ Mon-Sat, D££ Tues-Sat • Amex, MasterCard, Visa •

CORK

Cork is Ireland's largest county, so it's not surprising that it seems like a small country in its own right. Its highly individualistic people will happily go along with this distinction as they reflect on the variety of a large territory which ranges from the rich farmlands of East Cork, away westward to the handsome coastline of West Cork where the mighty light of the famous Fastnet Rock swings across tumbling ocean and spray-tossed headland. Like Cork city itself, the county is a repository of the good things of life, and the county is a treasure chest of the finest farm produce and the very best of seafood. As Ireland's most southerly county, Cork enjoys the mildest climate of all, and it's a place where they work to live, rather than live to work. The arts of living, in fact, are probably seen at their most skilled in County Cork, and they are practised in a huge territory of such variety that it is difficult to grasp even if you devote your entire vacation to this one county. But when you remember that your mind has to absorb the varieties of experience offered by, for instance, the stylish sophistication of Kinsale as set against the lively little ports further west, or the reviving bustle of Clonakilty as matched with the remote mountains above Gougane Barra in the northwest of the county, then you really do begin to wonder that so much can be crammed into this one place called County Cork.

Local Attractions and Information

Cork

Cork Tourist Information	021 273251
Guinness Cork Jazz Festival (late October)	021 278979
Cork International Choral Festival (April/May)	021 308308
Cork International Film Festival (October)	021 271711
Crawford Gallery, Emmett Place	021 966777
The English Market (covered, speciality food stalls Mon-Sat)	

Co Cork

Ballylickey	Mannings Emporium (specialist food products) 027 50456
Bantry	Bantry House, 027 50047
Bantry	Irish International Morris Minor Week (July) 023 44864
Bantry	Murphy's International Mussel Fair (May) 027 50360
Blarney	Blarney Castle 021 385252
Cape Clear Island	International Storytelling Festival (early Sept) 028 39157
Carrigtwohill	Fota Estate (Wildlife Park, Arboretum) 021 812728
Castletownroche	Annes Grove (gardens) 022 26145
Cobh	The Queenstown Story, 021 813591
Glandore	Glandore Regatta (mid July) 021 543333
Glanmire	Riverstown House (Lafrancini plasterwork) 021 821205
Glengariff	Garinish Island 027 63040
Glounthane	Ashbourne House Gardens 021 353319
Kinsale	Gourmet Festival (October)
Kinsale	Vintage Classic International Rally 021 774362
Kinsale	Charles Fort 021 772263
Kinsale	Desmond Castle 021 774855
Mallow	National Ploughing Championships (September) 0507 25125
Midleton	Jameson Heritage Centre 021 613594
Mizen Head	Signal Station 028 35591
Shanagarry	Ballymaloe Cookery School Gardens 021 646785
ShanagarryStephen Pearse's pottery and nearby 'Emporium'	
Skibbereen	Creagh Gardens 028 22121
Youghal	Myrtle Grove 024 92274

Ahakista

Ahakista Bar

Ahakista nr Bantry Co Cork

PUB **Tel: 027 67203**

Just across the road from the Shiro Japanese Dinner House, Anthony and Margaret Whooley run one of the most relaxed bars in the country. Known affectionately as "the tin pub" because of its corrugated iron roof, it has a lovely rambling country garden going down to the water at the back, where children are very welcome to burn off excess energy. Margaret does light snacks (soup and sandwiches from "lunchtime to 6 pm"). It's been in the family for three generations now and, although finally succumbing to the telephone after years of resistance, it's a place that just doesn't change. Normal pub hours don't apply in this part of the world, but they're open afternoon and evenings all year, except Xmas day and Good Fri. • No credit cards •

Ahakista   Hillcrest House

Ahakista Durrus nr Bantry Co Cork

FARM STAY   **Tel: 027 67045**

Hospitality comes first at Agnes Hegarty's working dairy farm overlooking Dunmanus Bay, and guests are welcomed with a cup of tea and home-baked scones on arrival. Her traditional farmhouse attracts many types of visitor, including walkers, who revel in the 55 mile "Sheep's Head Way". Families are very well catered for as there's a large games room, swing and a donkey on the farm – and comfortably furnished rooms are big enough for an extra child's bed or cot. There is also a ground-floor room suitable for less able guests, with parking at the door and direct access to the dining room. Evening meals by arrangement (7 pm; £13.50); light meals also available. • Acc£ • Closed Nov-Apr • No credit cards •

Ahakista   Shiro Japanese Dinner House

Ahakista Durrus nr Bantry Co Cork

RESTAURANT   **Tel: 027 67030**   **027 67206**

Since Kei and Werner Pilz first opened their unique restaurant in 1982, a visit to Shiro Japanese dinner house has always been a very special treat. Though Japanese food has become more familiar in recent years, this serene experience is as different from city restaurants as could be imagined. Shiro is in a beautifully maintained Georgian house overlooking Dunmanus Bay. Although it has grown somewhat – almost double the size of a few years ago, when it could only seat 12 guests in two groups of five and seven – this is still a very small restaurant, perfectly in keeping with the very detailed, fine nature of Kei's authentic classical Japanese cuisine. First there will be zensai (seasonal appetizers with azuke-bachi, egg and sushi snacks), then suimono (a seasonal soup, served in a traditional lidded bowl topped with a little origami bird). A choice of about seven main courses will probably include tempura (seasonal fish and vegetables, lightly-battered and deep-fried) beef teriyaki (gently cooked strips of steak, with teriyaki sauce and fresh vegetables), sashimi (finely sliced raw fish, served with soy sauce and wasabi, a very hot green mustard used for dipping) and combinations such as tempura-sahimi which provide an opportunity to try a wider range if the group is small. It is most interesting to choose as wide a variety as possible, including the sushi (raw fish and vegetables rolled with rice in dried seaweed, served sliced with wasabi and soy sauce for dipping). Presentation of food follows a precise pattern and is very beautiful. The meal is rounded off by a selection of home-made ice creams colourfully garnished with fresh fruit and arranged dramatically against black plates, followed by a choice of teas and coffees. No children under 14. Self-catering accommodation for two is available in a traditional cottage in the grounds. • D££££ 7 days • Closed Jan-Feb & 23-31 Dec • Amex, Diners, MasterCard, Visa •

Ballinadee   Glebe Country House

Ballinadee Bandon Co Cork

COUNTRY HOUSE   **Tel: 021 778294**   **Fax: 021 778456**

email: glebehse@indigo.ie   www.indigo.ie/glebehse/

Church records provide interesting detail about this charming old rectory near Kinsale which dates back to 1690 (when it was built for £250; repairs and alterations followed at various dates, and records show completion of the present house in 1857 at a cost of £1,160). More recently, under the hospitable ownership of Gillian Good Bracken, this classically proportioned house has been providing a restful retreat for guests since 1989. The house, which is set in large, well-tended gardens (including a productive kitchen garden) has spacious reception rooms and large, stylishly decorated en-suite bedrooms (2 shower only). Dinner for residents is at 8 pm by arrangement (please book by noon). Although unlicensed, guests are encouraged to bring their own wine. The whole house may be rented by parties by arrangement and several self-catering apartments are also available. • Acc££ • Closed 25 Dec • MasterCard, Visa •

Ballycotton   Bayview Hotel

Ballycotton Co Cork

HOTEL/RESTAURANT   **Tel: 021 646746**   **Fax: 021 646075**

Overlooking Ballycotton harbour, Bayview Hotel enjoys a magnificent location on the sea side of the road and with a path to the beach through its own gardens. Since 1971 the hotel has been owned by John and Carmel O'Brien, who completely rebuilt it – fairly low, and sympathetic to the traditional style and scale of the surrounding buildings and harbour – in the early 1990s. Major changes occurred again in 1996, when Stephen Belton (previously at Park Hotel Kenmare) joined as manager and soon had a well-trained team, including a new head chef, Ciaran Scully, working well together. Comfortable, homely public areas are complemented by spacious well-furnished bedrooms with good bathrooms; they open onto small balconies and include two corner suites (with jacuzzi) and some particularly cosy top floor rooms.

Restaurant

Head chef Ciaran Scully's daily changing menus could be described as creative modern Irish, built on a classic French base with contemporary international overtones. This, in the sure hands of this talented chef, makes for an interesting and satisfying dining experience, especially when complemented by an elegantly appointed restaurant with lovely sea and harbour views and good service. In fine weather light meals may be served in the garden. • D££ daily, L£ Sun • Acc£££ • Closed Nov-Easter • Amex, Diners, MasterCard, Visa •

Ballycotton   Spanish Point Seafood Restaurant
Ballycotton Co Cork

RESTAURANT/ACCOMMODATION   Tel: 021 646177   Fax: 021 646179

Halfway through the village of Ballycotton you suddenly come upon the entrance to Spanish Point, an attractive old building on the seaward side of the road with a clear view across the bay. John and Mary Tatton have been running this relaxed seafood restaurant since 1991 and have built up a considerable reputation locally. Mary takes pride in using local produce, especially fish, to produce creative but not over-elaborate meals. In a little lounge/bar at the back, aperitifs are served and orders taken from interesting menus that change weekly and offer a good choice – majoring on local seafood, of course, but also several meat and poultry dishes. Lunch menus are shorter; vegetarian options are usually available – ask if this is not mentioned on the menu. The restaurant is in two rooms overlooking the harbour – a fitting setting for good food, cooked and presented with care, and with service to match. A good wine list includes an interesting house selection under £15. • Meals daily£-££ low season weekends only. • Diners, MasterCard, Visa •

Accommodation

There are four comfortable, well-furnished en-suite bedrooms (all shower-only) and all with sea views. • Acc£ high season • Closed 2 Jan-14 Feb •

Ballydehob   Annie's Restaurant
Main Street Ballydehob Co Cork

RESTAURANT   Tel: 028 37292

Anne and Dano Barrie have been running their tiny cottagey restaurant since 1983 – and, for many, a visit to west Cork is unthinkable without a meal here. Annie makes a great host, welcoming everybody personally, handing out menus – and then sending guests over to Levi's pub across the road for an aperitif. Annie then comes over, takes orders and returns to collect people when their meals are ready. Annie's does have a wine licence but there certainly isn't any spare room for 'reception' and this famous arrangement works extremely well. As to the food at Annie's, everything is freshly made on the day, using local ingredients – fish is delivered every night, meat comes from the local butcher (who kills his own meat), farmhouse cheeses are local and all the breads, ice creams and desserts for the restaurant – and for the sister daytime coffee shop, 'Clara', up the road – are made on the premises. As for the cooking, it is simple and wholesome, the nearest to really good home cooking you could ever expect to find in a restaurant. Dano cooks fish like a dream. This place is magic. • D££ Mon-Sat • Closed Oct-Nov • MasterCard, Visa •

Ballydehob   Levi's Bar
Corner House Main Street Ballydehob Co Cork

PUB   Tel: 028 37118

Julia and Nell Levis have run this 150-year-old bar and grocery for as long as anyone can remember. It is a characterful and delightfully friendly place, whether you are just in for a casual drink or using the pub as the unofficial 'reception' area for Annie's restaurant across the road. • Closed 25 Dec & Good Fri •

Ballylickey

COUNTRY HOUSE/RESTAURANT

Ballylickey Manor House

Ballylickey Bantry Bay Co Cork
Tel: 027 50071   Fax: 027 50124
email: ballymh@tinet.ie

Located a few miles north of Bantry, on the N71 Kenmare road, this white painted house was built some 300 years ago by Lord Kenmare as a shooting lodge, and has been home to the Franco-Irish Graves family for four generations. It enjoys a stunning, romantic setting overlooking Bantry Bay, with moors and hills behind. There are ten acres of gardens, through which the Ouvane river (trout and salmon fishing) flows. Choose between the elegant and grand bedrooms in the manor, all lavishly furnished, or more rustic accommodation in the garden – cottages and chalets, some grouped around the outside swimming pool. Residents can dine either in the house or at the poolside restaurant.

Le Rendez-Vous

This weatherboard building next to the pool is remarkably comfortable and smart inside, with an entrance lounge and colourful dining room, decorated and furnished in a pleasing country house style. There's a definite air of France about it. The menu, whether à la carte or table d'hôte, is unashamedly French, almost classical, featuring starters such as foie gras with a Sauternes jelly, clear consommé with chicken liver ravioli, crusted local Bantry Bay scallops with a hint of orange or lightly smoked wild Atlantic salmon served with tapenade pancakes. For a main course, roast rack of west Cork lamb, fillet of beef with a sauce bordelaise and wild mushrooms or steamed John Dory should satisfy, and when available, lobster Thermidor. For dessert, a French apple tart, crème caramel, poached pears in red wine served with rice pudding, or, alternatively, a limited cheese selection.• L£ & D£££ daily except Wed • Acc£££ • Closed mid Nov-mid Feb • Amex, Diners, MasterCard, Visa •

Ballylickey

RESTAURANT/ACCOMMODATION

Larchwood House

Pearsons Bridge nr Bantry Co Cork
Tel: 027 66181

Coming from Kealkil, look out for the sign just before the bridge; however, if you go too far, there's another larger sign – it's worth stopping here and getting out of the car to admire the magnificent gardens sloping down to the river – all the work of Aidan Vaughan who has created everything himself in the last ten years, from building the summer house, paths and bridges to planting trees and shrubs. There are acres to explore, river boulders to cross and nothing prettier than the wild bluebell wood in spring. The house itself is relatively modern with both the traditionally-furnished lounge (afternoon tea and scones served here) and dining room enjoying fantastic views. Sheila Vaughan's very accomplished five-course dinner menus are priced according to the choice of main course, with a typical selection being seafood risotto, an unusual but very successful lettuce and rhubarb soup, pear and melon cup, loin of lamb (twelve slices would you believe!) with all the trimmings, and crème brûlée with a passionfruit sauce – quite wonderful food, for those with large appetites only!

Rooms

Accommodation is offered in two comfortable en suite letting bedrooms upstairs and a further two in an adjacent building. Rooms at the back overlook the garden. At the time of going to press plans were afoot to convert an old cowshed on the other side of the hill to make extra rooms. Excellent breakfasts offer a wide choice, including several fish options and a local cheese plate. • Mon-Sat D££-£££ • Acc££ • Closed Xmas wk • Amex, Diners, MasterCard, Visa •

Ballylickey

HOTEL/RESTAURANT

Sea View House Hotel

Ballylickey Bantry Co Cork
Tel: 027 50462   Fax: 027 51555

Personal supervision and warmth of welcome are the hallmarks of Kathleen O'Sullivan's renowned country house hotel close to Ballylickey Bridge. Peacefully located in private grounds, with views over Bantry Bay, it makes a very restorative base for business or pleasure. Spacious, well-proportioned public rooms include a graciously decorated drawing room, a library, cocktail bar and television room, while generously-sized bedrooms – some with sea views – all have good bathrooms and are individually decorated. Family furniture and antiques enhance the whole hotel and standards of maintenance and housekeeping are consistently high. A ground floor room is suitable for less able guests.

Restaurant

Furnished with antiques and fresh flowers and overlooking the garden, with views over Bantry Bay, the restaurant is elegant and well-appointed with plenty of privacy. Set five-course dinner menus change daily and offer a wide choice on all courses, with the emphasis firmly on local produce, especially seafood, in dishes ranging from warm smoked salmon with a pink peppercorn sauce or fresh ravioli with fresh herbs and tomato sauce, to dover sole on the bone with lemon butter or roast stuffed farmyard duckling with port and orange. Desserts are generally classic – glazed lemon tart, crème brûlée – or there are local cheeses to finish. Tea or coffee and petits fours may be served out of doors on fine summer evenings. • D££-£££ Mon-Sun, L£ Sun • Acc££ • Closed mid Nov-Mid Mar • Amex, Diners, MasterCard, Visa •

Baltimore

Baltimore Harbour Resort Hotel & Leisure Centre

Baltimore Co Cork

HOTEL   Tel: 028 20361   Fax: 028 20466

email: info@bhrhotel.ie

Since the Cullinane family took over this old hotel they have done a prodigious amount of work, beginning with the complete refurbishment of the original building prior to re-opening in 1995 and, most recently, adding on a block of suites (incorporating the traditional arch which now leads through to the carpark) and a new leisure centre. This has a wide range of facilities including a 16 metre swimming pool and gymnasium. The hotel enjoys a lovely position overlooking Roaring Water Bay and is well located for deep sea fishing and visits to nearby islands, including Sherkin and Cape Clear. Modern furnishings, with plenty of light wood and pastel colours, create a sense of space in public areas and the accommodation includes family rooms, junior suites and the new luxury suites. All rooms are comfortably furnished, with neat bathrooms and sea views, and the larger ones have double and single beds. Public areas include a bar that can be reversed to serve the Sherkin Room (banqueting/conferences for 130) and a bright semi-conservatory Garden Room for informal meals and drinks. • Acc££ • Closed Nov-Mar except 23 Dec-2 Jan • Amex, Diners, MasterCard, Visa •

Baltimore

Bushe's Bar

The Square Baltimore Co Cork

PUB/ACCOMMODATION   Tel: 028 20125

Everyone, especially visiting and local sailors, feels at home in this famous old bar – which is choc-a-bloc with genuine maritime artefacts such as charts, tide tables, ships' clocks, compasses, lanterns, pennants et al – but it's the Bushe family's hospitality that makes it really special. Since Richard and Eileen took on the bar in 1973 it's been "home from home" for regular visitors to Baltimore, for whom a late morning call is de rigeur (in order to collect the ordered newspapers that are rolled up and stacked in the bar window each day). Now there's a new generation of Bushes involved with the business, so all will be well for some time. Simple, homely bar food starts early in the day with tea and coffee from 9.30 , moving on to home-made soups and a range of sandwiches including home-cooked meats (turkey, ham, roast beef), salmon, smoked mackerel or – the most popular by far – open crab sandwiches, served with home-baked brown bread.

Accommodation

Over the bar there are three big, comfortable rooms, all with bath/shower, TV and a kitchenette with all that is needed to make your own continental breakfast. There are also showers provided for the use of sailors and fishermen. • Meals£ • Acc£ •Closed 25 Dec & Good Fri • MasterCard, Visa •

Baltimore

Casey's of Baltimore

Baltimore Co Cork.

HOTEL   Tel: 028 20197   Fax: 028 20509

email: baltimorecaseys@tinet.ie   www.indigo.ie/ipress/caseys-hotel/welcome.htm

Just outside Baltimore, on the Skibbereen road, with dramatic views over Roaring Water Bay to the islands beyond, this attractively developed hotel has recently grown from the immaculately maintained bar/restaurant that had been run by the Caseys for twenty years. The old back bar and restaurant have been ingeniously developed to extend the ground floor public areas and to make best use of the view. Bedrooms are spacious and well-furnished, with neat bathrooms and views – and there are four designed for disabled guests. As always, the staff are friendly and helpful, there's a relaxed atmosphere and, in addition to a fine dining room overlooking the bay, there are well organised outdoor eating areas for fine weather. On less favoured days the open fires are very welcome – and there's traditional music at weekends. •Acc££ • L£ & D££ daily • Closed 25 Dec • Amex, Diners, MasterCard, Visa •

Baltimore   Chez Youen

The Pier Baltimore Co Cork
RESTAURANT   Tel: 028 20136   Fax: 028 20495
Since 1979 Youen Jacob's Breton restaurant has been a major feature in Baltimore. Although other eating places have sprung up around him, Youen is still doing what he does best: simple but dramatic presentation of seafood in the shell. Lobster is very much a speciality and available all year round. The Shellfish Platter (£32 with dessert and coffee) is a complete meal of Dublin Bay Prawns, crab and often velvet crab as well as lobster – all served in shell. Only minor concessions are made to non-fish eaters – starters of leek and potato soup at lunch or melon with port on the dinner menu and, correspondingly, roast lamb or steak with green peppercorn sauce for main course. • L£ & D£ daily • Closed Nov & Feb • Amex, Diners, MasterCard, Visa •

Baltimore   La Jolie Brise

The Square Baltimore Co Cork
RESTAURANT/ACCOMMODATION   Tel: 028 20600   Fax: 028 20495
Just along from Bushe's Bar, La Jolie Brise has brought a breath of fresh air to eating out in Baltimore. Run by Youen Jacob the younger, this cheerful continental-style café spills out onto the pavement and provides holiday-makers with good, inexpensive meals to be washed down with moderately priced wines (four under £10). Breakfast menus include regular continental and full Irish breakfast and several fish choices, including hot smoked salmon, plus a range of drinks including hot chocolate. Generous, well-made pizzas (also available to take away) and pastas are available and for lunch and dinner there are "European & Irish " specialities like traditional mussels & chips and char-grilled sirloin steaks with salad & chips. There's also a special which is particularly good value – 2 main courses and a bottle of wine for £20.

Accommodation

Above the restaurant the Jacobs have opened eight very attractive, well-equipped bedrooms in a guesthouse overlooking the harbour known as "Baltimore Bay". Everything in it is big – the rooms, the beds, the bathrooms. There is one room suitable for disabled guests (the only one with shower only). Furniture is modern, with a light sprinkling of Georgian and Victorian pieces and, in addition to a good sitting area in each room, there's a comfortable residents' lounge. • L£ & D£-££ daily • Acc££ • Open all year • MasterCard, Visa •

Baltimore   The Mews

Baltimore Co Cork
RESTAURANT   Tel/Fax: 028 20390
Owner-chef Lucia Carey runs this well-appointed restaurant. It is hidden in a laneway just behind the square and occupies the ground floor and adjacent conservatory of an attractive stone building. Menus are contemporary and the cooking combines the admirable qualities of generosity and lightness. Meals start off with freshly-baked breads and tapenade and prompt service means that starters like Thai seafood chowder of prawn, crab and coriander parcels will not be far behind. Main courses could include a variation on traditional themes such as rack of lamb with a redcurrant & port sauce and minted onion. There will always be a delicious vegetarian dish such as oriental vegetable parcels with roasted pepper sauce, all served with imaginative and well-cooked vegetables. Good home-made ices are among the desserts, or you could finish with a local cheese plate and freshly brewed coffee. • D££-£££ Tues-Sun • Closed Oct-May •

Bandon   The Munster Arms Hotel

Oliver Plunkett Street Bandon Co Cork
HOTEL   Tel: 021 346800   023 346789
email: kingsley@tinet.ie   www.kingsleyhotels.com
This substantial town-centre hotel has spacious public areas and, unlike many of the hotels in the area, is as popular with business guests and locals as it is with holiday-makers. It is well-situated for touring the area and there is plenty to do, including angling

and riding (there is an equestrian centre nearby). Bedrooms are generally quite big and well-furnished with generous beds and stylish, well-fitted bathrooms (four of the older ones are shower only), providing a good standard of comfort and amenities at a reasonable rate. Five bedrooms are designated no-smoking. No private parking, but safe street parking is available beside the hotel. • Acc££ • Closed 24-26 Dec • Amex, Diners, MasterCard, Visa •

Bantry   O'Connor's

The Square Bantry Co Cork

RESTAURANT   Tel: 027 50011

Approaching town from the south on the N71, Matt and Ann O'Connor's seafood restaurant is right on the main square (site of the annual early-May mussel festival). Long established, with a front room, booths and a seated bar in the back (note the seafood tapas selection displayed here), all decorated in a nautical theme, there's also a lobster and oyster fish tank by the entrance door. Mussels, cooked all ways, are a speciality – a starter of them grilled with herbs and lemon butter fits the bill perfectly, followed perhaps by fresh scallops and salmon mornay in shells, served with an abundance of vegetables, or else mussels marinière with a fish pie as a main course. There are some non-fish dishes available, such as local lamb, beef and chicken, and at lunchtime you can have a soup and sandwich or daily-changing dishes off the blackboard. • Mon-Sat L£-££, Mon-Sun D££ • Telephone off season • MasterCard, Visa •

Bantry   The Westlodge Hotel

Bantry Co Cork

HOTEL   Tel: 027 50360   Fax: 027 50438

Easily spotted on an elevated site above the main road into Bantry, the Westlodge Hotel seems to have thought of all the possible requirements to make a family holiday successful, regardless of weather conditions. A wide range of outdoor activities can be organised, including golf, water sports, horse riding and pony trekking. But – and this is the hotel's greatest strength – there's also plenty to keep energetic youngsters happy if the weather should disappoint, including a 16m swimming pool in the leisure centre. Bedrooms, which have all been fairly recently refurbished, include three suites and there is 24 hour room service. The restaurant is well-positioned to take advantage of the view of the bay. Banqueting/conference facilities for 400. • Acc£££• Open all year • Amex, Diners, MasterCard, Visa •

Bere Island   Lawrence Cove House

Lawrence Cove Bere Island nr Bantry Co Cork

RESTAURANT   Tel: 027 75063

Seafood Restaurant of the Year   email: cove@indigo.ie

Surprise and delight are the usual reactions from first time visitors to the seafood restaurant that Mike and Mary Sullivan have run on Bere Island since 1995: surprise that a restaurant could succeed at all in this unlikely spot – it's just a short ferry ride from Castletownbere, but there certainly isn't too much passing trade – and delight at its professionalism and the warmth of the Sullivans' hospitality. But a loyal following is building up and the island's fine new marina encourages sailing people to tailor their cruising plans to fit in a comfortable and well-fed overnight stay. And perhaps it isn't quite so surprising that this restaurant has come into being, when you realise that Mike is the fisherman who supplies many of the country's top restaurants with fresh West Cork fish and shellfish. The menu is not over-long, yet it embraces a wide range of fish and seafood, including some unusual varieties unlikely to be found elsewhere, such as grouper and coryphene ("sunfish"), when in season. And Mike will even bring guests over to the restaurant in his fishing boat and deliver them back to the mainland after dinner if the ferry times aren't convenient – now these are people who really know the meaning of the word service. • Mon-Sun D££ • Closed Oct-early Mar • MasterCard, Visa •

* Bere Island Ferry Service (15 car capacity): Tel: 027-75009
* Comfortable, hospitable accommodation on the island is available at "Harbour View" B&B. Contact: Ann Sullivan : 027-75011

At the time of going to press we had information that new accommodation might be built in the Lawrence Cove area for the 1999 season; contact Lawrence Cove House for information.

Blarney

HOTEL

Blarney Park Hotel

Blarney Co Cork

Tel: 021 385281   Fax: 021 381506
email: info@blarneypark.com   www.blarneypark.com

Blarney may be best known for its castle (and the famous Blarney Stone) but for many people this modern hotel is the reason for the visit. There is always something going on at Blarney Park and its excellent facilities for both conferences and leisure are put to full use. Close proximity to Cork city (just half an hour on the Limerick road) makes this a very convenient location for business. The hotel also attracts steady all-year business through an energetic programme of short breaks and special interest holidays covering a wide range of topics (such as matching wine and food, learning to swim, rambling and the ever-popular golf). It's a bright, friendly hotel with open fires in spacious public areas and overlooking pleasant grounds. Very family-friendly rooms are arranged with doubles along one side of corridors and smallish twins more suitable for children opposite. Children's rooms have fun packs. Excellent back-up services, including an all-year crèche, make this a very relaxing place for a family break. And, of course, everyone loves the leisure centre which has a 40-metre water slide. • Acc££-£££ • Closed 25 Dec • Amex, Diners, MasterCard, Visa •

Butlerstown

ACCOMMODATION

Atlantic Sunset

Dunworley, Butlerstown Co Cork

Tel: 023 40115

Just along the road from Katherine Noren's Dunworley Cottage Restaurant, Mary Holland provides comfortable accommodation and a genuinely warm welcome in her neat modern house with views down to the sea at Dunworley. The breakfast room and some bedroom windows have sea views and, weather permitting, the sight of the sun setting over the Atlantic can indeed be magnificent. • Acc£ • Open all year • No credit cards •

Butlerstown

ACCOMMODATION

Butlerstown House

Butlerstown Bandon Co Cork

Tel: 023 40137

Elisabeth Jones' classic late eighteenth century house is set in ten acres of private grounds with long views over the rolling west Cork countryside to the Dunmanway Mountains. Guests are welcomed on arrival with tea in the drawing room, allowing a little time to wind down to the pace appropriate to a house characterised by peace and tranquillity. Elegant reception rooms are comfortably furnished in period style; the drawing room opens onto south facing gardens, and if the weather should disappoint there are open fires throughout. The staircase is a fine example of Georgian craftsmanship, leading to four bedrooms which include a master bedroom with four-poster bed. (All rooms are en-suite, although two have shower-only.) Breakfast is a major event ("a neglected repast we consider as the principal meal of the day") and is taken in style at the "Butlerstown Table" in the dining room. Full catering facilities are available for house parties and small conferences, ie parties of up to 10 people for 2-3 nights. • Acc££ • Closed mid Dec-Mar • Amex, Diners, MasterCard, Visa •

Butlerstown

RESTAURANT

Dunworley Cottage Restaurant

Dunworley Butlerstown Bandon Co Cork

Tel: 023 40314

The warmth of Katherine Noren's uniquely Swedish style of hospitality (and the cosiness of open fires when required) contrasts magnificently with the windswept coastal location of her famous west Cork restaurant. The quality of food at Dunworley is, in Katherine's own words, "defined by two principles – the best raw materials have to be used and the preparation has to be performed by a highly skilled cook". These principles are adhered to with admirable consistency by Katherine and her team: all ingredients are sourced locally and as many as possible are organic or wild – that means no intensively farmed fish on the menu, for instance, and much of the fresh produce comes from their own organic garden, which is patrolled by ducks to keep the slugs down. Catering for special dietary requirements is a matter of routine at Dunworley and children can choose from their own menu or have dishes from the à la carte menu at half price. Cooking skills are always of the highest quality at Dunworley, making even the simplest dishes special – the Swedish meatballs, for example, which were originally intended for children but were moved to the main menu by popular demand, and also the nettle soup, which has become a signature dish. Ultra fresh seafood, salads that sing with vitality and delicious home-made breads all contribute to the very special experience at Dunworley. Self-catering holidaymakers can also book ready made dinners to take away. Scandinavian languages, German and French spoken. • Wed-Sun L & D£-££ • Closed Oct-Mar • Diners, MasterCard, Visa •

Butlerstown   O'Neill's
Butlerstown Bandon Cork
PUB   **Tel: 023 40228**
Butlerstown is a pretty pastel-painted village, with lovely views across farmland to Dunworley and the sea beyond. Dermot and Mary O'Neill's unspoilt pub is as pleasant and hospitable a place as could be found to enjoy the view – or to admire the traditional mahogany bar and pictures that make old pubs like this such a pleasure to be in. • Closed 25 Dec & Good Fri •

Carrigaline   Glenwood House
Ballinrea Road Carrigaline Co Cork
ACCOMMODATION   **Tel/Fax: 021 373878**
This excellent, professionally run guesthouse is in purpose-built premises, very conveniently located for Cork airport and the ferry. Comfortable, well-furnished rooms (including one designed for disabled guests) have all the amenities normally expected of hotels, including well-designed bathrooms. Very good breakfasts too. • Acc££ • Closed 1 wk Xmas • Diners, MasterCard, Visa •

Carrigaline   Gregory's Restaurant
Main Street Carrigaline Co Cork
RESTAURANT   **Tel: 021 371512**
Owner-chef Gregory Dawson and his partner and restaurant manager Rachelle Harley opened here in 1994 and the restaurant was an immediate success. Bright, comfortable and friendly, with plenty of buzz, the restaurant provides a good setting for Gregory's menus which change weekly and, except for Sunday lunch, have always been based on a sensibly short à la carte (including some tempting vegetarian options). Typical dishes from a summer menu might include carrot and coriander soup or fresh crab salad to start, then fish of the day or Madras lamb curry with basmati rice and accompaniments. Desserts could include hot apple crumpets with vanilla ice cream or tiramisu with chocolate sauce – or there's an Irish cheese plate. Home-baked breads, good coffee and helpful service complete a very good all-round package. • L£ Mon-Fri & Sun, D£-££ Mon-Sat • Closed Bank Hols • Amex, MasterCard, Visa •

Castlelyons   Ballyvolane House
Castlelyons Co Cork
COUNTRY HOUSE 🏛   **Tel: 025 36349   Fax: 025 36781**
email: ballyvol@iol.ie   www.iol.ie/ballyvolane
Jeremy and Merrie Greene's lovely country house is a gracious mansion surrounded by its own farmland, magnificent wooded grounds, a recently restored trout lake and formal terraced gardens. The Italianate style of the present house – including a remarkable pillared hall with a baby grand piano and open fire – dates from the mid19th century when modifications were made to the original house of 1728. This is a very lovely house, elegantly furnished and extremely comfortable, with central heating and big log fires; the five bedrooms are varied, but all are roomy and, like the rest of the house, are furnished with family antiques and look out over attractive gardens and grounds. Ballyvolane has private salmon fishing on 15 km of the renowned River Blackwater, with a wide variety of spring and summer beats. Fishing is Merrie's special enthusiasm (a special brochure is available outlining the fishing services she provides) and she's also a great cook, providing guests with delicious country house dinners which are served in style around a long mahogany table. There is much of interest in the area – the beautiful Blackwater valley is well worth exploring, with its many gardens and historic sites, and Lismore, the Rock of Cashel and Waterford Crystal are among the many interesting places which can easily be visited nearby. The standard of hospitality, comfort and food at Ballyvolane are all exceptional, making this an excellent base for a peaceful and very relaxing break. French is spoken. • D££ • Acc££ • Closed 23-28 Dec • Amex, Diners, MasterCard, Visa •

Castletownbere   MacCarthy's

The Square Castletownbere Co Cork

PUB   Tel: 027 70014

Dating back to the 1870s, and currently run by Adrienne MacCarthy, this famous old pub and grocery store really is the genuine article. Fortunately, it shows no signs of changing. Atmosphere and live traditional music are the most obvious attractions but the grocery is real and provisions the local fishing boats. Simple bar food – seafood chowder, open seafood sandwiches – is available from 9.30 am – 9.30 pm. • Closed 25 Dec & Good Fri • No credit cards •

Castletownbere   The Old Presbytery

Brandy Hall House Castletownbere Co Cork

ACCOMMODATION   Tel: 027 70424   Fax: 027 70420

On the edge of Castletownbere and well-signposted from the road, this very pleasant old house on 4 acres is in a magnificent position – on a little point with the sea on two sides and clear views of Berehaven Harbour. The house dates back to the late 1700s and has been sensitively restored by the current owners, David and Mary Wrigley. The five bedrooms vary in size and outlook but all are en-suite and furnished to a high standard, in keeping with the character of the house. Breakfast – which includes a vegetarian menu – is served in a pleasant conservatory overlooking the sea. • Acc£ • MasterCard, Visa •

Casteltownshend   Bow Hall

Casteltownshend Co Cork

ACCOMMODATION   Tel 028 36114

A very comfortable 17th century house, with a pleasant outlook, excellent home-cooking and a warm welcome by enthusiastic hosts. A visit to this lovely home is a memorable experience. Breakfasts a highlight. • Closed Xmas wk • Advance bookings only in winter • No credit cards •

Castletownshend   Mary Ann's Bar & Restaurant

Castletownshend nr Skibbereen Co Cork

PUB/RESTAURANT ⭐   Tel: 028 36146   Fax: 028 36377

email: golfer@indigo.ie

Mention Castletownshend and the chances are that the next words will be 'Mary Ann's'. For, half way up the steep hill of this picturesque west Cork village, just below the tree, this welcoming landmark has been the source of happy memories for many a visitor over the years. (For those who have come up the hill with a real sailor's appetite from the little quay, the sight of its gleaming bar seen through the open door is one to treasure.) The pub is as old as it looks, going back to 1846, and has been in the energetic and hospitable ownership of Fergus and Patricia O'Mahony since 1988. Even the best old bars need a bit of attention occasionally, however, and 1998 saw refurbishments at Mary Ann's – but with the original character left intact. The O'Mahony's have built up a great reputation for food at the bar and in the restaurant, which is split between an upstairs dining room and The Vine Room, which can be used for private parties. Seafood is the star, of course, and comes in many guises, usually along with some of the lovely home-baked brown bread which is one of the house specialities. Another is the Platter of Castlehaven Bay Shellfish and Seafood – a sight to behold, and usually including langoustine, crab meat, crab claws, and both fresh and smoked salmon. Much of the menu depends on the catch of the day, although there are also good steaks and roasts, served with delicious local potatoes and seasonal vegetables. Desserts are good too, but local west Cork cheeses are an excellent option. • L£ & D£-££ Mon-Fri • Closed 25 Dec & Good Fri • MasterCard, Visa •

Cloghroe   Blairs Inn

Cloghroe Blarney Co Cork

PUB   Tel: 021 381470   Fax: 021 382353

email: Blair@tinet.ie   www.homepage.tinet.ie/~blair

John and Anne Blair's delightful riverside pub is in a quiet, wooded setting just 5 minutes drive from Blarney. Sitting in the garden in summer, you might see trout rising in the Owennageara river (or see a heron out fishing) while winter offers welcoming open fires in this comfortingly traditional pub. It's a lovely place to drop into for a drink or a session – there's traditional music on Sunday nights all year round and on Mondays from April to October – and the Blairs have built up a special reputation for their food. Anne supervises the kitchen personally, and care and commitment are evident in menus offering a wide (but not over-extensive) range of interesting but fairly traditional dishes based on seafood (from Kenmare and Dingle), local lamb, beef and poultry, and game in season. à la carte menus are available in the bar from lunchtime onwards; lunch and dinner can be booked in the candlelit Snug or Pantry dining areas. • Mon-Sun L£ & D££ • Closed 25 Dec & Good Fri • MasterCard, Visa •

Clonakilty   An Sugan

Wolfe Tone Street Co Clonakilty Co Cork

PUB   **Tel: 023 33498**

An Sugan is one of the country's best loved pubs, so it was with trepidation that we heard that this colourful, characterful place was to be "re-located" because of traffic congestion in Clonakilty and the impossibility of providing parking. The O'Crowley family have owned An Sugan since 1980 and they have done a great job: it's always been a really friendly, well-run place and their reputation for good food is well-deserved. So we wish them luck – and look forward, with great interest, to seeing the new 'out-of-town' An Sugan. • Mon-Sun L£ & D£-££ • Closed 25-26 Dec & Good Fri • MasterCard, Visa •

Clonakilty   Dunmore House Hotel

Muckross Clonakilty Co Cork

HOTEL   **Tel: 023 33352   Fax: 023 34686**

email: dunmorehousehotel@tinet.ie

The magnificent coastal location of Jeremiah and Mary O'Donovan's family-owned and managed hotel has been used to advantage to provide sea views for all bedrooms and to allow guests access to their own stretch of foreshore. Comfortable public areas include a bar and lounges, and there are conference and function facilities available for international and Irish visitors. Bedrooms – all of them with full bathrooms en-suite – are furnished to a high standard and include two mini-suites and a room especially suitable for disabled guests. Numerous leisure activities in the area include angling and golf – green fees are free to residents on the hotel's own (highly scenic) nine hole golf course. Cycling, horseriding and watersports are also popular and packed lunches are provided on request. • Acc ££ • Closed 22-27 Dec • Amex, MasterCard, Visa •

Clonakilty   Emmet Hotel

Emmet Square Clonakilty Co Cork

HOTEL   **Tel: 023 33394   Fax: 023 35058**

Pat Pettit's Emmet Hotel, which opened in 1997, is hidden away in the centre of Clonakilty on a lovely serene Georgian square that contrasts unexpectedly with the hustle and bustle of the nearby streets; it's a most unusual location. Car parking is an obvious potential difficulty but the hotel has an arrangement with a nearby car park. The standard of furnishing and comfort is high throughout, with management in the capable hands of Tony and Marie O'Keeffe (who ran their own successful restaurant in Cork for a number of years). Marie is responsible for both restaurant and bar food; her cooking is based on the best of seasonal local produce, much of it organic, and The Bistro is already earning a reputation for good, creative cooking.• Meals £-££ • Acc ££ • Closed 25 Dec • MasterCard, Visa •

Clonakilty   Kicki's Cabin

53 Pearse Street Clonakilty Co Cork

RESTAURANT   **Tel: 023 33884**

Sister restaurant to Katherine Noren's Dunworley Cottage, Kicki's may be very different in location – it's on a busy street in the centre of Clonakilty – but the principles of Dunworley apply here too. That means that nothing but the best fresh local produce goes into the kitchen – as much as possible being wild or organic – and the cooking will be very good. The maritime decor is delightful, details – such as the freshly baked breads – are just right and it's nice to see the most famous local product, Clonakilty pudding, put to such good use only a few doors down from Edward Twomey's butchers, where it is made. Delicious ready-made meals to take away are also available from Kicki's – and they'll make up picnic baskets to order too. • L£ Mon-Fri, D££ Mon-Sat • Closed Xmas & New Year • Visa •

Cloyne

COUNTRY HOUSE/RESTAURANT

Barnabrow Country House

Cloyne Midleton Co Cork
Tel/Fax: 021 652534
email: barnabrow@tinet.ie

It takes a brave person to open a country house just down the road from Ballymaloe House, but John O'Brien -a competent professional with a keen knowledge of the local market – is just the man for the job. His sensitive conversion of an imposing seventeenth century house makes good use of its stunning views of Ballycotton, and the decoration is commendably restrained. Innovative wooden furniture (commissioned from local craftsmen) and comfortable, spacious bedrooms provide a motif of sorts, and the service is discreet but efficient.

Mór Chlúana Restaurant

The attractive restaurant, Mór Chlúana (in a courtyard behind the main house) features starters like grilled, marinated Thai prawns with a chilli dipping sauce (£5.95) and a tasty salad of seared beef with a blue cheese dressing. The selection of main courses includes lamb shanks braised in tomato and garlic and roast cod with chive butter sauce. Like many chefs in the area, David Smith trained at the Ballymaloe Cookery School, and he was clearly a good student. Smith uses free-range and organic ingredients wherever possible, and most of his produce is sourced locally. The four course Sunday Lunch is particularly good, and at £12.95 it certainly represents decent value. At the time of going to press a barbecue 'verandah' was due to open shortly. Note: the restaurant is a no-smoking zone. • D££ Tues-Sun, L£ Sun only • Acc£-££ • Closed Xmas wk • Amex, Diners, MasterCard, Visa •

Cobh

PUB

Mansworth's

Cobh Co Cork
Tel: 021 811965

Cobh's oldest established family-owned bar dates back to at least 1895 and is currently in the capable hands of John Mansworth, who is a great promoter of the town. Bar snacks are available but it's really as a character pub that Mansworth's is most appealing. It's a bit of a climb up the hill to reach it but well worth the effort, especially for anyone with an interest in the history of Cobh as a naval port – the photographs and memorabilia on display here will provide hours of pleasure. • Closed 25 Dec & Good Fri •

Cork

HOTEL/RESTAURANT

Arbutus Lodge

Cork Co Cork
Tel: 021 501237   021 502893
email: arbutus@iol.ie

Approaching Cork city from the main Dublin road, the hotel is signposted off to the right – this will save you driving into town and then back up to the Montenotte area. Established by Patsy and Declan Ryan over 35 years ago, the hotel is perhaps best described as a 'country house', with an award-winning garden in which grows, amongst other lovely trees and shrubs, an Arbutus tree, hence the name. Once the home of the Lord Mayor of Cork, the house overlooks the River Lee and surrounding hills, a spectacular sight at night, but not quite the view enjoyed 150 years earlier before the city became industrialised and built up – one of the master bedrooms has old prints of what the view used to look like. Inside, the house is a veritable treasure trove of antiques, fine art (old and new) – some of the modern Irish paintings are much in demand by galleries and museums for exhibitions – even a book singed by W.B. Yeats in the library. Guests can relax in the panoramic bar (with sliding glass doors to the terrace) or in the lounge. There are elegant, individually-designed bedrooms boasting period furniture and fine fabrics, and smart bathrooms with quality towels, robes and toiletries. Several rooms have canopied beds, one a magnificent carved four-poster. There are also lavish self-contained suites across the road. Staff are terrific, a tribute to the Ryan's own professionalism and dedication in bringing on young trainees. Breakfast is a splendid affair, more so now that Arbutus has gone into the bread-making business! • Amex, Diners, MasterCard, Visa •

Restaurant ★

A marvellous traditional dining room, Arbutus continues to set standards that many others try to follow. Many fine chefs have worked here at some time in their career, having been schooled by Declan (no mean chef himself!). There are strong hints of French classicism and discipline (that is to say, correct procedures are maintained – real stocks, properly-made sauces, long marinades), but the cooking cannot be described as strictly French since there's a perceptible nod to modernism and Irishness. Thus, a crispy confit of duck on a bed of Puy lentils, an escalope of salmon served with braised leeks cream sauce, and a true caramelised apple tart represents a table d'hôte luncheon. There are starters such as simple but plump Galway oysters, Irish Atlantic smoked salmon or foie gras terrine with home-made toasted sourdough bread served with baby greens. Produce is local, herbs and soft fruit from their own garden, fish ultra-fresh (note the tank in the bar) and Irish farmhouse cheeses top notch. Desserts are displayed on the trolley and include three silver ice cream/sorbet holders. Bar meals, featuring some rustic Irish dishes, are served lunchtime only (not Sunday). The wine list is unquestionably one of the finest in Ireland: Declan has built up his cellar over many years, criss-crossing the channel to seek out the finest from France and, more recently, from Australia and New Zealand. Prices are keen throughout, with plenty of very good wines for under £20. Service is spot on, friendly and unobtrusive. • L£, D££-£££ Mon-Sat • Acc££ • Closed Xmas week • Amex, Diners, MasterCard, Visa •

Cork   Bully's

40 Paul Street Cork Co Cork

RESTAURANT   Tel: 021 273555   Fax: 021 273427

A small buzzy restaurant in one of the busiest little shopping streets in the city centre, Bully's has built up a strong reputation over the years for good food at reasonable prices. A speciality is pizzas, which had ultra light, crisp bases long before they began to show up in fashionable restaurants; the dough is made on the premises every day using Italian flour, then baked in a special wood-burning oven. They serve lots of other things too – freshly made burgers, steaks, omelettes, chicken dishes and pasta – and there's a short, reasonably priced wine list.

Branches at: *Bishopstown*, Cork (021-546838) and *Douglas*, Cork (021-892415).

• L£, D£ Mon-Sun • Closed 25-26 Dec & 1 Jan • MasterCard, Visa •

Cork   Café Paradiso

16 Lancaster Quay Western Road Cork Co Cork

RESTAURANT   Bookings: 021 277939/Other: 021 274973   Fax: 021 307469

Denis Cotter opened his mould-breaking restaurant near Jurys Hotel in 1993 and it has gone on to become a huge success. Vegetarian food never seems the same after eating at Café Paradiso, and many a committed carnivore has had to give serious consideration to choosing meatless dishes on menus henceforth. It's a lively place with a busy atmosphere and the staff, under the direction of Bridget Healy, are not only friendly and helpful but obviously enthusiastic about their work. Seasonal menus, topped up by daily specials, might include asparagus gratin with a tangy Gabriel cheese crust; peperonata with olive-grilled ciabbatta, basil & parmesan; fresh tagliatelle in basil oil with mangetout, broad beans, cherry tomatoes and parmesan. Lovely desserts too – pear & almond frangipani with blackcurrant coulis perhaps – and some organic wines on a seriously global list. • L£, D££ Tues-Sat • Closed Xmas wk, First 2 wks Sept • Amex, Diners, MasterCard, Visa •

Cork   Crawford Gallery Café

Emmet Place Cork Co Cork

RESTAURANT   Tel: 021 274415

In the city centre, next to the Opera House, stands the Crawford Art Gallery, a fine 1724 building which houses an excellent collection of 18th- and 19th-century landscapes. This is also home to the Crawford Gallery Café, one of Cork city's favourite informal eating places. An outpost of Ballymaloe House at Shanagarry (since 1988), the menu offers Ballymaloe breads and many of the other dishes so familiar to Ballymaloe fans (who will also recognise the importance of "Fish of the Day, landed on the pier in Ballycotton last night"). The menu changes weekly, but the style – a judicious mixture of timeless country house fare and trendier international dishes featuring lots of roasted vegetables – remains reassuringly constant. Interesting choice of drinks includes homemade lemonade, fresh orange juice, Cappoquin apple juice and a house wine. • Meals£, daytime Mon-Sat • Closed Bank Hols, Xmas wk & Good Fri • Diners, MasterCard, Visa •

Please note that price indications are intended only as a guideline - always check current prices (and special offers) when making reservations.

Cork

Dan Lowrey's Tavern

13 MacCurtain Street Cork Co Cork

PUB   Tel: 021 505071

This smashing pub just across the road from Isaacs was established in 1875 and has been run by Anthony and Catherine O'Riordan since 1995. Long before the arrival of the "theme pub", Lowrey's was famous for having windows which originated from Kilkenny cathedral, but it also has many of its own original features, including a fine mahogany bar. Bar food has become a point of pride under the current ownership, with Catherine O'Riordan and Eleanor Murray in the kitchen There's also a nice little quarter-bottle wine list representing France, Chile, Italy and Romania, all at £2.60.
• Meals£ • Closed 25 Dec & Good Fri •

Cork

Farmgate Café

Old English Market Princes Street Cork Co Cork

CAFE BAR   Tel: 021 278134   Fax: 021 632771

A sister restaurant to the Farmgate Country Store and Restaurant in Midleton, Kay Harte's Farmgate Café shares the same commitment to serving fresh food – and, as it is located above the English Market, where ingredients are purchased daily, it doesn't come much fresher than this. They serve traditional food, including some famous old Cork dishes with a special market connection – tripe & drisheen and corned beef & champ with green cabbage. Another speciality is " the freshest of fish". All this and homebaked cakes and breads too. • Meals£-££ daytime Mon-Sat • Diners, MasterCard •

Cork

Fitzpatrick Cork Hotel

Tivoli Cork Co Cork

HOTEL   Tel: 021 507533   Fax: 021 507641

Situated on a bank above the main Dublin road (and clearly signed off it) about five minutes drive from the city centre (courtesy coach service all day), this modern tower block hotel has an eye-catching external glass lift and overlooks the River Lee. Two self-contained conference/banqueting suites can each accommodate up to 700 guests and a well-equipped leisure centre has indoor tennis as well as a 25-metre pool. • Acc££-£££
• Closed 25-26 Dec •

Cork

Flemings

Silver Grange House Tivoli Cork Co Cork

RESTAURANT   Tel: 021 821621   Fax: 021 821178

Clearly signed off the main Cork-Dublin road, this large Georgian family house is set in well-maintained grounds, including a kitchen garden which provides most of the fruit, vegetables and herbs required for the restaurant during the summer. The light, airy double dining room is comfortably furnished and, in contrast to the current wave of designer decor, has a pleasant air of faded gentility. Well-appointed linen-clad tables provide a suitable setting for Michael Fleming's classical cooking. Seasonal table d'hôte and à la carte menus offer a good selection of classics, slightly influenced by current international trends – a vegetarian dish of crispy vegetable wontons with tossed leaf salad, Atlantic prawns & scallops with grilled polenta & a sweet pepper jus – but the main thrust of the cooking style is classical French.. Vegetables are imaginative in selection and presentation, desserts include a beautiful tasting plate. Lunch and dinner are served every day.

Rooms

Accommodation is available (£35 pps/£14 single supplement), in four spacious en-suite rooms, comfortably furnished in a style appropriate to the age of the house. • L£, D£-££ Mon-Sun • Acc££ • Closed 25 Dec • Amex, Diners, MasterCard, Visa •

Cork

Harold's

Tramway House Douglas Village East Cork Co Cork

RESTAURANT   Tel: 021 361613 /891155   Fax: 021 891155

When Euro-Toques chef Harold Lynch and front-of-house partner Beth Haughton opened this stylish little place just off the busiest shopping area of Douglas in August 1993 it was an immediate hit. The interesting modern interior sets the right tone for Harold's lively Cal-Ital influenced food. On a sensibly limited, moderately priced à la carte menu, old favourites like twice-baked cheese souffle jostle for space with starters such as tapas or warm salad of smoked chicken with sundried tomatoes, pinenuts, parmesan shavings and balsamic dressing. Main courses range from reassuringly familiar, perfectly cooked noisettes of spring lamb with warm mint dressing through to fish of the day – a gleaming white fillet of John Dory, perhaps, on a light buttery sauce – or a flavoursome vegetarian option like fettucine with wild and fresh mushrooms. Desserts favour classics with a modern twist – crème brûlée with plum salad, perhaps – and there's always a selection of Irish farmhouse cheeses. Delicious brown soda bread, good coffee by the cup.• L£ Sun Sep-Apr only, D££ Tue-Sat • Closed 25 Dec • MasterCard, Visa •

Cork   Hayfield Manor Hotel

Perrott Avenue College Road Cork Co Cork
HOTEL   **Tel: 021 315600   Fax: 021 316839**
email: hayfield@indigo.ie   www.indigo.ie/~hayfield

Set in two acres of gardens next door to University College Cork, Hayfield Manor Hotel provides every comfort and a remarkable level of privacy and seclusion just a mile from the city centre. Although newly built – it only opened in 1996 – it has the genuine feel of a large period house. Conference rooms of varying sizes include a library/boardroom beside the drawing room that doubles as a private dining room. Spacious bedrooms vary in decor, are beautifully furnished to a very high standard with antiques and have generous marbled bathrooms with individual tiling, heated towel rails and quality toiletries. Accommodation includes two suites, six junior suites, fifteen non-smoking rooms, two rooms designed for disabled guests and a further two ground floor rooms which are "wheelchair friendly". Housekeeping is immaculate. Conference facilities for up to 120 delegates. Tennis, golf and fishing nearby. Beauty and massage therapies by arrangement. • L££ Mon-Thur, D£££ daily • Acc££££ • Open all year • Amex, Diners, MasterCard, Visa •

Cork   Hotel Isaacs

48 MacCurtain Street Cork Co Cork
HOTEL   **Tel: 021 500011   Fax: 021 506355**

Opposite the theatre and approached through a cobbled courtyard, the rustic charm of the bedrooms (polished stripped wood floor and free-standing pine furniture) at this city-centre hotel would be better appreciated had walls and windows been sound-proofed, especially those overlooking the busy main street. Beware – some rooms can be noisy. Also, a note to explain how to operate the shower would be helpful (there's a switch outside the bathroom). Otherwise, it's a simple hotel offering basic comforts at a reasonable price. There's no lift (rooms go up to the third floor) and no car park, though there's a secure park at the end of the street a few minutes' walk away. Greene's Restaurant (not to be confused with the long-standing Isaacs in the same building) offers breakfast and some food at other times. Note the man-made waterfall cascading down rocks outside – an unusual feature for a city-centre hotel. • Acc££ • Closed 27-30 Dec • Amex, Diners, MasterCard, Visa •

Cork   Imperial Hotel

South Mall Cork Co Cork
HOTEL   **Tel: 021 274040   Fax: 021 275375**

Near the river and just a couple of minutes walk from the St Patrick Street shopping area, this thriving hotel in Cork's main commercial and banking centre dates back to 1813 and has a colourful history – Michael Collins spent his last night here, no less, and that suite now bears his name. Today, however, this well-run hotel is equally suited to business or pleasure and has free car parking available for residents. Rooms are all en-suite, with a mixture of furnishings, and there are conference facilities for up to 600 (banqueting 350). Attractive weekend rates. Private car park. • Acc££-£££ • Closed 24 Dec-4 Jan • Amex, Diners, MasterCard, Visa •

Cork   Isaacs

48 MacCurtain Street Cork Co Cork
RESTAURANT   **Tel: 021 503805   Fax: 021 551348**

Since its opening in 1992 this large, atmospheric modern restaurant in an 18th-century warehouse has been one of the great restaurant success stories, not just in Cork but throughout the country. The culinary pedigree is impeccable – the co-owners are Michael and Catherine Ryan (of Arbutus Lodge) and head chef Canice Sharkey; together they make a magnificent team. There's a set menu at lunch (2/3 course £9.50/£12) and dinner (2/3 courses £12.50/£17) plus a short à la carte and daily blackboard specials, with plenty to interest vegetarians. Canice Sharkey's cooking is consistently excellent in tempting, colourful dishes which cleverly combine sunny Mediterranean influences and comforting Irish traditions – sometimes separately, as in bruschetta with roast peppers, tapenade, goats cheese & pesto, or lamb casserole with flageolet beans, at other times together, as in salmon & potato cakes with provençale sauce. A short list of world wines at friendly prices is carefully chosen; house wines are £9.10 and four wines of the month are offered at £10.50-£12.50. • L£ Mon-Sat, D££ daily • Closed Xmas wk • Amex, Diners, MasterCard, Visa •

Cork   The Ivory Tower

Exchange Buildings Princes Street Cork Co Cork
RESTAURANT   Tel:021 274665

Upstairs in an early Victorian commercial building is not the place you'd expect to find a controversial restaurant, but that's where you'll find the Ivory Tower – and the owner-chef Seamus O'Connell, a talented and creative cook. Very best quality ingredients, interesting – possibly even inspired – menus, excellent details like delicious home-baked breads, imaginative` presentation – all these can be taken as read at The Ivory Tower. The problem is slow service, and by this we mean really slow – an hour's wait before starters arrive is not uncommon (and, as on the guide's visit, the "surprise starter" mentioned on the menu may be overlooked), followed by up to another hour before the main course arrives. Add to this an off-hand "take it or leave it" attitude and it seems in our view that there is "room for improvement". On the other hand, it's an interesting establishment and the food, when it eventually arrives, is worth waiting for. Just make sure you aren't in a hurry in case it's a slow night. • D only ££ Tues-Sat • Closed 25 Dec & 1 Jan • MasterCard, Visa •

Cork   Jacques Restaurant

9 Phoenix Street Cork Co Cork
RESTAURANT   Tel: 021 277387   Fax: 021 270634

This restaurant near the GPO has been an integral part of Cork life since 1982. It has changed with the years, evolving from quite a traditional place in the earlier years to a dashing Mediterranean-toned bistro. Jacqueline Barry's menus – lunch, early dinner and dinner – are based on carefully sourced ingredients in a network of suppliers built up over 18 years. They are refreshingly short, allowing her to concentrate on the delicious cooking that is her forte. There are starters such as organic spinach with beetroot jelly, Orla cheese & walnut dressing, main courses like roast breast of duck with confit of leg, apricot sauce & potato stuffing. Desserts could be lemon tart or almond cake with plums in red wine & mascarpone cheese. This is really good cooking – and excellent value too, especially the early dinner (6-7 pm, £10.90 for 2 courses). • L£ Mon-Fri, D££ Mon-Sat • Closed Bank Hols & Xmas wk •

Cork   Jurys Cork Inn

Anderson's Quay Cork Co Cork
HOTEL   Tel: 021 276 444   Fax: 021 276144
email: margaret_nagle@jurys-hotel.ie

In a fine central riverside site, this budget hotel has all the features that Jurys Inns have now become well known for: room prices include accommodation for up to four (including a sofa bed) and there is space for a cot (which can be supplied by arrangement). No room service. Limited parking (22 spaces), plus arrangement with nearby car park. Rooms 133 (7 suitable for disabled guests). Café/restaurant 7-10am, 6-9.30pm.The Inn Pub bar serves lunch every day and there's a late bar (residents only) every night. (Bar closed on Good Friday). • Acc£-££ • Closed 25 Dec • Amex, Diners, MasterCard, Visa •

Cork   Jurys Hotel

Western Road Cork Co Cork
HOTEL   Tel: 021 276622   Fax: 021 274477

Consistently popular with both business and leisure guests since it opened in 1972, this comfortable hotel has a relaxed atmosphere and is in an attractive riverside setting half a mile from the city centre. Bedrooms include 20 designed for disabled guests, four suites/mini-suites and 30 executive rooms, 10 of which are designated lady executive. All rooms are a good size and have both double and single beds • Acc££££ • Closed 25 Dec & 1 Jan • Amex, Diners, MasterCard, Visa •

Cork

Lotamore House

Tivoli Cork Co Cork

ACCOMMODATION   Tel: 021 822344   Fax: 021 822219

email: lotamoreiol.ie

Just 5 minutes from the city centre and clearly signed from the main Dublin/Waterford road out of Cork, this large period house is set in mature gardens. Although not grand it was built on a large scale, with big, airy rooms comfortably furnished to sleep three, with room for an extra bed or cot (baby-sitting by arrangement). A large drawing room has plenty of armchairs and an open fire and, although only breakfast and light meals are offered, Fleming's Restaurant (see entry) is next door. • Acc£-££ • Closed 20 Dec-7 Jan • Amex, MasterCard, Visa •

Cork

Lovetts

Churchyard Lane off Well Road Douglas Cork Co Cork

RESTAURANT   Tel: 021 294909   Fax: 021 294024

One of the finest restaurants in Cork, Lovetts is in a late Georgian house situated in mature grounds (home to both the restaurant and the Lovett family since 1977). Committed to serious cooking, using the best of fresh, free range and local products, head chef Marie Harding is a talented and creative cook and has been a finalist in the Restaurants Association of Ireland/Bord Bia "New Irish Cuisine" competition. The restaurant has many sides to its character, including a fully licensed bar (the extensive wine list is Dermod Lovett's particular passion), private dining for parties of 8 to 24 in the 'Wild Geese' Room and, in addition to the main restaurant, more informal dining in the Brasserie. Marie's lunch and dinner menus are consistently interesting and always offer a separate vegetarian menu. • L£-££ Mon-Fri, D££ Tues-Sat • Closed Xmas week, 1 wk Aug • Amex, Diners, MasterCard, Visa •

Cork

Maryborough House Hotel

Maryborough Hill Douglas Cork Co Cork

HOTEL 🏛   Tel: 021 365555   Fax: 021 365662

email: maryboro@indigo.ie

The Maryborough House Hotel opened in autumn 1997; at its heart is a fine country house set in its own grounds and gardens developed with sensitivity. The original house, which is beautifully proportioned, has many fine features, restored with care and furnished in period style with antiques. The main entrance is via the original flight of steps up to the old front door and, although there is no conventional reception area, guests receive a warm welcome at the desk just inside the front door. The new section of the hotel is modern and blends comfortably with the trees and gardens surrounding it. The new wing includes excellent leisure facilities and, better still, accommodation which is exceptionally good in terms of design – simple, modern, bright, utilising Irish crafts. Rooms are generously-sized, with a pleasant outlook, good amenities and extras including complimentary mineral water. Bathrooms are well-finished and well-lit, with plenty of marbled shelf space, generous towels and a robe; they have environmentally friendly toiletries and suggestions on saving water by avoiding unnecessary laundry. Some public areas are less successful: the bar (lower ground floor, Arctic temperature caused by misuse of air conditioning) and restaurant, which has no clear definition of area, or proper system of reception. We found the menu, furniture, lighting, air conditioning, service and, alas, the food itself to be disappointing for a hotel of this quality. • Acc£££ • Closed 24-26 Dec • Amex, Diners, MasterCard, Visa •

Cork

Metropole Hotel

MacCurtain Street Cork Co Cork

HOTEL   Tel: 021 508122   Fax: 021 506450

email: enq@metropoleh.com   www.metropoleh.com

This imposing city-centre hotel next door to the Everyman Palace and backing on to the River Lee, celebrated its centenary last year. Many of the original features remain, such as the marble facade, outside carved stonework and plaster ceilings inside. Always popular with those connected with the arts and entertainment industry, there are many displays (photos and press cuttings) of stars past and present in the public areas and the atmospheric, traditionally-styled Met Tavern. The hotel has recently completed a refurbishment programme, noticeably in the bedrooms that now combine a period feel with modern facilities. Unusually for an old city-centre hotel, there's a splendid leisure club with a large (and unconventionally shaped) indoor swimming pool, overlooked by the Waterside Café. There's also a 'serious' gym with some fierce-looking training equipment. Extensive conference facilities (for up to 350). • Acc££ • Open all year • Amex, Diners, MasterCard, Visa •

Cork

Michael's Restaurant

71/72 Patrick Street Cork Co Cork
RESTAURANT ☆
Café of the Year
Tel: 021 277716

In Cork's main shopping street, Michael Clifford makes a welcome return, though in much less formal surroundings than his previous restaurant. Here you can relax in a large and bright first-floor room without frills. What has not changed is his enthusiasm for cooking (he still crosses over to France to undertake unpaid 'stages' learning new techniques from the hands of some of France's greatest chefs) or his talent to bring out all the flavours from top-quality ingredients. The menu is not overly long – start with a chili and sweetcorn chowder, local smoked salmon or chicken (deep-fried pieces) with Milleens cheese and a red onion marmalade, to be followed by roast monkfish with a carrot and orange risotto, sirloin of beef with a whiskey cream, or oven-baked baby chicken with a bread and clove sauce. Desserts might include a caramelised banana pancake with butterscotch sauce and a scoop of ice cream, chocolate truffle and rum slice with Baileys cream or just a bowl of fresh strawberries. Alternatively, there's a plate of Irish farmhouse cheeses. Lunchtime sees simpler dishes at bargain prices, so it's no surprise to see the place packed with a lively crowd of workers and shoppers alike. As usual, accompaniments for meals are excellent – breads, vegetables and splendid coffee. Service, too, is excellent: swift, friendly and professional. The wine list reflects the atmosphere of this award- winning establishment, unpretentious and inexpensive. •L£ & D££ Mon-Sat • Closed Xmas & New Year •

Cork

Proby's Bistro/Deanshall

Crosses Green St Finbarr's Cathedral Cork Co Cork
RESTAURANT/ACCOMMODATION   Tel: 021 316531   Fax: 021 316523
This restaurant is handier to the city centre than it first appears and is a pleasant spot for a bite to eat during the day (tables outside for fine weather) as well as in the evening. The style – established before the current wave and competently executed – is global cuisine, with an emphasis on things Mediterranean. Accommodation arrangements are unusual, in that rooms occupied by students during the academic year become available for visitors in summer (and consequently Proby's is open for breakfast from June to September). • L£ & D£-££ daily • Acc£ • Closed 25 Dec & 1 Jan • Amex, Diners, MasterCard, Visa •

Cork

Quality Hotel

Morrisons Quay Cork Co Cork
HOTEL   Tel: 021 275858   Fax: 021 275833
Very central and right on the river bank, this compact hotel aims to provide the luxury of hotel suites but at an affordable price. The richly coloured foyer, although small, makes a good impression with its oriental rugs. Of the 42 rooms, 28 are suites, each well-equipped with its own lobby and kitchenette in addition to a bedroom with seating area or separate sitting room. Simple modern decor is pleasant and quality materials have been used throughout. • Acc£££ • Closed 25 Dec & 1 Jan • Amex, Diners, MasterCard, Visa •

Cork

Rochestown Park Hotel

Cork Co Cork
HOTEL   Tel: 021 892233   Fax: 021 892178/918052
Close to both Cork airport and the ferry port, this attractive hotel stands in lovely grounds and, although it has developed and changed in many ways since opening in 1989, remains under the same general management of Liam Lally. Formerly a home of the Lord Mayors of Cork, the original parts of the building feature gracious, well-proportioned public rooms. Facilities include excellent conference/banqueting facilities (recently extended up to 800/450 respectively) and a fine leisure centre with a Roman style 20 metre swimming pool. It also features the country's premier Thalasso Therapy Centre. Bedrooms include three rooms designed for disabled guests and a new executive wing.• Acc££-£££ • Amex, Diners, MasterCard, Visa •

Cork

ACCOMMODATION

Seven North Mall

7 North Mall Cork Co Cork
Tel: 021 397191   Fax: 021 300811
email: sevennorthmall@tinet.ie

Angela Hegarty runs one of the city's most pleasant guesthouses, on a tree-lined south-facing mall overlooking the River Lee. Rooms in this 1750s townhouse are all spacious, individually furnished in keeping with the house (with new bathrooms skilfully incorporated). Some rooms have river views and there is a ground floor room specially designed for disabled guests. Excellent breakfasts. Secure parking. Many of the city's best restaurants, pubs, museums, galleries and theatres are within a short walk. • Acc££ • Closed 17 Dec-8 Jan • Amex, MasterCard, Visa •

Cork

ACCOMMODATION

Victoria Lodge

Victoria Lodge Victoria Cross Cork Co Cork
Tel: 021 542233   Fax: 021 542572

This unusual guesthouse is about five minutes' drive from the city centre. It was built early this century as a Capuchin monastery and opened as a guesthouse in 1988. The refectory, which still has its panelling and benches intact, is used for breakfast and the old common room has become a television lounge for guests. Comfortably furnished bedrooms include one designed for disabled guests. There are five designated non-smoking. Bedrooms, which are generously sized, with en-suite bath and shower, have been recently renovated. Ample private parking. • Acc£-££ • Open all year • Amex, MasterCard, Visa •

Cork

The Wine Vault

Lancaster Quay Western Road Cork Co Cork
Tel: 021 275751

Situated just across the road from the entrance to Jurys Hotel, Reidy's Wine Vault is a stylish contemporary pub and makes a convenient meeting place or a good choice for an informal bite to eat. Originally a wine warehouse, it has been imaginatively converted to its present use, with a high vaulted ceiling and an attractive mixture of old and new fixtures and furnishings. Noelle Reidy supervises the food personally and early visitors will be greeted by the aroma of bread baking at the back, shortly followed by soups, pies and casseroles (shepherd's pie, Irish stew) for lunch, all marked up on the blackboard as they come on stream. Seafood choices are particularly strong but don't overlook the home-cooked Cork spiced beef, which is a local speciality. • Closed 25 Dec, Good Fri • Amex, Diners, MasterCard, Visa •

Courtmacsherry

HOTEL/RESTAURANT

Courtmacsherry Hotel

Nr Bandon Co Cork
Tel: 023 46198   Fax: 023 46137

Family-run by Terry and Carole Adams since 1973, this unpretentious homely hotel offers simple comfort and a relaxed atmosphere. Spacious, pleasantly old-fashioned public rooms provide plenty of places for guests to relax. By comparison, bedrooms are on the small side, but they have direct-dial phones, satellite TV and tea/coffee trays and all except three are en-suite. Traditional family holiday activities are well catered for, with boats and bikes available nearby, lawn tennis in the grounds and there is also Carole Adams' riding school which is on the premises and offers riding and qualified instruction for all ages.

Restaurant

Overlooking Courtmacsherry Bay, the restaurant is in a pleasant traditionally furnished room. Local fish is the speciality and cooking is supervised personally by Terry Adams. The wine list, which offers over 100 wines from throughout the world, from over a dozen suppliers, is a particular source of pride. Regular visits are made to vineyards.
• L£ Sun, D££ Mon-Sun • Acc££ • Closed Oct-Easter • MasterCard, Visa •

Establishments recommended in the guide are entitled to display the current year's plaque or certificate. However, we strongly recommend that you also read the guide's entry as some establishments may be praised for certain aspects of their operation and criticised for others.

Courtmacsherry

Travara Lodge

Courtmacsherry Co Cork

ACCOMMODATION   **Tel: 023 46493   Fax: 023 46045**

email: travara@tinet.ie

This modernised Georgian house enjoys an attractive seafront location. Bedrooms, which are all non-smoking, vary in size and outlook but are all very comfortable and well-appointed. All have en-suite facilities (5 shower-only), one room has wheelchair access and the three front bedrooms have a view over Courtmacsherry harbour. High standards of maintenance and housekeeping; no phones or TVs in rooms. No evening meals, but there are two restaurants nearby. • Acc£ • MasterCard, Visa •

Crookhaven

Journey's End

Crookhaven Co Cork

RESTAURANT   **Tel: 028 35183**

At the time of going to press Ina Manahan – who has run this tiny waterside cottage restaurant for over 20 summers now – is uncertain whether she will re-open in 1999. We hope she does and suggest a phone call to check might be worthwhile; she normally opens from 1 June – 31 August.

Crookhaven

O'Sullivans

Crookhaven Co Cork

PUB   **Tel: 028 35319**

This long-established family-run bar is in one of the most attractive situations in the country. Situated right on the harbour at Crookhaven, with tables beside the water, it can be heaven on a sunny day. Angela O'Sullivan supervises all the food served in the bar personally – home-made soups and chowders, shrimps, open sandwiches, home-baked bread, scones and desserts – all good homely fare. • Closed 25 Dec & Good Fri • Diners, Visa •

Crosshaven

Whispering Pines

Crosshaven Co Cork

HOTEL   **Tel: 021 831843   Fax: 021 831679**

A particular favourite of fishing people and the sailing community, this hospitable, laid-back family-run hotel is in a sheltered position overlooking the Owenabue River. Accommodation is modest but comfortable and reasonably priced. The hotel owns three boats, custom-built for sea angling. • Acc£ • Closed Dec • Amex, Diners, MasterCard, Visa •

Durrus

Blairs Cove House

Durrus Co Cork

RESTAURANT/ACCOMMODATION   **Tel: 027 61127   Fax: 027 61487**

In a stunning waterside location at the head of Dunmanus Bay, visual sensations at Sabine and Philippe de Mey's remarkable restaurant are so intense that you feel you can almost touch the images that remain in the mind. Although additions over the years have enlarged the restaurant considerably – and now include the option of enjoying the view from an elegant conservatory while you dine – the original room is lofty, stone-walled and black-beamed: but, although characterful, any tendency to rusticity is immediately offset by the choice of a magnificent chandelier as a central feature, gilt-framed family portraits on the walls and the superb insouciance of using their famous grand piano to display an irresistible array of desserts. They have things down to a fine art at Blairs Cove – and what a formula: an enormous central buffet groans under the weight of the legendary hors d'oeuvre display, a speciality that is unrivalled in Ireland. Main course specialities of local seafood or the best of meat and poultry are char-grilled at a special wood-fired grill right in the restaurant and, in addition to those desserts, full justice is done to the ever-growing selection of local farmhouses cheese for which West Cork is rightly renowned. Contrast is the key at Blairs Cove: closeness to and awareness of the elements is emphasised by the comfort and protection indoors; the rough background of stone and beam defuse any potential pomposity; the simplicity of superb main course ingredients prepared at the grill, or farmhouse cheeses laid out for the taking, highlights the caring preparation of speciality displays. This place is truly an original – and what a blessing that there is a small apartment above the restaurant for the use of lucky diners who may have the foresight to book it in time. • D£££ Tues-Sat • Acc£££ • Closed Nov-Mar • MasterCard, Visa •

Fermoy

La Bigoudenne

28 McCurtain Street Fermoy Co Cork

Tel: 025 32832

RESTAURANT

What a joy it is to discover this little piece of France in the main street of a County Cork town. Noelle and Rodolphe Semeria's hospitality is matched only by their food, which specialises in Breton dishes, especially crêpes – both savoury (made with buckwheat flour) and sweet (with wheat flour). But they do all sorts of other things too, like salads that you only seem to get in France, soup of the day served with 1/4 baguette & butter, a plat du jour and lovely French pastries. The bill is a pleasant surprise too. Highly recommended. • L£ Tues-Sat, D££ Tues-Sun • Closed 2 wks Nov • MasterCard, Visa •

Fermoy

Castlehyde Hotel

Castlehyde Fermoy Co Cork

Tel/Fax: 025 31865/31924

email: cashyde@iol.ie

HOTEL

Opened in 1998, shortly before we went to press, Erik Speekenbrink's new hotel is in a beautifully restored 18th century courtyard building, with all the original features preserved and the hotel retained within the original buildings. The restaurant had not opened at the time of our visit but is very pleasantly situated overlooking a lawn and mature woodland, and has a conservatory extension. Bedrooms, which are individually furnished to a high standard with antiques, have a private home feeling. There is a heated outdoor swimming pool.

* The restaurant has since opened, under the direction of head chef Clive Connors, who presents both lunch and dinner menus. A phone call is advised to check details.

• Acc££ • Amex, Diners, MasterCard, Visa •

Glandore

Hayes Bar

Glandore Co Cork

Tel: 028 33214/021 293308

PUB

Hayes Bar overlooks the harbour, has outdoor tables – and Ada Hayes' famous bar food. The soup reminds you of the kind your granny used to make and the sandwiches are stupendous. A written description will not suffice, everything that goes to makes Hayes' special – including the wines and crockery collected on Declan and Ada's frequent trips to France – has to be seen to be believed. Just order a simple cup of coffee and see what you get for £1.10. • Meals£ • Closed weekends Sept-Jun except Xmas & Easter • No credit cards •

Glandore

The Rectory

Glandore Co Cork

RESTAURANT   **Tel: 028-33072   Fax: 028-33600**

In a prime location overlooking Glandore harbour, this fine Georgian residence makes a very good restaurant. The spacious reception rooms along the front of the house have converted well to a linking bar/reception room. The table d'hôte menu is good value at £26 for four courses; there are some supplements but that is to be expected unless the price is very high or there is also an à la carte. Ciaran Woods, head chef since 1995, presents a fine array of dishes in a well-balanced and imaginative menu. Interesting dishes included a starter of venison sausage, grilled and served with caramelised red onions and blue cheese sauce. Desserts include a number of variations on traditional themes – individual sticky toffee pudding with maple-flavoured Anglaise sauce – but when in west Cork, farmhouse cheeses are hard to resist. Service, especially reception, can sometimes be a weak point.• D££-£££ Mon-Sun • Closed Nov-Apr •

Glanmire

The Barn Restaurant

Glanmire nr Cork Co Cork

RESTAURANT   **Tel: 021 866211   Fax: 021 866525**

Just outside Cork, on the old Youghal road, this long-established neighbourhood restaurant has a devoted local clientele. It is comfortably old-fashioned, with uniformed waiters and food with a real home-cooked flavour. Dinner menus offer a wide choice on all courses – roast fillet of local salmon with sorrel sauce indicates the style. Vegetarians are well looked after, saucing is good and accompaniments are carefully selected. Finish with Irish cheeses or something from the traditional dessert trolley. Sunday lunch is very popular and menus are similar in style. Car parking is available behind the restaurant. • L£ Sun, D££ Mon-Sun • Amex, Diners, MasterCard, Visa •

Goleen Harbour

The Heron's Cove

Harbour Road Goleen nr Skibbereen Co Cork

RESTAURANT/ACCOMMODATION   Tel: 028 35225   Fax: 028 35422

email: suehill@tinet.ie   www.westcork_web.ie

When the tide is in and the sun is out there can be few prettier locations than Sue Hill's restaurant overlooking Goleen harbour. She does tasty, inexpensive day-time food – which can be served on a sunny balcony – like hearty soups and home-baked bread, home-cooked ham, farmhouse cheeses and seafood specials. Delicious desserts – tangy lemon tart or a wicked chocolate gateau – are also available with afternoon tea (also freshly brewed coffee). The Heron's Cove philosophy is to use only the best of fresh, local ingredients – typically in wholesome starters like fisherman's broth or warm duckling salad and main courses such as Goleen lamb cutlets with a port & redcurrant sauce. Lobster and Rossmore oysters are available fresh from a tank and prices are refreshingly reasonable.

Rooms

Five good-sized en-suite rooms have bathrooms, satellite TV, phones, tea/coffee-making facilities and hair dryers. The three doubles have private balconies with sea views and two smaller rooms have a woodland view. Open for B&B all year except Christmas week , but it is always advisable to book, especially when the restaurant is closed (although evening meals are available for residents off-season). • L£££, D££ Mon-Sun • Closed Nov-mid Mar • B&B closed only Xmas wk (meals available for residents) • Amex, MasterCard, Visa •

Gougane Barra

Gougane Barra Hotel

Gougane Barra Ballingeary Co Cork

HOTEL   Tel: 026-47069   Fax: 026-47226

In one of the most peaceful and beautiful locations in Ireland, this delightfully old-fashioned family-run hotel is set in a Forest Park overlooking Gougane Barra Lake (famous for its monastic settlements). The Lucey family have run the hotel since 1937, offering simple, comfortable accommodation as a restful base for walking holidays. Rooms are comfortable but not over-modernised, all looking out onto the lake or mountain. There are quiet public rooms where guests often like to read; breakfast is served in the lakeside dining room. No weddings or other functions are accepted. • Acc££ • Closed mid Oct-May • Amex, Diners, MasterCard, Visa •

Heir Island

Island Cottage

Heir Island Skibbereen Co Cork

RESTAURANT   Tel/Fax: 028 38102

email: islandcottage@tinet.ie   www.indigo.ie/ipress/heir

This place is unique – just a short ferry ride from the mainland yet light years away from the "real" world. Hardly a likely location for a restaurant run by two people who have trained and worked in some of Europe's most prestigious establishments – but, since 1989, that is exactly what John Desmond and Ellmary Fenton have been doing at Island Cottage. Everything about it is different from other restaurants, including the booking policy: a basic advance booking for at least six people must be in place before other smaller groups of 2 to 4 can be accepted – not later than 3 pm on the day; changes to group numbers require 24 hours notice and a booking deposit of £5 per head is required to reserve a table. The no-choice menu consists of a starter, home-made brown bread, main course, dessert and filter coffee; everything depends on the availability of the fresh local, organic (where possible) and wild island ingredients of that day. A vegetarian dish can be accommodated with advance notice. An early autumn menu that earned special praise for John at a recent Irish Restaurants Association/Bord Bia "New Irish Cuisine" competition will give an idea of John's attachment to the island and the kind of meal to expect: roast duck legs on a bed of turnip with duck jus (using hand-reared ducks "of exceptional quality" from Ballydehob), Cape Clear turbot with shrimp sauce on a bed of sea beet or spinach (the turbot is farmed on Cape Clear Island and the shrimp is caught by local fishermen; sea beet is a wild foreshore vegetable, rather like spinach) and a classic terrine of vanilla ice cream with meringue served with a blackberry sauce, using berries picked by children holidaying on the island. Cookery courses and demonstrations can be arranged, also private dinner parties (October-May). Details of cottages for rent also available from the restaurant. • No credit cards •

The best – independently assessed

Innishannon

HOTEL/RESTAURANT

Innishannon House Hotel

Innishannon Co Cork
Tel: 021 775121   Fax: 021 775609
email: inishannon@tinet.ie

The O'Sullivans call Innishannon House "the most romantic hotel in Ireland", and both the riverside location and the early 18th century house certainly have great charm. Public rooms include a residents' bar, sitting room and conservatory, all very comfortably furnished but mainly remarkable for the family's astonishing collection of Irish and American paintings. Bedrooms include one suitable for disabled guests and all have en-suite bath and shower. They vary in shape and character but are all individually decorated with antiques; the best rooms have river views, while others overlook the lovely gardens and all have original wooden shutters and are thoughtfully furnished. Rooms 13. Garden, fishing, boating.

Restaurant

Conal and Vera O'Sullivan's son, Pearse, returned to Innishannon after gaining experience in kitchens abroad – including a 2-star restaurant in Brussels – and with Michael Clifford in Cork. Since 1997 he has been head chef and is doing an excellent job, presenting classical French/new Irish menus at lunch and dinner and cooking with great flair. In addition to formal lunch and dinner in the restaurant every day, he is also responsible for an imaginative bar menu and special afternoon teas are served in the drawing room (or in the garden) from 3-7pm daily. • L£ & D££ Mon-Sun • Acc£££ • Closed mid Jan-mid Mar • Amex, Diners, MasterCard, Visa •

Kanturk

COUNTRY HOUSE/RESTAURANT 🏛

Assolas Country House

Kanturk Co Cork
Tel: 029 50015   Fax: 029 50795
email: assolas@tinet.ie

Home to the Bourke family for generations, this gracious 17th century manor house was first opened to guests in 1965 by Hugh and Eleanor Bourke, founder members of the Irish Country Houses & Restaurants Association, now known as the "Blue Book". Although still very much involved, day-to-day management has passed to their son Joe, who now runs the house jointly with his wife Hazel, the genius in the kitchen. Generous, thoughtful hospitality, impeccable housekeeping and wonderful food are three of the many attractions that bring guests back to Assolas. Rooms vary according to their position in this lovely old house – some are very spacious and overlook the garden and river and there are some courtyard rooms which are especially suitable for families. All are comfortably and elegantly furnished in genuine country house style with good bathrooms and many thoughtful details. In addition, there is the charm of a lovingly maintained walled kitchen garden, a little river with tame swans and a couple of boats for guests to potter about in – even boots kept beside the front door for the use of anyone who may feel like looking up the local otters at dusk. Another nice touch at Assolas – applying to accommodation, food and wine – is the service charge policy: "We do not apply a service charge and gratuities are not expected." Would that more establishments would think the same way.

Restaurant ★

Hazel Bourke is renowned for imaginative and skilled use of produce from their own garden and the surrounding area, offered in a seasonal menu and a daily dinner menu (both £30). Like the rest of the house, the dining room – which is high-ceilinged and elegantly proportioned with deep red walls, antique furniture and crisp white line – is not overdecorated, providing an appropriate setting for food that is refreshingly natural in style. Seafood features regularly, typically in starters like warm Kenmare mussels served in a toasted brioche or Rosscarbery oysters grilled with garden herbs. Garden produce usually takes over for the soup course – sorrel, perhaps, or potato and leek. Main course seafood dishes are heartier – oven-baked monkfish for example – or there could be Kanturk lamb served with Hazel's mint jelly, or tender local roast duckling. Vegetables are a predictable strength and there is always a good vegetarian choice. Desserts tend to be classic – lemon tart or blackcurrant fool with vanilla shortbread – and local farmhouse cheeses are superb. The wine list concentrates on European wine, notably Maison Guigal, which has supplied the house wines since 1983. The famous Blackwater Valley Reichensteiner, made locally by Dr Billy Christopher, is also listed (£18). • D£££ • Acc£££ • Closed Nov-Apr• Amex, Diners, MasterCard, Visa •

Kanturk

The Vintage
O'Brien Street Kanturk Co Cork
Tel: 029 50549   Fax: 029 51209

PUB

In a terrace of houses alongside the river in Kanturk, Stephen Bowles has been running this fine pub since 1985, and the experienced pub visitor will quickly recognise all the signs of a well-run establishment. The attractive, well-maintained exterior draws people in and, once through the door, the comfortable, pleasingly traditional interior keeps them there. Be sure to stay for a pint or a quick bite of bar food, even if it's only a bowl of home-made soup. Other regulars include a roast of the day, a catch of the day and something special for vegetarians, as well as freshly prepared sandwiches. • Meals£ • Closed 25 Dec & Good Fri • MasterCard, Visa •

Kilbrittain

Casino House
Coolmain Bay Kilbrittain Nr Kinsale Co Cork
Tel: 023 49944   Fax: 023 49945

RESTAURANT
Farmhouse Cheese Award Winner

While Kerrin and Michael Relja's delightful restaurant is just a few miles west of Kinsale it's one of the country's best kept secrets. The couple's cool continental style makes a pleasing contrast to their lovely old house, and the warmth of Kerrin's hospitality is matched only by the excellence of Michael's food. Michael cooks with verve and confidence, in soups like saffron-scented fish with aioli and starters such as garlic prawns on a mixed leaf salad or risotto of lobster. Well-balanced main course choices include meats – fillet steak with a burgundy sauce, saddle of lamb with rosemary jus or spicy pork kebabs with pesto noodles – but also local seafood, such as cod in a sesame crust on creamed spinach and classic grilled salmon steak with sauce hollandaise, all with their own vegetable garnish and simple seasonal side vegetables. Their attention to detail in every aspect of the restaurant is admirable and the way they handle cheese reflects the perfectionism that is evident throughout – and is one of the reasons they have been chosen for our Farmhouse Cheese Award. The selection does not aim to be comprehensive, but it is perfectly tailored to the scale of their operation and presented with great care: on the Guide's most recent visit we found a quartet of farmhouse cheeses – Desmond, Durrus and Gubbeen from west Cork plus Cashel Blue from Tipperary – all in excellent condition, served charmingly plated with herb-sprinkled sliced tomatoes and a choice of home made bread or crackers. While Irish farmhouse cheeses are now well known and widely available, it is still all to rare to find them handled with such respect. • L£ daily July & Aug & Sun, D££ Mon-Sun • Closed Feb-mid Mar • MasterCard, Visa •

The guide aims to provide comprehensive recommendations of the best places to eat, drink and stay throughout Ireland. We welcome suggestions from readers. If you think an establishment merits assessment , please write or email us.

Killeagh

Ballymakeigh House
Killeagh Youghal Co Cork
Tel: 024 95184   Fax: 024 95370
email: ballymakeigh@tinet.ie

FARM STAY
Farmhouse of the Year

Winner of our Farmhouse of the Year Award, Ballymakeigh House provides an exceptional standard of comfort, food and hospitality in one of the most outstanding establishments of its type in Ireland. Set at the heart of an east Cork dairy farm, this attractive old house is immaculately maintained and run by Margaret Browne, who is a Euro-Toques chef and author of a recent cookery book. The house is warm and homely with plenty of space for guests, who are welcome to use the garden and visit the farmyard. The individually decorated bedrooms are full of character and equally comfortable – and, needless to say, the food is outstanding. Margaret's hospitality is matched only by her energy – as if all this were not enough, plans are afoot to build an equestrian centre on the farm as well.

Restaurant

Non-residents may also sample Margaret's excellent cooking, in a personal blend of traditional and new Irish cuisine with international influences, all based on the very best of fresh local ingredients. • D££ • Closed Dec-Jan • Diners, MasterCard, Visa •

Kinsale

PUB

1601

Pearse Street Kinsale Co Cork
Tel: 021 772529

Named in honour of the battle of Kinsale – the story is chronicled on the walls inside the pub – James Gahan took over the pub in 1989 and has proceeded to build up a reputation for good food which draws people from far around. Like many other establishments in the area, the 1601 specialises in seafood – oysters, mussels, real scampi, Kinsale salmon (fresh and smoked). But they also look after vegetarians, with quiches and stir-fries, and use other local produce imaginatively – Clonakilty black pudding, for example, is presented unusually in a salad. Live music is also a feature – details from the pub. • Meals£ • Closed 25 Dec & Good Fri • MasterCard, Visa •

Kinsale

HOTEL

Actons Hotel

Pier Road Kinsale Co Cork
Tel: 021 772135   Fax: 021 772231
email: actonsh@indigo.ie

Overlooking the harbour and standing in its own grounds, this attractive quayside establishment is Kinsale's most famous hotel, dating back to 1946 when it was created from several substantial period houses. It has recently undergone extensive renovations. The leisure facilities are possibly the best in the area and there are also good conference/banqueting facilities for up to 300. • Acc££ • Open all year • Amex, Diners, MasterCard, Visa •

Kinsale

HOTEL/RESTAURANT

The Blue Haven Hotel

Kinsale Co Cork
Tel: 021 772209/06   Fax: 021 774268
email: bluhaven@iol.ie

Brian and Anne Cronin's attractive hotel is right at the heart of Kinsale – some would say it is the heart. After recent major refurbishments all the well-appointed bedrooms are new or redone, with double glazing offsetting the street noise that is inevitable with a central location. Both the rooms and their neat bathrooms make up in thoughtful planning what they lack in spaciousness. Due to the nature of the building public areas are also quite compact, but the lounge/lobby and the bar areas are well-planned and comfortable. The wine shop/delicatessen off the lobby is an enjoyable place to browse for picnics or presents. The hotel has its own sea angling boat, the 'Peggy G', for shark fishing in summer and catching the likes of conger eel, pollock, ray, ling and whiting all year round.

Restaurant

The strong maritime theme of this well-appointed restaurant reflects its specialities, while helpful and discreet service and a particularly good pianist add to the atmosphere. Head chef Peter Wood, who joined the hotel in 1998, is responsible for both the restaurant and bar food menus, all of which are based on local produce, especially seafood. The wine list is also of note, as the wines of the Irish "Wine Geese" families are Brian Cronin's particular passion – their chateaux are honoured in the naming of rooms in the hotel and well represented on the list and in the wine shop. A visit to Desmond Castle is recommended to learn the full story. • Meals£-££ • Acc£££ • Closed 24-25 Dec & 4-29 Jan • Amex, Diners, MasterCard, Visa •

Kinsale

PUB

The Bulman

Summercove Kinsale Co Cork
Tel: 021 772131   Fax: 021 773359

The emphasis at The Bulman has shifted more towards food since the first floor restaurant was opened, but it is still very much a pub. The bar is characterful and maritime (though this is definitely not a theme pub) and a great place to be in fine weather, when you can wander out to the seafront and sit on the wall beside the carpark. The plan for 1999 is to encourage more live music, in both the restaurant and bar. • Meals£-££ • Closed 25 Dec & Good Fri • MasterCard, Visa •

Visit our web site - www.ireland-guide.com

Kinsale — Man Friday

Scilly Kinsale Co Cork

RESTAURANT   Tel: 021 772260   Fax: 021 772262

High up over the harbour, Philip Horgan's popular, characterful restaurant is housed in a series of rooms. It has recently grown, with a new extension – there is now seating for about 50, overlooking Kinsale and the harbour. It has a garden terrace which makes a nice spot for drinks and coffee in fine weather. Abdu LeMarti, who has been head chef since 1990, presents seasonal à la carte menus that major on seafood but offer plenty else besides, including several vegetarian choices and duck, steak and lamb. While geared to fairly traditional tastes, the cooking is sound and can include imaginative ideas. Simple, well-made desserts include good ice creams. Service is cheerful and efficient. • L£ Sun, D££ daily • Closed 25 Dec & Good Fri • Amex, Diners, MasterCard, Visa •

Kinsale — Max's Wine Bar

Main Street Kinsale Co Cork

RESTAURANT   Tel: 021 772443

As long as Wendy Tisdall's delightful little restaurant remains unchanged there can't be too much wrong with the world. Since 1975 it has maintained consistently high standards, never ceasing to charm with its trademark mirror-varnished tables, fresh flowers and creative menus. These make special use of seafood and have particularly tempting starters. Grilled mussels with garlic butter and breadcrumbs, roast duck with orange & ginger sauce and monkfish chunks simmered in cream & tarragon indicate the style. Vegetarians are well looked after too. The early bird menu is especially good value. • L£ & D£-££ daily • Closed Nov-Feb • MasterCard, Visa •

Kinsale — The Moorings

Scilly Kinsale Co Cork

ACCOMMODATION   Tel: 021 772376   Fax: 021 772675

Pat and Irene Jones' superbly appointed, purpose-built guesthouse has its own car park (a very big plus in Kinsale), spacious bedrooms with good en-suite bathrooms (bath and shower) and balconies with views across the marina. Downstairs there's a large conservatory that is used for breakfast (although room service is available) and just lounging around harbour-watching There is one bedroom equipped for disabled guests. Children over 9 are welcome and dogs are allowed.• Acc££ • Closed Xmas wk • Diners, MasterCard, Visa •

Kinsale — The Old Bank House

Pearse Street Kinsale Co Cork

ACCOMMODATION   Tel: 021 774075   Fax: 021 774296

Marie and Michael Riese's townhouse in the middle of Kinsale has earned a high reputation for quality of accommodation and service – it has an elegant residents' sitting room, a well-appointed breakfast room and comfortable country house-style bedrooms with good amenities, antiques and quality materials. Now the news is that the Old Bank House is expanding into the Post Office next door. Work should be completed by spring 1999.This will provide a further seven bedrooms and a 2-bedroom suite (with a little kitchen) for long-stay guests. Also – and this will be a very big improvement – they will be including a lift in the new development. ("American guests don't realise that a Georgian house is 'all up and down'!") Well-behaved children over 3 and small dogs are welcome by arrangement. • Acc£££ • Closed 23-27 Dec • Amex, MasterCard, Visa •

Kinsale — The Old Presbytery

43 Cork Street Kinsale Co Cork

ACCOMMODATION   Tel: 021 772027   Fax: 021 772144

email: oldpres@iol.ie   www.ireland.iol.ie/Kinsale/presbyt.htm

Philip and Mary McEvoy have been doing great things to this old house in the centre of the town (which has provided excellent accommodation for many years during both the current and previous ownership). At the time of going to press they were completing the construction of three new self-catering suites, each with two en-suite bedrooms, sitting room, kitchenette and an extra bathroom. The new rooms are well-proportioned and furnished in the same style as the original bedrooms (with stripped pine country furniture and antique beds) and will be available on a nightly basis, sleeping up to six adults. The top suite is to have an additional lounge area leading from a spiral staircase, with magnificent views over the town and harbour • Acc£-££ • Closed mid Dec-early Jan •

Kinsale

The Old Rectory

Rampart Lane Kinsale Co Cork
Tel/Fax: 021 772678

ACCOMMODATION

Set in large secluded gardens overlooking the town, this fine Georgian house offers luxurious accommodation in three very spacious rooms. It is an unusual set-up for Kinsale, being very quiet and private, with plenty of parking and lots of space. The reception rooms are very big too, and there's even a wine bar. However, Martha and Dave Pringle are anxious to impress on guests the informality of their home – don't be surprised if they answer the door in their pyjamas! • Acc££ • Closed Xmas • MasterCard, Visa •

Kinsale

Perryville House

Kinsale Co Cork

ACCOMMODATION   🏛

Tel: 021 772731   Fax: 021 772298
email: sales@perryville.iol.ie

Laura and Andrew Corcoran have renovated this characterful house on the harbourfront in Kinsale to a very high standard, opening it to guests in 1997. It is one of the prettiest houses in Kinsale and now, under the management of Barry McDermott, provides luxuriously appointed accommodation. Gracious public rooms are beautifully furnished, as if for a private home. Spacious, individually decorated bedrooms vary in size and outlook, but all have extra large beds and thoughtful extras such as fresh flowers, complimentary mineral water, quality toiletries, robes and slippers. Accommodation includes seven suites and three rooms especially suitable for disabled guests, all with exceptionally well-appointed bathrooms (5 shower only). Breakfasts include home-baked breads and local cheeses.Morning coffee and afternoon tea are available to residents in the drawing room and there is a wine licence. No smoking. • Acc££ • Closed Dec-Mar • Amex, Diners, MasterCard, Visa •

Kinsale

Scilly House

Scilly Kinsale Co Cork

ACCOMMODATION   Tel: 021 772413   Fax: 021 774629

Scilly House is one of the finest traditional houses in Kinsale, with views over an extensive garden down to the sea. Reception rooms, which are impressive in an informal style, include a bar/library with grand piano, a second (cosy) sitting room and a dining room with the lovely view. The proprietors are Bill Skelly and Karin Young, who is Californian. Karin's influence is seen in the charming American country decor throughout the house and in the standard of accommodation. The whole house is bright, airy and immaculately maintained and the bedrooms, which nearly all have views, have great individuality and good bathrooms. The Californian influence can also be seen in the breakfast, which can be served in the garden in fine weather. • Acc£££ • Closed Nov-Apr • Amex, MasterCard, Visa •

Kinsale

Sovereign House

Newman's Mall Kinsale Co Cork

ACCOMMODATION   Tel: 021 772850   Fax: 021 774723

In the heart of old Kinsale, the McKeown family's Queen Anne townhouse dates from 1708. It offers a high level of comfort in elegant and fascinating surroundings. Fourposter beds are at home in this historic house, but so too are the modern amenities – good bathrooms, direct dial phones and tea & coffee trays. The house also has a reading room and a full size snooker room. And, if Mrs McKeown isn't too busy, ask to see the workshop at the top of the house. •Acc£££ • Closed 20 Dec-6 Jan • Amex, MasterCard, Visa •

Kinsale

The Spaniard

Scilly Co Cork

PUB   Tel: 021 772436   Fax: 021 773303

Who could fail to be charmed by The Spaniard, that characterful and friendly old pub perched high up above the town? Although probably best known for music (nightly), they do a good job on the food side too. Much of their wholesome, tasty fare is traditional but it occasionally strays into the international zone – Cajun chicken and peppers, for example – and, of course, local seafood is especially important. There's a daily special for vegetarians and evening meals are quite elaborate affairs – sirloin steak with three pepper sauce, or farmhouse duckling with plum brandy sauce for instance. • Meals£ • Closed 25 Dec & Good Fri • Diners, MasterCard, Visa •

Kinsale   Trident Hotel
World's End Co Cork

HOTEL   Tel: 021 772301   Fax: 021 774173
email: tridentk@iol.ie   www.indigo.ie/ipress/trident

This blocky, concrete-and-glass 1960s waterfront building might not win any architectural awards today, but it certainly wins on location and, under the excellent management of Hal McElroy, is a well-run, hospitable and comfortable place to stay. The pubby Fisherman's Wharf bar is a good meeting place and Gerry O'Connor, head chef for the main restaurant, also has responsibility for the bar food. Bedrooms include two suites, with private balconies directly overlooking the harbour. • Acc£££ • Closed 24-26 Dec • Amex, Diners, MasterCard, Visa •

Kinsale   The Vintage Restaurant
50 Main Street Kinsale Co Cork

RESTAURANT   Tel: 021-772502   Fax: 021-774828
email: Raoul@vintagerestaurant.ie   www.vintagerestaurant.ie

Since 1994 Raoul and Seiko de Gendre have run this famous old restaurant with great professionalism. There has been a lot of work put into the restaurant without spoiling its traditional cottagey style – Raoul's fine paintings would probably be the most obvious change to a casual observer who had not visited for some time. From the start this restaurant has operated an unusually democratic kitchen, where a number of chefs of equal standing take turns. But, whoever is cooking, the best of Irish ingredients are used with pride, in dishes that tend towards the classical but are also influenced by world cuisines (as well as by the special qualities of individual ingredients). Wide-ranging, à la carte menus change with the seasons, tending to be especially strong on seafood in summer and game in the winter. Details are good – tasty little amuse-bouches are served with aperitifs, tables are beautifully appointed, service excellent. Wine appreciation evenings and other special events are held regularly. Private dining is available. • D£££ daily except Sun low season • Closed Jan & Feb • Amex, MasterCard •

Macroom   The Castle Hotel
Main Street Macroom Co Cork

HOTEL   Tel: 026-41074   Fax: 026-41505
email: castlehotel@tinet.ie   www.castlehotel.ie

Big changes have been going on behind the neat frontage of this hotel on the main street of Macroom. In the ownership of the Buckley family since 1952, it is currently under the management of Don and Gerard Buckley, who are maximising its potential; first through gradual refurbishment and, more recently, through thoughtfully planned reconstruction. Public areas gleam welcomingly, and the bar and dining room, especially, are most attractive. Bedrooms are on the small side but all have recently been refurbished; there are slight variations – some older rooms are shower-only, newer ones have trouser presses – but all have phone, TV and tea/coffee trays. The back of the building has recently been demolished and replaced with an impressive 2-storey extension which has a new leisure centre on the ground floor (with fine swimming pool and updated gym) with new bedrooms above it. • Acc££ • Closed 25-27 Dec • Amex, Diners, MasterCard, Visa •

Macroom   The Mills Inn
Ballyvourney Macroom Co Cork

PUB/ACCOMMODATION   Tel: 026 45237   Fax: 026 45454

One of Ireland's oldest inns, The Mills Inn is in a Galetacht (Irish-speaking) area and dates back to 1755. It was traditionally used to break the journey from Cork to Killarney but is now clearly popular with locals as well as travellers. It has old-world charm (despite the regrettable conversion of real fires to gas) and there is a real sense of hospitality.

Accommodation

Rooms vary considerably due to the age of the building, but all are comfortably furnished with neat bathrooms and good amenities. Superior rooms even have jacuzzi baths, and there is a large, well-planned ground-floor room suitable for less able guests (who can use the residents' car park right at the door – in a courtyard shared with a vintage car and an agricultural museum!). Full room service is available for drinks and meals.• Acc££ • Closed 25 Dec • Amex, Diners, MasterCard, Visa •

Mallow   Longueville House

Mallow Co Cork.

HOTEL/RESTAURANT   **Tel: 022 47156   Fax: 022 47459**

email: longueville_house_eire@msn.com

Longueville House opened its doors to guests in 1967 – it was one of the first Irish country houses to do so. Its history is wonderfully romantic, "the history of Ireland in miniature", and it is a story with a happy ending. Having lost their lands in the Cromwellian Confiscation (1652-57), the O'Callaghans took up ownership again some 300 years later. The present house, a particularly elegant Georgian mansion of pleasingly human proportions, dates from 1720, (with wings added in 1800 and the lovely Turner conservatory – which is still in good order – in 1862) overlooks the ruins of their original home, Dromineen Castle. Many things make Longueville special, most importantly the warm, informal hospitality and charm of the O'Callaghans themselves – Michael and Jane, now joined by their son (and talented chef) William and his wife Aisling. The location, overlooking the famous River Blackwater, is lovely. The river, farm and garden supply fresh salmon in season, the famous Longueville lamb and all the fruit and vegetables. In years when the weather is kind, the estate's crowning glory (and Michael O'Callaghan's great enthusiasm) is their own house wine, a light refreshing white fittingly named "Coisreal Longueville". Graciously proportioned reception rooms include a bar and drawing room, both elegantly furnished in country house style. Accommodation is equally sumptuous and bedrooms – which include seven mini-suites and five rooms designated non-smoking – are spacious, superbly comfortable and stylishly decorated to the highest standards (under the personal supervision of Jane O'Callaghan). As well as being one of the finest leisure destinations in the country, this all adds up to a good venue for small conferences and business meetings (max 30). A range of back-up services is available to business guests.

Presidents' Restaurant ★

This is named after the family collection of specially commissioned portraits of all Ireland's past presidents, which made for a seriously masculine collection until the recent addition of Mary Robinson. The main dining room opens into the conservatory – very pleasant on summer evenings or at breakfast – and there is a smaller, inner room for those who wish to smoke. William O'Callaghan's well-balanced dinner menus (£30) offer a sensibly limited choice of four or five dishes on each course, plus an intriguing Tasting Menu (£40) for complete parties. Local ingredients star, in a starter of Ardrahan cheese pastry with avocado salad & hazelnut sauce, for example, followed by fish of the day (which might be Blackwater salmon, or a sea fish such as turbot baked in crepinette with a garden herb purée and tomato sauce). Longueville lamb comes in many guises – roast loin filled with parsley purée, perhaps, with a mint & chive sauce. Garden produce influences the dessert menu too, as in gooseberry tart with elderflower ice cream (a magic combination) and it is hard to resist the local farmhouse cheeses. Home-made chocolates and petits fours come with the coffee and service, under Jane or Aisling O'Callaghan's direction, is excellent. A fine wine list includes many wines imported directly by Michael O'Callaghan • D£££ & light bar L daily • Acc£££ • Closed 20 Dec-mid Feb • Amex, Diners, MasterCard, Visa •

Midleton   The Clean Slate Restaurant

Distillery Rd Midleton Co Cork

RESTAURANT   **Tel/Fax: 021 633655**

Colm Falvey, previously at the impressive Earl of Orrery in Youghal, moved into this striking modern restaurant close to the Jameson Heritage Centre in spring 1998. He presents interesting and very reasonably priced à la carte lunch menus – which include simple things such as open sandwiches as well as stuffed mussels and salade tiede of lamb's kidneys – and more adventurous and wide-ranging evening menus, which are also à la carte. Although the cooking style is international, local produce features strongly – Kenmare Bay sea trout, Rossmore mussels, Ardsallagh goats cheese. Desserts are very tempting, service friendly and the wine list wide-ranging but not overlong (with most wines under £20). • L£ & D££ daily, except Sun low season • MasterCard, Visa •

Midleton   The Farmgate

Coolbawn Midleton Co Cork

RESTAURANT   **Tel/Fax: 021 632771**

This unique shop and restaurant has been drawing people to Midleton in growing numbers since 1985 and it's a great credit to sisters Marog O'Brien and Kay Harte. Kay now runs the younger version at the English Market in Cork while Marog looks after Midleton. The shop at the front is full of wonderful local produce – organic fruit and vegetables, cheeses, honey – and their own super home baking, while the evocatively decorated, comfortable restaurant at the back, with its old pine furniture and modern sculpture, is regularly transformed from bustling daytime café to sophisticated evening restaurant (on Friday and Saturday) complete with string quartet. • Meals£ all day Mon-Sat, D££ Fri & Sat • Closed Bank Hols • MasterCard, Visa •

Midleton   Finins

75 Main Street Midleton Co Cork

PUB   **Tel: 021-631878   Fax: 021 633847**

Finin O'Sullivan's thriving bar in the centre of the town has long been a popular place for locals to meet for a drink and to eat some good wholesome food. An attractive, no-nonsense sort of a place. • L£ & D££ daily • Closed 25-26 Dec • Amex, Diners, MasterCard, Visa •

Midleton   Jameson Heritage Centre

Midleton Co Cork

CAFÉ/BAR   **Tel: 021 613594   021 613642**

The Jameson Heritage Centre is a fascinating place to visit – that such visiting can be thirst-encouraging work is acknowledged at the door (a whiskey tasting is part of the tour) but it can also be hungry work. Sensibly, the Centre has an informal little restaurant where you can get simple home-made food – typically, freshly-made sandwiches such as Irish Cheddar and homemade chutney or baked ham & wholegrain mustard. Alternatives are ploughman's lunches or quiche and salad. There are also afternoon teas with tempting home-made cakes and scones & jam. • Daily meals£ • Closed mid Oct-mid April • Amex, MasterCard, Visa •

Midleton   Midleton Park Hotel

Old Cork Road Midleton Co Cork

HOTEL   **Tel: 021 631767   Fax: 021 631605**

email: kingsley@tinet.ie

This pleasant hotel close to the Jameson Heritage Centre is roomy with good business facilities. Although the decor may seem a little dated, the bedrooms – which are all en-suite with TV, video, phone, hair dryer and trouser press – include 8 rooms suitable for disabled guests and 6 non-smoking rooms as well as a 'presidential suite' for VIP guests. Although it is used a lot by the business community, the hotel also makes a good base for touring east Cork – Fota Island wildlife park, Cobh harbour (last port of call for the Titanic) are nearby and golf packages are arranged. Banqueting/conferences 400. Ample free parking. • Acc££-£££ • Closed 25 Dec • Amex, Diners, MasterCard, Visa •

Monkstown   The Bosun Restaurant & Bar

Monkstown Co Cork

RESTAURANT/ACCOMMODATION   **Tel: 021-842172   Fax: 021-842008**

Nicky and Patricia Moynihan's waterside establishment close to the Cobh car ferry, has grown a lot over the years, with the restaurant and accommodation now more important features than the original bar (15 new rooms next door). Bar food is still something they take pride in, however; seafood takes pride of place and the afternoon/evening bar menu includes everything from chowder or garlic mussels through to real scampi and chips, although serious main courses for carnivores such as rack of lamb and beef stroganoff are also available. Next to the bar, a well-appointed restaurant provides a more formal setting for wide-ranging dinner and à la carte menus – and also Sunday lunch, which is especially popular. Again seafood is the speciality, ranging from popular starters such as crab claws in garlic butter, served with delicious home-baked bread or oysters with caviar, and main courses that include steaks and local duckling as well as seafood every which way, from grilled sole on the bone to medallions of soy marinated monkfish or a cold seafood platter. There's always a choice for vegetarians and vegetables are generous and carefully cooked. Finish with home-made ices, perhaps, or a selection of Irish farmhouse cheeses. • L£, D££ • Acc££ • Closed 25-26 Dec & Good Fri • Amex, Diners, MasterCard, Visa •

Oysterhaven   Finders Inn

Nohoval Oysterhaven Co Cork

RESTAURANT   **Tel/Fax: 021 770737**

Very popular with local people (but perhaps harder for visitors to find) the McDonnell family's characterful restaurant is in a row of traditional cottages above Oysterhaven, en route from Crosshaven to Kinsale. It is a very charming place, packed with antiques and, because of the nature of the building, broken up naturally into a number of dining areas (which gives it an air of mystery). Seafood stars, of course – smoked salmon, Oysterhaven oysters, bisques, chowders, scallops and lobster are all here, but there are a few other specialities too, including steaks, lamb and lovely tender crisp-skinned duckling with an orange-sage sauce. Good desserts, charming service and a great atmosphere. Well worth taking the trouble to find. • D££-£££ Mon-Sat & D Sun July & Aug • Closed Xmas wk • Amex, Diners, MasterCard, Visa •

Rathpeacon   Country Squire Inn

Rathpeacon Old Mallow Rd

PUB   .   **Tel: 021 301812**

The County Squire is just a couple of miles outside Cork city on the Old Mallow road, the N20. It's a very old pub, dating back to the early 1800s. Pat and Regina bought it in 1987 and converted it into half a pub half a restaurant. It's an immaculately kept place and full of character, with old Singer sewing machine tables (and stools). Pat likes to cook a blend of traditional Irish and classic French food, and the bar food is quite ambitious – garlic mussels, stuffed sole, salmon with prawns and fillet and sirloin steaks are all typical, with vegetarian food available on request. In the evening similar food is presented more formally in the cosy little restaurant. • L£ Mon-Sat, D££ Mon-Sun • Closed Good Fri & 25 Dec • Amex, MasterCard, Visa •

Rosscarbery   Celtic Ross Hotel

Rosscarbery Co Cork

HOTEL   **Tel: 023 48722   Fax: 023 48723**

email: info@celticrosshotel.com

Opened in 1997, this new hotel is close to the sea, overlooking Rosscarbery Bay (although not on the sea side of the road). It's an attractive modern building with an unusual tower feature containing a bog oak, which is quite dramatic. Public areas are attractive and spacious, with the restaurant (and many of the bedrooms) overlooking the sea. It is also well placed as a base for touring west Cork, and offers facilities in the leisure centre for alternative activities if the weather should disappoint. • Acc£££ • Amex, Diners, MasterCard, Visa •

Schull   Adèle's

Main Street Schull Co Cork

RESTAURANT   **Tel: 028 28459   Fax: 028 28865**

Adèle Connor's bakery and coffee shop in Schull works like a magnet – if you happen to be in Schull early in the morning, you'll find it hard to squeeze in to buy some of her wonderful home bakes, never mind trying to find a table for a cup of coffee and a home-baked scone. There are delicious savoury things too, such as ciabatta specials served with small tossed salads – traditional and smoked Gubbeen with chutney perhaps – or an omelette with roasted red pepper and garlic. In the evening Simon Connor presents a different kind of menu in the first floor restaurant; a short à la carte might include a roast tomato, fennel and mozzarella salad, roast poussin with dried cepes, sundried tomatoes, rosemary scented potatoes and tossed salad, followed by luscious puddings such as rum soaked raisins with mascarpone. Officially, they say bookings are 'accepted'; 'advised' might be wiser. • Open all day L£ & D££ daily • Closed Nov-Xmas & 1 Jan-Easter • MasterCard, Visa •

Schull   The Bunratty Inn

Schull Co Cork

PUB   Tel: 028 28341

This comfortable pub serves home-cooked bar food and there is outside eating in summer. Call ahead off-season. • Closed 25 Dec & Good Fri • MasterCard, Visa •

Schull   La Coquille

Schull Co Cork

RESTAURANT   Tel: 028 28642   Fax: 028 28573

Jean-Michel Cahier's chic little restaurant is situated in the main street, convenient to the harbour. Unlike the majority of restaurants in the area, it sets seafood in context on a wide-ranging menu which includes more red meats and poultry than most places. Competently handled classics are the main feature, in starters like smoked salmon and crab mayonnaise, well-made soups and main courses such as quail with brandy and raisins, fillet steak in pepper sauce and sole on the bone. Desserts include an excellent tarte tatin and M. Cahier's cheeseboard does justice to the quality of local produce. Professional service is provided by French staff. Disappointingly, they no longer serve lunch, inscrutably explaining that "it's to do with the weather". Pity – it's a great place to spend an afternoon when the weather's bad. • D££ Mon-Sat • Closed 25 Dec & Feb • Diners, MasterCard, Visa •

Schull   Corthna Lodge Country House

Schull Co Cork

ACCOMMODATION   Tel: 028 28517   Fax: 028 28032

Situated up the hill from Schull, commanding good countryside and sea views, this roomy modern house has been one of the best places to stay in the area since opening in 1991. All of the six rooms are suitable for disabled guests, all are non-smoking and, despite the fact that they are all shower-only, the bedrooms are very comfortable with good amenities. The atmosphere is hospitable and easy-going, with plenty of space for guests to sit around and relax (both indoors, in a pleasant and comfortably furnished sitting room and outdoors, on a terrace overlooking the lovely garden towards the islands of Roaring Water Bay). • Acc£-££ • Closed Oct-Mar •

Schull   East End Hotel

Main Street Schull Co Cork

HOTEL   Tel: 028 28101   Fax: 028 28012

This modest hotel on the main street overlooks Schull harbour, is family-run and very friendly. Non-resident sailors and fishing people are welcome to come and have showers. Most bedrooms have en-suite facilities (some shower only) and each year sees some improvements – in 1998 direct dial phones were installed in all rooms and a large paved area completed at the back of the hotel. • Acc£-££ • Open all year • Amex, Diners, MasterCard, Visa •

Schull   Restaurant In Blue

Crookhaven Road Schull Co Cork

RESTAURANT   Tel/Fax: 028-28305

About two miles outside Schull (near Corthna Lodge), Burvill Evans and Christine Crabtree's Restaurant in Blue is on the R592 to Toormore. Thick walls, small windows and homely antique furnishings create a relaxed cottagey atmosphere. The dining room is divided between a high room which was originally a barn and an adjoining conservatory which overlooks a very natural garden. His ingredients are carefully sourced and he is adamant about the care to be taken: local seafood stars on the menu with all fish bought on the bone and filleted by him; similarly, breast of local free-range chicken is also bought whole and boned out then, perhaps, rolled and stuffed with spring onions and oyster mushrooms, and served with delicious organic vegetables. Finish with local cheeses or a quartet of desserts (in "Guess What? Pots") – small servings of four daily desserts, served in ramekins on a large plate. • D££ daily • Closed Nov-Apr • Amex, Diners, MasterCard, Visa •

Schull

T J Newman's

Corner House Main Street Schull Co Cork

PUB

Tel: 028 28223

"As was" is the record of our most recent visit to Newman's – a remark that will please and reassure the many who have come to love this characterful and delightfully old-fashioned little pub. Just up the hill from the harbour, it's a special home-from-home for visiting sailors. • Closed 25 Dec & Good Fri • No credit cards •

Shanagarry

Ballymaloe House

Shanagarry Midleton Co Cork

COUNTRY HOUSE/RESTAURANT 🏛

Tel: 021 652531   Fax: 021 652021

email: bmaloe@iol.ie

Ireland's most famous country house hotel, Ballymaloe was one of the first country houses to open its doors to guests when Myrtle and her husband, the late Ivan Allen, opened The Yeats Room restaurant in 1964. Accommodation followed in 1967 and since then a unique network of family enterprises has developed around Ballymaloe House – including not only the farmlands and gardens that supply so much of the kitchen produce, but also a craft and kitchenware shop, a wine company, a company producing chutneys and sauce, the Crawford Gallery Café in Cork city and, of course, Tim and Darina Allen's internationally acclaimed Cookery School. Yet, despite the fame, Ballymaloe is still most remarkable for its unspoilt charm: Myrtle – now rightly receiving international recognition for a lifetime's work "recapturing forgotten flavours, and preserving those that may soon die"- is ably assisted by her children and now their families too. The house, modestly described in its Blue Book entry as "a large family farmhouse" is in the middle of the family's 400 acre farm, but the description fails to do justice to the gracious nature of the original house, or the sensitively designed later additions. The intensely restorative atmosphere of Ballymaloe is still as strong as ever; there are few greater pleasures than a fine Ballymaloe dinner followed by the relaxed comforts provided by a delightful, thoughtfully furnished (but not over decorated) country bedroom. Groundfloor courtyard rooms are suitable for wheelchairs.

Restaurant ★

A food philosophy centred on using only the highest quality ingredients is central to everything done at Ballymaloe, where much of the produce comes from their own farm and gardens. The rest, including seafood from Ballycotton and Kenmare, and meats from the trusted local butcher, comes from leading local producers. Rory O'Connell (who is Darina Allen's brother) has been head chef at Ballymaloe since 1995 and has proved himself supremely suited to translating the Ballymaloe philosophy into cooking which takes account of international trends but is utterly true to itself. Although based on skilful interpretations of classic French and Irish country cooking, the style is light and colourful, occasionally witty; presentation is creative but not over-complicated, allowing the beauty of the food to speak for itself. The restaurant is in a series of domestic-sized dining rooms (some for non-smokers) and guests are called to their tables from the conservatory or drawing room, where aperitifs are served. Rory presents a daily 5-course dinner menu (£31.50 at the time of going to press) with vegetarian dishes given a leaf symbol. A good beginning in early summer might be Ballycotton crab soup with rouille and croutons, while second courses might include classics like lobster mayonnaise and asparagus with hollandaise sauce – local lobster, home grown asparagus and skilfully made sauces based on free range eggs. Then, half a dozen main courses will include two or three imaginative fish dishes plus, perhaps, succulent, crisp-skinned roast duck (from a local farmyard) with a Madeira sauce and wonderful fresh peas. There is always a strong vegetarian choice, typically courgette blossoms stuffed with Ardsallagh goats cheese & parsley pesto. Lovely simple side dishes – Shanagarry new potatoes, young carrots and a green salad – accompany. A cheese course follows – Irish farmhouse cheeses, of course, in excellent condition – then the famous dessert trolley is wheeled to the table, laden with irresistible things like lemon souffle, fresh raspberries, chocolate hazelnut tart and praline ice cream (served from the ice bowl – a Ballymaloe invention). Finish with coffee or tea and home-made petits fours, served in the drawing room – and perhaps a drink from the small bar before retiring contentedly to bed. • Acc£££ • L££ & D£££ daily • Closed 24-26 Dec • Amex, Diners, MasterCard, Visa •

Shanagarry

The Garden Café

Ballymaloe Cookery School Shanagarry Co Cork

RESTAURANT   Tel: 021 646422   Fax: 021 646909

When this colourful little addition to the Ballymaloe empire opened on Easter Saturday, 1998 it was full within half an hour. It has stayed like that ever since, and it is not hard to see why. Simple, well prepared food (with the Ballymaloe imprimatur) at rock bottom prices is difficult to resist. In addition to the many other visitors, the café also has a captive market of students from the famous cookery school nearby. The menu takes its cue from the fabulous gardens which surround the café and school (there is a £3 entry charge if you want to tour them). Organic fruit and vegetables feature prominently, while meat and fish are sourced locally and cooked in a wood burning oven. For breakfast there are plenty of freshly squeezed fruit juices and a superb selection of Frittatas at £3. The Mexican Frittata, with onion, chilli, cherry tomatoes and coriander, is particularly good, although the Full Irish, with bacon, mushrooms, parsley and chives, will accommodate more pedestrian tastes. At lunchtime the Thai fish cakes with cucumber relish are surprisingly mild but very tasty, while another starter, the spinach and mushroom pancake (£4.95) is big enough to suffice as a meal in itself. Home made elderflower cordial makes a delicious accompaniment, although there is also a commendable array of quarter-bottles of wine. Service is excellent. There is a lovely view over fields and down to the sea. At the time of going to press the café was only open for breakfast and lunch but is due to open for dinner at the beginning of 1999. • L£ & D£-££ daily • Closed Oct-Apr •

Skibbereen

Liss Ard Lake Lodge

Skibbereeen Co Cork

HOTEL   Tel: 028 40000   Fax: 028 40001

email: lissardlakelodge@tinet.ie   www.lissard.com

This Victorian lodge opened in 1994 as a most unusual small luxury hotel. It is set in extensive gardens (which are open to the public) and has been designed and renovated with oriental simplicity, thereby enhancing the garden and water views framed by every window. Rooms – all suites except 1 double – combine clean-lined simplicity with unexpected amenities: mini-bars,TV units with video, and hi-fi. Equally unusual bathrooms are finished to a very high standard. • D£££ Wed-Mon • Acc££££ • Closed Jan & Feb • Amex, Diners, MasterCard, Visa •

Timoleague

Lettercollum House Restaurant

Timoleague Co Cork

RESTAURANT   Tel: 023 46251   Fax: 023 46276

email: conmc@iol.ie   www.clon.ie/letterco.html

Con McLoughlin and Karen Austin's restaurant is in the Chapel of their Victorian house. The Chapel retains its stained glass windows, thereby providing a striking contrast to the lively modern food for which the restaurant has earned its reputation, both locally and further afield. Carefully sourced ingredients include organic produce from the walled garden as well as the best of local meats and seafood. This is cooked and presented in a style that is described as "based on classical French cuisine but with strong ethnic and vegetarian influences." The result is exciting food. Karen also runs cooking classes and there are all sorts of special events, including theatre and music nights. • L£ Sun, D££ Mon-Sun high season • Closed Jan-mid Mar • Amex, Diners, MasterCard, Visa •

Toormore

Fortview House

Gurtyowen Toormore Goleen Skibbereen Co Cork

FARM STAY   Tel/Fax: 028 35324

Violet & Richard Connell's remarkable farmhouse in the hills behind Goleen is immaculate. It is beautifully furnished, with country pine and antiques, brass and iron beds in en-suite bedrooms (that are all individually decorated) and with all sorts of thoughtful little details to surprise and delight. Violet loves cooking, and provides guests with a remarkable choice at breakfast, including Tom & Giana Ferguson's Gubbeen cheese, made down the road. • Acc£ • Closed Nov-Mar • No credit cards •

Union Hall

The Baybery

Gladore Bay Union Hall **Co Cork**

RESTAURANT

Tel/Fax: 028 33605

email: baybery@iol.ie   www.interactsi/baybery

Francis and Kathleen Broadbery opened this stylish little restaurant in Union Hall village in the spring of 1998. It's a pleasant room, with interesting slightly crafty furniture, fresh flowers, good tableware and a welcoming open fire on a chilly day. Menus offer a mixture of simple dishes highlighting the goodness of local and organic produce, especially seafood, and lively Mediterranean/global cuisine style dishes which are competently cooked and well presented. Service is charming and helpful and there's a pleasant relaxed atmosphere. • D££ daily high season • Closed Xmas & New Year • MasterCard, Visa •

Union Hall

Shearwater

Keelbeg Union Hall **Co Cork**

ACCOMMODATION

Tel/Fax: 028 33178

Adela Nugent's B&B is located close to Keelbeg pier, on an elevated site overlooking Glandore harbour and the surrounding countryside. All bedrooms are good-sized and comfortably furnished with en-suite facilities (only one with bath); most rooms overlook the harbour. The breakfast room and TV room also have views, and there's a patio for guests' use in fine weather. • Acc£ • Closed Nov-Apr •

Youghal

Aherne's Seafood Restaurant

163 North Main Street Youghal Co Cork

RESTAURANT/ACCOMMODATION

Tel: 024 92424   Fax: 024 93633

email: ahernes@tinet.ie

Now in its third generation of family ownership, one of the most remarkable features of Aherne's is the sheer warmth of the FitzGibbon family's hospitality (and their enormous enthusiasm for the business) which, since 1993, has included seriously luxurious accommodation. It is for its food – and, especially, the ultra-fresh seafood which comes straight from the fishing boats in Youghal harbour – that Aherne's is best known, however. While John FitzGibbon supervises the front of house his brother David reigns over a busy kitchen, catering for full meals at lunch and dinner (in the dining room), as well as lighter food served in both bars. The bar food tends towards simplicity, – oysters, chowder, smoked salmon (all served with the renowned moist dark brown yeast bread) – relying on its sheer freshness to make its own statement.

Rooms

The stylish en-suite rooms at Aherne's are generously sized and individually decorated to a very high standard; all are furnished with antiques and have luxurious, beautifully finished bathrooms. Housekeeping is exemplary and excellent breakfasts are served in a warm and elegantly furnished residents' dining room. Newer rooms, recently added, bring the total to 12 and are equipped to give the option of self-catering if required. • L£-££. D££-£££ daily • Acc£££ • Closed Xmas wk • Amex, Diners, MasterCard, Visa •

DONEGAL

Donegal is big country. It may not have Ireland's highest mountains, it may not be Ireland's biggest county, but there's still a largeness of spirit about this rugged northwestern corner which lingers long and fondly in the memory of those who visit it. For many folk, particularly those from Northern Ireland, Donegal is the holiday area par excellence. But in recent years the development of industries in the eastern part of the county, and the strengthening of the fishing industry, particularly at the hugely busy port of Killybegs, has led to a more balanced economy which actually makes Donegal a more attractive place for the modern visitor, even if some of today's international industries can come and go with alarming rapidity. However, much and all as Donegal county aspires to be a place where people can live and make a living on a year-round basis, nevertheless it still is witness to nature on the grand scale, a place assaulted by the winds and weather of the Atlantic Ocean if it is given the slightest chance. But that is part of Donegal's enduring attraction. For the fact is that here, in some of Ireland's most rugged territory, you will find many sheltered and hospitable little places whose comforts are emphasised by the challenging nature of their broader environment. And, needless to say, it is simply, startlingly utterly beautiful as well.

Local Attractions and Information

Glenveagh National Park (castle, gardens, parkland)	074 37088
Carrick Carr Memorial Traditional Music w/e (June)	073 39009
Donegal Highlands Hillwalking/Irish Language (adults)	073 30248
Church Hill Letterkenny Glebe House & Gallery	074 37071

Annagry   Danny Minnie's Restaurant

Annagry The Rosses Co Donegal
RESTAURANT/ACCOMMODATION   Tel/Fax: 075 48201

The O'Donnell family have run Danny Minnie's since 1962, and it never fails to please. Hidden behind a frontage of overgrown creepers a surprise awaits, where guests are suddenly surrounded by antiques and elegantly appointed tables, receive a warm welcome from Terri O'Donnell and helpful service from attentive waitresses. The menu is presented in both Irish and English (but not the wine list, mercifully) and Michael O'Donnell's cooking is a fine match for the surroundings – fine, with imaginative saucing, but not at all pompous. On a wide-ranging à la carte menu, seafood stars in the main courses – lobster and other shellfish, availability permitting, and baked fillet of turbot with prawn sauce and pesto, perhaps, or monkfish and courgette with a ginger & herb cream. There is also a strong selection of meats and poultry, including Donegal lamb, typically served with caramelized onions and a rich dark basil sauce. Vegetables are a strength and desserts can be relied on to create an appropriately dramatic finale.

Rooms

Accommodation is also available in eight non-smoking rooms, five of them en-suite and one suitable for disabled guests. Although not viewed for the guide, they are ITB registered. • D££ Mon-Sun, L summer only • Acc££ • Closed 1 wk Xmas & Feb, also Mar • MasterCard, Visa •

Ardara   Nancy's

Front Street Ardara Co Donegal
PUB   Tel: 075 41187

This famous pub, in the village renowned for its tweeds and handknits, is a cosy, welcoming place, with five or six small rooms packed with bric a brac and plenty of tables and chairs for the comfortable consumption of good home-made food, especially seafood. The renowned soups – chowder in summer and a wonderful vegetable broth in the colder months – head up a good choice of food, including mussels, smoked salmon, oysters, excellent burgers (made by the local butcher), vegetarian choices like ploughman's or veggie-burgers – and home-made apple pie & cream for pudding. Live music too. • L£ & D£ daily • Closed 25 Dec & Good Fri • No credit cards •

Ballybofey

Kee's Hotel

Stranorlar Ballybofey Co Donegal

HOTEL/RESTAURANT   Tel: 074 31018   Fax: 074 31917

This centrally located, all-year hotel is popular with business and leisure guests. It has an unusually long line of continuous family ownership, having been in the Kee family since 1892. Major changes have been taking place over the last few years and public areas have undergone radical renovations. These include a new foyer, meeting rooms and a lift, all completed in 1998. Bedrooms, of which 18 were newly built last year, include a suite, a mini-suite, one room suitable for disabled guests and 20 executive rooms, some with views of the Blue Stack mountains. Rooms are regularly refurbished and very comfortable with good bathrooms, fresh flowers and complimentary mineral water. The hotel's excellent leisure facilities are available free to residents, who have direct access from their rooms. Children are welcome – cots and high chairs are available and there's a crèche at certain times in the leisure centre. Special breaks offered by the hotel include a novel "Post Christmas Recovery Break".

The Looking Glass

Lovely hand-worked tapestries are the most striking decoration in this pleasant warm-toned restaurant, which is in two areas with plenty of alcoves for privacy. Since his arrival in 1994, head chef Frederic Souty has made big changes to what was a country hotel menu. His stylish, confident cooking is seen through seasonal menus, plus daily specials which particularly emphasise seafood. The style is indicated in starters such as blini of oyster with balsamic vinaigrette and tartelette of lambs kidney and bacon. The main courses such as roast rack of lamb with garlic confit and spring vegetables and the catch of the day which, if you're lucky, might be grilled shelled lobster with a lemon cream and baby vegetables. There's a cheese trolley and desserts, which are taken from the à la carte menu, could include a "Tasting Plate", the perfect choice for the undecided. • Bar L£, D££ daily • Open all year • Amex, Diners, MasterCard, Visa •

Bruckless

Bruckless House

Bruckless Co Donegal

FARM STAY   Tel: 073 37071   Fax: 073 37070

email: bruc@iol.ie   www.iol.ie/bruc/bruckless.html

Since 1984 Clive and Joan Evans have been welcoming guests to their home 12 miles west of Donegal town. Although on a working farm, and registered as a farmhouse, the term doesn't do justice to this lovely 18th-century building, which is set in 19 acres of woodland and gardens overlooking Bruckless Bay. Family furniture collected through a Hong Kong connection add an unexpected dimension to the elegant reception rooms and generous, comfortably furnished bedrooms. The four bedrooms are all non-smoking and include two single rooms and one bathroom. • Acc£-££ • Closed Oct-Apr • Amex, MasterCard, Visa •

Bunbeg

Ostan Gweedore

Bunbeg Co Donegal

HOTEL   Tel: 075 31177   Fax: 075 31726

email: boyle@iol.ie   www.celtic-internet.com/ostangweedore/index.htm

Although its architectural style may not be to today's taste, this hotel was built to make the most of the view – and this it does very well. Most of the comfortable en-suite bedrooms (plus three suites) and all the public areas, including the recently refurbished restaurant and the Library Bar ("the most westerly reading room on the Atlantic seaboard") have superb views over the shoreline and Mount Errigal. It's ideal for families, with its wonderful beach and outdoor activities, including tennis, pitch & putt and day visits to nearby Tory Island. Wet days are looked after too, with indoor leisure facilities, including a 17 metre swimming pool, jacuzzi and gym, all supervised by qualified staff. This romantic setting means weddings are popular (functions from 10-350 are catered for banqueting-style, up to 250 for conferences) and at the time of going to press the hotel was offering an imaginative "Flybreak", including a return flight Dublin to Donegal, overnight stay and dinner "on the edge of a continent', from IR£145. Check for latest offers. • Acc££ • Closed Dec-Feb • Amex, Diners, MasterCard, Visa •

Please note that price indications are intended only as a guideline - always check current prices (and special offers) when making reservations.

Bundoran

Le Chateaubrianne

Sligo Road Bundoran Co Donegal

Tel/Fax: 072 42160

RESTAURANT

Since opening here in 1993 Brian and Anne Loughlin have established this welcoming and very professionally run establishment as the leading restaurant in the area. Brian's cooking is classic French with New Irish overtones and he is a strong supporter of local produce. Imaginative dinner menus (sensibly priced according to the choice of main course) offer a well-balanced selection with local seafood well-represented, also game in season, with interesting vegetarian options available. Sunday lunch provides something for everyone by offering a clever combination of traditional roasts and more adventurous fare; the same high standard of cooking applies and the meal will be nicely finished off with coffee and petits fours. • L£ Sun, D££ Mon-Sat • Closed all Jan, Bank Hols • Amex, MasterCard, Visa •

Donegal

St Ernan's House Hotel

Donegal Town Co Donegal

Tel: 073 21065   Fax: 073 22098

COUNTRY HOUSE

Set on its own wooded island connected to the mainland by a causeway, tranquillity is the main characteristic of Brian and Carmel O'Dowd's unique country house hotel. Spacious public rooms have log fires and antique furniture and, while they vary in size and outlook, the individually decorated bedrooms are furnished to a high standard. All are en-suite (2 shower only) and have good amenities including (surprisingly perhaps) television, while most also have lovely views. • Acc£££-££££ • Closed Nov-Easter •

Restaurant

The dining room is mainly intended for resident guests, but reservations may be taken from non-residents if there is room. Gabrielle Doyle has been Head Chef since 1992 and produces daily 5-course country house-style dinner menus based on local produce. Vegetarian dishes on request. • D£££ • MasterCard, Visa •

Dunkineely

Castle Murray House Hotel

Dunkineely Co Donegal

Tel: 073 37022   Fax: 073 37330

HOTEL/RESTAURANT

Just a mile off the main Killybegs-Donegal road, Thierry and Clare Duclos' beautifully located clifftop hotel has wonderful sea and coastal views over the ruined castle after which it is named. Since they opened in 1991, the Duclos have made numerous improvements, including the addition of a little bar and a residents' sitting room. More recently, the seating for summer meals was extended by the addition of a large verandah complete with awning. Bedrooms are all quite large and fairly comfortably furnished with a mixture of utilitarian modern units and a sprinkling of antiques; all have a double and single bed, most have sea views and there are extra beds and cots available for families on request. Good breakfasts are served in bedrooms or the restaurant.

Restaurant

The restaurant is on the seaward corner of the hotel and maximises the impact of the dramatic view, including the castle (which is floodlit at night). Tweed curtains and an open fire make for real warmth in this exposed location, even in winter. Owner-chef Thierry Duclos' multi-choice menus (basically 3-course, plus options of soup and sorbet), are sensibly priced according to the choice of main course and offer a wide choice, including vegetarian dishes. Seafood is the speciality of the house in the summer months; in winter there are more red meats, poultry and game. • L£ Sun, D££ daily • Acc££ • Closed 1st 2 wks Feb & Mon, Tues low season • MasterCard, Visa •

Fahan

Restaurant St John's

Fahan Inishowen Peninsula Co Donegal

Tel: 077 60289   Fax: 077 60612

RESTAURANT/COUNTRY HOUSE

Irish Lamb Award Winner

Since 1980 Reggie Ryan and Phil Mcafee have run Restaurant St John's, in their substantial period house overlooking Lough Swilly, to growing acclaim. The restaurant has grown of late and now has a large conservatory with Lough views in addition to the original rooms. Phil's cooking combines a respect for tradition and understanding of the value of simplicity with a willingness to experiment, ensuring that the many guests who regularly return always have a meal that is both stimulating and relaxing. Given the location, seafood is very popular but Phil's table d'hôte and à la carte menus are based on a wide range of local ingredients, including game in winter. Donegal mountain lamb, which she cooks in many different ways, is an established favourite. A fairly priced wine list includes nine house wines, a special seasonal selection and a good choice of half bottles. Restaurant St John's "Rack of Donegal Mountain Lamb with Rosemary and Mascarpone Risotto" is the winner of our Bord Bia Irish Lamb Award • D££ daily, L£ Sun • Closed Feb, 25 Dec, New Year & Good Fri •

Accommodation
Five en-suite rooms, comfortably furnished with antiques, were recently added. • Acc££ • Closed Feb, 25 Dec, New Year & Good Fri •

Greencastle   Kealys Seafood Bar

The Harbour Greencastle Co Donegal
PUB/RESTAURANT   **Tel/Fax: 077 81010**
email: kealys@iol.ie

James and Tricia Kealy's excellent seafood restaurant has more than doubled in size since it opened in 1989, but it has remained true to its original character. Under-stated quality is probably a fair description of the tone of a place that has always valued simplicity – the restaurant is a key establishment in a major fishing port and still retains the original bar at its heart. Lunch menus are shortish and the dishes offered simple; however the choice is very adequate and the quality of food and cooking admirable. Dinner is more ambitious and, in addition to a wide selection of ultra-fresh seafood, James includes a fair selection of meat and poultry – steaks, Inishowen lamb, duck – as well as vegetarian dishes. James bakes a variety breads and uses local organic vegetables and farmhouse cheeses – typically Gubbeen, St Killian, Boilie and Cashel Blue.• L£, D££ daily • Closed 25 Dec & Good Fri • Amex, Diners, MasterCard, Visa •

Letterkenny   Castle Grove Country House

Ballymaleel Letterkenny Co Donegal
COUNTRY HOUSE/RESTAURANT   **Tel: 074 51118   Fax: 074 51384**

Parkland designed by "Capability" Brown in the mid 18th-century creates a wonderful setting for Raymond and Mary Sweeney's lovely period house overlooking Lough Swilly. The last few years have seen major changes, including a new conservatory and a larger new restaurant. Most recently, the adjoining coach house has been developed to make seven new bedrooms and a small conference room, and the original walled garden is currently being restored. Bedrooms (all now non-smoking) are generally spacious and furnished to a high standard; all have en-suite or private shower and/or bathroom and good amenities. Very good breakfasts include a choice of fish as well as traditional Irish breakfast, home-made breads and preserves. There is a high standard of maintenance and housekeeping and staff are friendly and helpful. Two boats belonging to the house are available for fishing on Lough Swilly.

Restaurant
Dawn Bagnall has been head chef at Castle Grove since 1997. She offers several menus -table'd'hôte, à la carte and vegetarian – at dinner, plus 2 or 3-course set lunch menus. The style is "New Irish Cuisine" with international overtones and menus are based on local ingredients, including home grown herbs, vegetables and soft fruit, as well as local seafood including wild salmon and Swilly oysters. • L£ Sun, D££ daily • Closed 23-27 Dec & Good Fri • Amex, Diners, MasterCard, Visa •

Lough Eske   Ardnamona House

Lough Eske Co Donegal
COUNTRY HOUSE   **Tel: 073 22650   Fax: 073 22819**
email: ardnamon@tempoweb.com   www.tempoweb.com/ardnamon

It's hard to credit that Kieran and Annabel Clarke's secluded Victorian house overlooking Lough Eske is only a couple of miles from Donegal town. Its sense of other-worldliness is partly due to the location, but it's also an effect achieved by the glorious gardens, which were first planted by Sir Arthur Wallace in the 1880s. This is a very gentle, hospitable house and draws people who value its peace and beauty. Front rooms have lovely views over the lough to the mountains beyond, but all are individualistic with private bathrooms (and a peaceful outlook through rhododendrons and azaleas which have received international acclaim). Gardeners will enjoy doing the garden trail (guide leaflet provided and all plants labelled) and special interest groups are welcome to visit the gardens by arrangement. There are also miles of walks through ancient oak forests full of mosses and ferns and private boating and fishing on the lough. Except on

Sundays, communal dinner is available for residents, by arrangement, at 8 pm.(£18; nice wine list from £10.50). • Acc££ • Closed Dec-Feb • Amex, Diners, MasterCard, Visa •

Lough Eske   Harvey's Point Country Hotel

Lough Eske Co Donegal

HOTEL/RESTAURANT Tel: 073 22208   **Fax: 073 22352**

email: harveyspoint@tinet.ie   www.commerce.ie//harveys.tt/

In a stunning location on the shores of Lough Eske, this unusual hotel has a distinctly alpine atmosphere, with chalet-style buildings, pergolas and covered walkways joining the residential area to the main bars and restaurant. Rooms, which include executive suites with four-posters and which have all been refurbished recently, are based on a Swiss design; they have good amenities and direct access to verandah and gardens. Dinner dances and special breaks are often offered at Harvey's Point; telephone for details.

Restaurant

Original paintings by a talented family member, well-appointed tables and the beautiful view make a promising start to the meal, and Marc Gysling's cooking – which is based on Swiss training with Irish influences – does not disappoint. Menus are imaginative but not over-fussy, local produce is used to good effect, the saucing is good and so are details – for example farmhouse cheeses, which are served plated, come with a delicious home-made nut bread. Service is attentive and professional. The wine list includes a range of 'everyday easy drinking' wines (all under £20) and a good selection of half bottles. • L£ Tues-Sun, D££ daily • Acc££ • Closed mid-week Nov-Mar • Amex, Diners, MasterCard, Visa •

The best – independently assessed

Portsalon   Croaghross Cottage

Portsalon Letterkenny Co Donegal

ACCOMMODATION   **Tel/Fax: 074 59548**

email: jkdeane@iol.ie

John and Kay Deane's new single-storey house was purpose built and enjoys a lovely location on the Fanad peninsula, overlooking Lough Swilly. It's within 5 minutes walk of a great beach – and the renowned 100 year old Portsalon Golf Course – and very convenient to Glenveagh National Park. Three of the five bedrooms have full bathrooms and open onto a sun terrace, while the two side rooms overlook a landscaped rock garden – one of them is especially suitable for wheelchair users, who can park close to the room. Residents' dinner is, like breakfast, based on local ingredients and good home cooking, with home-made breads and farmhouse cheeses always available (£15 please book ahead; very reasonable short wine list). Barbecues are sometimes arranged when the weather is favourable and, although officially closed in winter, bookings can be made by arrangement. This is an attractive option for a group, as the house is centrally heated throughout and the living room has a big open fire. The Deanes also have a 3-bedroom self-catering cottage available nearby. • Acc££ • Closed Oct-mid- Mar • MasterCard, Visa •

Rathmullan   Fort Royal Hotel

Rathmullan Letterkenny Co Donegal

HOTEL   **Tel: 074 58100   Fax: 074 58103**

Overlooking the sea, and with easy access to sandy beaches, the Fletcher family's attractive Victorian hotel is set in 19 acres of lawn and woodland above Lough Swilly. Public rooms are spacious, well-proportioned and comfortably furnished in country house style, with big armchairs and open fires. Well-appointed bedrooms (all en-suite, most with bath and shower, a few bath only) are designed for relaxation and enjoy a pleasant outlook over wooded grounds. Much of the food at Fort Royal comes from the hotel's own walled gardens and is cooked by Robin and Ann Fletcher's son, Timothy, who has been head chef since 1995. Fort Royal also has croquet, tennis, squash and golf on the premises and activities such as riding and fishing nearby. It's a good base for family holidays or visiting places of local interest, including Glenveagh National Park and Glebe House, the artist Derek Hill's former home, which has a museum and gallery next door. • Acc£££ • Closed Nov-mid- Mar • Amex, Diners, MasterCard, Visa •

Rathmullan

HOTEL/RESTAURANT

Rathmullan House

Rathmullan Co Donegal

Tel: 074 58188   Fax: 074 58200

email: rathhse@iol.ie

Built as a summer house by the Batt banking family of Belfast in the 1800s, Rathmullan has been run by Bob and Robin Wheeler as a country house hotel since 1961, aided by their son Mark, manager since 1987. Set in lovely gardens on the shores of Lough Swilly, this gracious early nineteenth century house remains friendly and informal. Although on quite a large scale and furnished to a high standard, the public areas, which include three elegant sitting rooms, are not too formal – and there's a delightful cellar bar which can be very relaxed. Bedrooms vary in decor, facilities and cost to suit different requirements and budgets – there are luxurious garden suites (close to the Egyptian Baths, swimming pool and leisure facilities) as well as the unpretentious old-fashioned comforts of family rooms at the top of the house. Donegal has an other-worldliness that is increasingly hard to capture in the traditional family holiday areas, and the laid-back charm of Rathmullan House – albeit given invisible backbone by the professionalism of the Wheeler family and their staff – somehow symbolises that special sense of place.

Restaurant

The dining room with its unusual tented ceiling makes the most of the garden outlook and provides a fine setting for Seamus Douglas's country house cooking as well as the tremendous breakfasts for which Rathmullan is justly famous.• D££ daily • Acc£££ • Closed Jan-Mar • Amex, Diners, MasterCard, Visa •

Rossnowlagh

HOTEL/RESTAURANT

Sand House Hotel

Rossnowlagh Co Donegal

Tel: 072 51777   Fax: 072 52100

email: sandhoouse@tinet.ie

Mary and Brian Britton's famous crenellated hotel is perched on the edge of a stunning sandy beach two miles long. The wonderful sea views and easy access to the beach are great attractions of the Sand House. Many of the bedrooms have a superb outlook and all are very comfortable, with good bathrooms – and everyone can enjoy the view from the sun lounge (known as the Atlantic Conservatory). Immaculate maintenance and a high standard of furnishing have always been a special feature, and a major refurbishment of the ground floor, including reception, bars and lounges, will be completed for the 1999 season. But it is nevertheless the hospitality of the Britton family and staff (not to mention Mary Britton's reputation for exceptional housekeeping) which is the real appeal of this remarkable hotel.

Restaurant

The restaurant is rather unexpectedly at the front of the hotel (and therefore faces inland) but is well-appointed, in keeping with the rest of the hotel. Sid Davis, Head Chef since 1993, presents 5-course dinner menus that change daily. It is wholesome fare and simplest choices are usually the wisest; meals finish well with a choice of Irish cheeses or desserts that include very good fruit pies.• L£ Sun, D££ daily • Acc£££ • Closed Nov-Easter • Amex, Diners, MasterCard, Visa •

Rossnowlagh

PUB/ACCOMMODATION

Smugglers Creek Inn

Rossnowlagh Co Donegal

Tel: 072 52366

High up on the cliffs, overlooking Donegal Bay and the Blue Stack Mountains, this inn actually dates back to 1845. Most of what you see today is due to the efforts of the present owner, Conor Britton, who has undertaken a major refurbishment and extension programme since he took over in 1991. (And it's not over yet – as we go to press he's about to begin an extension and build a new kitchen, both due for completion by the 1999 season.) Developments to date have been very sympathetically done, with stonework, stone-flagged floors and open fires providing both atmosphere and comfort. Comforting traditional bar food – chowder, home-baked bread, garlic mussels – has always been good. However, items previously enjoyed in the bar – moules marinières, home-made pâté with hot toast – are also on the restaurant menu which is predictably strong on seafood but also provides a decent choice for carnivores and vegetarians too.

Accommodation

There are five en-suite rooms at the inn, two with full bathrooms, three shower only. (£24.50 pps, single suppl £10.50). • Meals£-££ • Acc£ • Closed Mon & Tues, Oct-Easter • MasterCard, Visa •

Tory Island

Ostan Thoraig (Hotel Tory)

West End Tory Island Co Donegal

HOTEL **Tel: 074 35920 Fax: 074 35613**

The Gaeltacht (Irish-speaking) island of Tory lies 5 miles off the north-west corner of Donegal and, in spite of its exposed position, has been inhabited for four thousand years. Perhaps not surprisingly, this other-worldly island managed quite well without an hotel until recently, but once Patrick and Berney Doohan's Ostan Thoraigh was built in 1994 it quickly became the centre of the island's social activities – or, to be more precise, The People's Bar in the hotel quickly became the centre. The hotel is beside the little harbour where the ferries bring in visitors from mainland ports. Although simple, it provides comfortable en-suite accommodation with telephone and television. A special feature of the island is its 'school' of primitive art (founded with the support of well-known artist Derek Hill of nearby Glebe House and Gallery, Church Hill). It even has a king as a founder member: the present King of the Tory is Patsy Dan Rogers, who has exhibited his colourful primitive paintings of the island throughout the British Isles and in America. A tiny gallery on Tory provides exhibition space for the current group of island artists. Tory is accessible by ferry (subject to weather conditions) from several mainland ports – telephone 075-31320 for details, or ask at the hotel. • Acc££ • Closed Oct-Easter • Amex, Diners, MasterCard, Visa •

GALWAY

Galway has to be Ireland's most generous county. You get two counties for the price of one, neatly divided by the handsome sweep of island-studded Lough Corrib. And as a bonus, where the Corrib tumbles into Galway Bay, you get one of Ireland's liveliest cities, a bustling place which cheerfully sees itself as being linked to Spain and the great world beyond the Atlantic. However much the Spanish links may have been romanticised as they filter through the mists of time, the fact is that today Galway city is a place confident of itself. Its strength in the west, when seen in the national context, is a welcome counterbalance to the inevitable domination of the greater Dublin area on the east coast. For although Galway city's population is only a fraction of Dublin's total, nevertheless the western capital is more than ready to stand fair square for the pride of Connacht and a positive assertion of the qualities of life beyond the Pale and west of the Shannon. It does so with pleasure and in the diversity of its territory. Lough Corrib is both a geographical and psychological divide. East of it, there's flatter country, home to hunting packs of mythic lore. West of the Corrib – which used itself to be a major thoroughfare and is now as ever a place of angling renown – you're very quickly into the high ground and moorland which sweep up to the Twelve Pins and other splendid peaks, wonderful mountains which enthusiasts would claim as the most beautiful in all Ireland. Their heavily indented coastline means this region is Connemara, the Land of the Sea, where earth, rock and ocean intermix in one of Ireland's most extraordinary landscapes. Beyond, to the south, the Aran Islands are a place apart, yet they too are part of the Galway mix in this fantastical county which has its own magical light coming in over the sea. And yet all its extraordinary variety happens within very manageable distances. For instance, in the western part of Galway city, the mature and leafy suburb of Taylor's Hill speaks eloquently of a quietly comfortable way of life which has been established for well over a century. Yet much less than an hour's drive away, whether along the shores of Galway Bay or taking the Corrib route via Oughterard, you'll quickly find yourself in the rugged heart of Connemara, where the scatter of cottages bespeaks a different way of life, an austere way of life which is every bit as significant a part of that remarkable Galway tapestry which enchants Galwegians and visitors alike.

Local Attractions and Information

Galway City

Galway Arts Festival (July)	091 583800
Island Ferries Teo	(Aran Islands from Rossaveal) 091 568903 / 561767
O'Brien Shipping Ltd	(Aran Islands ferries) 091 567283
Tourist Information	091 563081
Town Hall Theatre	091 569755

Co Galway

Aran Islands	Inis Mor, Ionad Arann (heritage centre) 099 61355
Aughrim	Ballinasloe, Battle of Aughrim Centre 0905 73939 / 565201
Clifden	Connemara Pony Show (mid August) 095 21863
Gort	Thoor Ballylee (Yeats' Tower) 091 631436 / 563081
Tuam	Little Mill (last intact cornmill in area) 093 25486

Aughrim   Aughrim Schoolhouse Restaurant

Ballinasloe Co Galway

RESTAURANT   **Tel: 0905 73622**

Just off the main Galway road, this charming country restaurant is well-located for people visiting the nearby Battle of Aughrim site. New owners Christophe and Caroline Pele took over the restaurant in March 1998, so it now has a distinctly French tone: pan-fried frog legs, terrine of rabbit, french onion soup, seafood pot-au-feu. The Peles are working on a front garden and conservatory, optimistically planning to have barbecues on summer evenings. More immediately, a "culinary tour de France" is planned for the winter months – Christophe will cook dishes from different parts of France to make a special evening and promote French food in Ireland at a very reasonable price. • L£, D££ Tues-Sun • Closed 25 Dec, 1 Jan • MasterCard, Visa •

Ballinasloe

Haydens Hotel

Dunlo Street Ballinasloe Co Galway

HOTEL   Tel: 0905 42347

Haydens is a long-established and much-loved family hotel, very much the centre of local activities in and around Ballinasloe – conference and wedding facilities are good, with a particularly pleasant banqueting room overlooking the courtyard garden at the back. It's also about halfway between Dublin and Galway, making it a handy place to break the journey. Great improvements have been taking place at the hotel lately, the most recent being complete redevelopment of the bar area – an imaginative new bar has been built, incorporating an extension into the building next door. Bedrooms, all recently refurbished and with neat en-suite bathrooms, are comfortably furnished. Staff are friendly and helpful and there's plenty of free parking. Special breaks, notably golf breaks, are worth inquiring about. • Acc££ • Closed 24-27 Dec • Amex, Diners, MasterCard, Visa •

Ballyconneely

Erriseask House Hotel

Ballyconneely Clifden Co Galway

HOTEL/RESTAURANT   Tel: 095 23553   Fax: 095 23639

email: erriseask@connemara-ireland.com

Irish Beef Award Winner   www.erriseask.connemara-ireland.com

This beautifully located shoreside hotel and restaurant seven miles south of Clifden has a low-key, continental atmosphere. With the notable exception of Christian and Stefan Matz's collection of extraordinary Gertrude Degenhardt pictures, the overall decorative approach in the hotel is – like their thoughtful hospitality – understated, allowing the wildness and the raw beauty of the surroundings to take centre stage. There is much light wood, in polished floors and furniture (but the black stuff on draught in the bar) and a generally low-key approach throughout most of the ground floor and the original bedrooms. These were quite simply decorated with en-suite showers (but were due to be refurbished – with bathroom improvements – for the 1999 season). There are also five quite dramatic newer rooms on the ground floor, with excellent bathrooms and a mezzanine level sitting area with stunning views over untamed fields to the sea and land beyond.

Restaurant ★

The restaurant has always been the heart of this unusual hotel. Overlooking fields running down to the white coral strand, it is well-appointed in classical style, with an open fire for chilly evenings, crisp linen, fine glasses and an attention to detail which complements the exceptionally fine food that Stefan Matz prepares for guests. Christian makes a fine host, quietly ensuring that no small detail is overlooked and explaining the wonderful menus – a Menu Degustation (for complete tables), a carte du jour, a table d'hôte and a vegetarian menu, none of them overlong but all changed almost daily. Using the best of local ingredients, Stefan enjoys working on the traditional themes of his adoptive country and brings a continental sophistication to the dishes he creates. His menus are always beautifully balanced and regularly feature an abundance of local seafood and Connemara lamb, as well as Irish beef. We selected Erriseask for our Irish Beef Award this year because of Stefan's consistently creative approach, and particularly for his wonderful dish of Fillet of Beef Freshly Smoked on Turf served with Potato Pancakes and Glazed Autumn Vegetables. This imaginative dish owes its inspiration to the Connemara landscape and was part of a menu that earned this talented and dedicated chef the title 'New Irish Cuisine Chef of the Year' in 1997. The wine list, which is interesting and far from static, includes a strong selection of half bottles and an unusual number available by the glass.• Acc££ • L by arr, D££ daily • Closed Nov-Easter •

Cashel

Cashel House Hotel

Cashel Co Galway

COUNTRY HOUSE/RESTAURANT 🏛   Tel: 095 31001   Fax: 095 31077

email: info@cashel-house-hotel.com   www.cashel-house-hotel.com

Dermot and Kay McEvilly were among the pioneers of the Irish country house movement when, as founder members of the Irish Country Houses and Restaurants Association (now known as The Blue Book) they opened Cashel House as an hotel in 1968. The following year General and Madame de Gaulle chose to stay for two weeks in 1969, an historic visit of which the McEvilly's are justly proud – look out for the photographs and other memorabilia in the hall. The de Gaulle visit meant immediate recognition for the hotel, but it did even more for Ireland by putting the Gallic seal of approval on Irish hospitality and food. Comfort abounds here, even luxury, yet it's tempered by common sense, a love of gardening and the genuine sense of hospitality that ensures each guest will benefit as much as possible from their stay. The gardens, which run down to their own private beach, contribute greatly to the atmosphere, and the accommodation includes especially comfortable ground floor garden suites with access onto the patio. Relaxed hospitality combined with professionalism have earned an international reputation for this outstanding hotel and its qualities are perhaps best seen in details – log fires that burn throughout the year, day rooms furnished with antiques and filled with fresh flowers from the garden, rooms that are individually decorated with many thoughtful touches. Service is impeccable and breakfast includes an interesting selection of home-made produce, from soda bread and marmalade to black pudding.

Restaurant

A large conservatory extension enhances this well-appointed split-level restaurant. Dermot McEvilly has overseen the kitchen personally since the hotel opened, providing a rare consistency of style in fixed-price five-course dinners (£32.00 + 12/5% service) that make imaginative use of the best of local produce. Local seafood – lobster (£8 supplement), oysters, fresh and home-smoked wild salmon, mussels, turbot, monkfish – is a great strength. Local meats include Connemara lamb, but less predictable ingredients also feature – rabbit, for instance (which is surprisingly little used in Irish restaurants) and ostrich (even less so, but which is becoming quite popular). Garden produce is also much in evidence throughout, in soups, salads, side dishes, fine vegetarian dishes and desserts, such as rhubarb tart or strawberries and cream. Farmhouse cheeses come with home-baked biscuits and a choice of coffees and infusions is offered to finish. Service, under the personal supervision of Kay McEvilly, is excellent. An interesting wine list includes four House Wines (£14.95). Lunch (12.30-2.30) and afternoon tea (2.30-5) are served in the bar. • Bar L££, L££ Sun, D£££ daily • Acc££ • Closed Jan • Closed Nov-Easter • Amex, Diners, MasterCard, Visa •

Cashel	Zetland House Hotel

Cashel Bay Connemara Co Galway

HOTEL   Tel: 095 31111   Fax: 095 31117

email: zetland@iol.ie   http://connemara.net/zetland

On an elevated site, with views over Cashel Bay, Zetland House Hotel was originally built as a sporting lodge in the early 19th century – and still makes a good base for fishing holidays. This is a charming house, with a light and airy atmosphere and an elegance bordering on luxury, in both its spacious antique-furnished public areas and bedrooms. The latter are individually decorated in a relaxed country house style. The gardens surrounding the house are very lovely too, greatly enhancing the peaceful atmosphere of the house. • D£££ daily • Acc£££ • Closed Nov-Apr • Amex, Diners, MasterCard, Visa •

Claddaghduff	Acton's Guesthouse

Leegaun Claddaghduff Co Galway

ACCOMMODATION/RESTAURANT   Tel: 095 44339   Fax: 095 44309

In one of the most stunning away-from-it-all locations in Ireland, this wonderful, professionally run guesthouse has direct access to a sandy beach and uninterrupted views of the sea and islands. It is just heavenly. The house – a modern bungalow – is neat and homely, with seven comfortable en-suite rooms (4 shower-only, 1 with jacuzzi bath), tea/coffee trays, phones and satellite TV. There's a cosy sitting room with a turf fire, and Rita Acton's home cooking to enjoy in the restaurant (which is placed to take full advantage of the view). The restaurant is open to non-residents by arrangement (reservation required); Rita's imaginative set menu dinners could include Connemara salmon with strawberries and lemon dressing, rack of Connemara lamb with fresh herb crust, and vegetarian dishes such as Castle farm goats cheese in filo pastry with red onion and raisin relish. • D££ • Acc££ • Closed Oct-Apr • Amex, Diners, MasterCard, Visa •

Clarenbridge	Oyster Manor Hotel

Clarenbridge Co Galway

Tel: 091 796777   Fax: 091 796770

Family-owned by Ned and Julianne Forde, this new hotel on the edge of Clarenbridge is popular for weddings and family celebrations (up to 60 for a sitdown meal) and conferences (up to 100) and the large bar at the back makes a focal point in the area, with live music most nights. Rooms have all the necessary amenities and are comfortably furnished in country style - very handy for the Oyster Festival. • Acc££ • Closed 25 Dec • Amex, Diners, MasterCard, Visa •

Clarenbridge   Paddy Burkes

Clarenbridge Co Galway

PUB   Tel: 091 796226   Fax: 091 796016

Established in 1650 and still going strong, Paddy Burkes' internationally famous pub and seafood bar is home to the Clarenbridge Oyster Festival – September 1999 will see its 45th birthday. Extensive renovations have recently brought many improvements. Although most famous for its seafood, this characterful old pub serves much else besides, including stir-fries, curries, steaks and vegetarian dishes, both on the regular bar menu and as daily specials. The visitors book reads like a Who's Who – an unbelievable array of the rich and famous. And that's not including the ones who "prefer not to be named". • Meals£-££ • Closed 24, 25 Dec & Good Fri • Amex, Diners, MasterCard, Visa •

Clifden   Abbeyglen Castle

Sky Road Clifden Co Galway

HOTEL   Tel: 095 21201   Fax: 095 21797

email: info@abbeyglen.ie   www.abbeyglen.ie

Set romantically in its own parkland valley overlooking Clifden and the sea, Abbeyglen is family-owned and run in a very hands-on fashion by Paul and Brian Hughes. It's a place that has won a lot of friends over the years and it's easy to see why: it's big and comfortable and laid-back – and there's a generosity of spirit about the place which is very charming. Public areas include a spacious drawing room for residents and a relaxing, pubby bar with open peat fire. Bedrooms (all with good bathrooms) are quite big and have been recently refurbished, as part of an ongoing improvement programme. • Acc££-£££ • Amex, Diners, MasterCard, Visa •

Clifden   Ardagh Hotel & Restaurant

Ballyconneely Road Clifden Co Galway

HOTEL/RESTAURANT   Tel: 095 21384   Fax: 095 21314

email: ardaghhotel@tinet.ie   www.commerce.ie/ardaghhotel

Beautifully located on the Ballyconneely road, overlooking Ardbear Bay, Stephane and Monique Bauvet's family-run hotel is well known for hospitality, comfort and good food. It has style, too, in a gentle sort of way – not "decorated" but furnished in a homely style with good fabrics and classic country colours. Turf fires, comfortable armchairs and a plant-filled conservatory area upstairs all indicate that peaceful relaxation is the aim here. Bedrooms vary according to their position but they are all well-furnished, with all the amenities required for a comfortable stay. (Not all have sea views – single rooms are at the back with a pleasant countryside outlook, and have shower only.) Bedrooms include some extra large rooms, especially suitable for families. • Amex, Diners, MasterCard, Visa •

Restaurant

The well-appointed restaurant is on the first floor and set up to take full advantage of the view, providing a fitting setting for Monique's fine cooking, which specialises in local seafood. She presents an imaginative nightly dinner menu (£26) offering four courses with plenty of choice. Typical dishes: warm salad with pot-roasted quail, fresh mussel soup, fresh fillet of turbot on a bed of spinach, coated with a saffron sauce and tomato concasse. • D£££ • Acc£££ • Closed Nov-Mar • Amex, Diners, MasterCard, Visa •

Clifden   Destrys Restaurant

Main Street Clifden Co Galway

CAFÉ/RESTAURANT   Tel: 095 21722   Fax: 095 21008

This wacky little restaurant was opened by Paddy and Julia Foyle a few years ago and, in addition to normal custom, head chef Dermot Gannon provides dinners for residents at their other establishment Quay House (see entry). It's a fun, buzzy restaurant; Dermot's new-wave cooking is superb and prices are reasonable, so a good time is sure to be had by all. At night they do an à la carte menu (main courses about £8.95-£14.95) and there's a lighter selection at lunchtime. Dishes typical of Dermot's style might be: mussels steamed in coconut, garlic and lime; smoked loin of pork, baked apples, meaux mustard, crème fraîche and a vegetarian choice such as tortellini with goat's cheese, roast pepper and peanut pesto. Home baking is a strong point, and they make great brown yeast bread as well as foccaccia. Another interesting point: Dermot's sister and her husband run Wings, a Chinese restaurant up the road. We haven't eaten there but it looks really promising (simple, great menu) and is highly spoken of locally. • L£, D£ daily • Closed Mar-Easter • Amex, Diners, MasterCard, Visa •

Clifden   O'Grady's Seafood Restaurant

Market Street Clifden Co Galway

RESTAURANT   **Tel: 095 21450**

O'Grady's was the first place to give Clifden a reputation as a good food town. In season (April-October) they're open for lunch and dinner and it's an education to see the French visitors flocking in – O'Grady's isn't trendy, but they know how to cook seafood and good old-fashioned service doesn't go amiss. Which is not to say that the food is old-fashioned, just that they do the classics well. Spinach and riccota tart or penne pasta tossed with mussels and smoked garlic cream are typical starters, and main course peppered fillet of salmon could come with Chinese noodles and a passion fruit coulis. Desserts might include a classic crème brûlée with ginger shortbread biscuits, or there will be farmhouse cheese – with a glass of dessert wine or vintage port perhaps. • L£, D££ Mon-Sat • Closed 25 Dec • Amex, MasterCard, Visa •

Clifden   The Quay House

Beach Road Clifden Co Galway

ACCOMMODATION   🏛   **Tel: 095 21360   Fax: 095 21608**

email: thequay@iol.ie

In a lovely location – the house is right on the harbour, with pretty water views when the tide is in – The Quay House was built around 1820. It has the distinction of being not only the oldest building in Clifden, but has also had a surprisingly varied usage: it was originally the harbourmaster's house, then a convent, then a monastery, was converted into a hotel at the turn of the century and finally, since 1993, has been enjoying its most recent incarnation as specialist accommodation in the incomparable hands of long-time hoteliers, Paddy and Julia Foyle. Accommodation is in a growing number (now 14) of airy, wittily decorated and sumptuously comfortable rooms, which includes not only two wheelchair-friendly rooms but a whole new development alongside the original house – seven stunning new studio rooms with small fitted kitchens and balconies overlooking the harbour. As in the older rooms, excellent bathrooms all have full bath and shower. Evening meals are no longer served at Quay House, but guests can be booked into the Foyles' restaurant, Destrys, just up the road. Breakfast, including delicious freshly-baked breads and scones straight from the Aga, is served in the conservatory, where Paddy also serves lunch and afternoon tea. (Open to non-residents). Although officially closed in winter it is always worth inquiring. • Acc££ • Closed mid Nov-mid Mar • Amex, MasterCard, Visa •

Clifden   Rock Glen Country House Hotel

Ballyconneely Road Clifden Co Galway

HOTEL/RESTAURANT   **Tel: 095 21035   Fax: 095 21737**

email: rockglen@iol.ie   www.connemara.net/rockglenhotel

Built in 1815 as a shooting lodge for Clifden Castle, Rock Glen is now run by the Roche family as a delightful hotel – beautifully situated in quiet grounds well away from the road, it enjoys views over a sheltered anchorage. The public rooms and some of the bedrooms have the full advantage of the view, but the whole hotel is very restful and comfortable, with a pleasing outlook from all windows. Rooms are furnished in country house style, with good bathrooms (all have a full bath and over-bath shower) and amenities – some, such as tea/coffee trays, are not in the rooms but available on request. In addition to local activities – fishing, pony trekking, golf – there's a putting green on site, also all-weather tennis and croquet; indoors there are plenty of places to read quietly and a full size snooker table.

Restaurant

John Roche has been in charge of the kitchen for many years and now has a head chef, Michael Rath to assist with this side of the hotel. Five-course menus are also available as individually priced courses (ie semi à la carte) and based on local ingredients, especially seafood, in an updated country house style. Thus Irish Beechwood salmon with potato cakes and crème fraîche, duo of farmed rabbit & prawns pan-fried with prawn cappuccino and apple crumble with vanilla ice cream or Irish farmhouse cheese & biscuits are all typical. Service is friendly and efficient and an excellent breakfast is served in the restaurant. • D££-£££ • Acc£££ • Closed Nov-mid Mar • Amex, Diners, MasterCard, Visa •

Clifden   Station House Hotel

Clifden Co Galway

HOTEL   Tel: 095 21699

Set on the site of the late lamented railway station this large new hotel comes complete with leisure centre and conference facilities for 250 people. Public areas are impressively spacious and modern while bedrooms are a good size, contemporary in style and comfortable. The old Station House has become a themed bar and restaurant and the complex includes a wide range of shops and boutiques. • Acc££ • Open all year • Amex, Diners, MasterCard, Visa •

Clifden   Sunnybank House

Clifden Co Galway

ACCOMMODATION   Tel: 095 21437   Fax: 095 21976

Set in its own mature gardens, with panoramic views, Sunnybank is owned and run by the O'Grady family, of O'Grady's restaurant. They offer exceptional facilities at reasonable prices: as well as very comfortably appointed en-suite bedrooms and day rooms for guests' use. There is also a heated swimming pool, sauna and tennis court.
• Acc££ • Closed Nov-Mar • Amex, Diners, MasterCard, Visa •

Costello   Fermoyle Lodge

Costello Co Galway

COUNTRY HOUSE   Tel: 091 786111   Fax: 091 786154

One of Ireland's best-kept secrets, Nicola Stronach's delightful sporting lodge seems to enjoy the best of all possible worlds. Although only 29 miles from Galway, it's hidden from the road in one of the wildest and most remote parts of Connemara. Protected by mature woodland and shrubs, it has stunning lake and mountain views, with both salmon and sea trout fishing on the doorstep. All this and creature comforts too. The spacious, well-proportioned house has been sensitively renovated and beautifully furnished and decorated. Nicola has used the best of materials wisely, in a warm, low-key style that allows for every comfort without detracting from the wonderful setting that is its greatest attribute. Bedrooms are all very comfortable, with private bathrooms. A set dinner (£22) is served at 7.30 – 24 hour notice is required and any particular dislikes or allergies should be mentioned on booking. • Acc££ • Closed Xmas • Amex, MasterCard, Visa •

Craughwell   St Clerans

Craughwell Co Galway

COUNTRY HOUSE   Tel: 091 846555   Fax: 091 846600

email: stcleran@iol.ie   www.merv.com/stcleran

Previously the home of John Huston, St Clerans is a magnificent manor house beautifully located in rolling countryside. It has been carefully restored by the current owner, the American entertainer Merv Griffin, and decorated with no expense spared to make a sumptuous, hedonistically luxurious country retreat, operating under the management of Richard Swarbrick. The decor, which is for the most part in an elegant style, with some regard for period tastes, does occasionally go right over the top – as evidenced in the carpets in the hall and drawing room. But, what the heck – there's a great sense of fun about the furnishing and everything is of the best possible quality. As to the accommodation, each room is individually decorated and most are done in what might best be described as an upbeat country house style. Others – particularly those on the lower ground floor, including John Huston's own favourite room, which opens out onto a terrace with steps up to the garden – are restrained, almost subdued, in atmosphere. All are spacious, with luxuriously appointed bathrooms (one has its original shower only) and a wonderful away-from-it-all feeling. Although not operational at the time of the guide's visit (shortly after the house opened), the restaurant is now up and running and open to non-residents. Head chef Hisashi Kumagai's cooking style – a mixture of Japanese and traditional Irish – sounds fascinating. Daily-changed menus are offered (L £18, D £30; House Wine £12-18). • Acc££££ • Amex, MasterCard, Visa •

Craughwell   Raftery's, The Blazers Bar

Craughwell Co Galway

BAR   Tel: 091 846708   Fax: 091 846004

Donald and Theresa Raftery's famous family-run establishment is on the main Galway-Dublin road and is the meeting place for the well-known Galway Blazers Hunt, who are kennelled close by. It can make a handy stopping place: bar food is served every day – house specialities are seafood chowder, smoked salmon and home-made brown bread. • Closed 25 Dec & Good Fri •

Furbo   Connemara Coast Hotel

Furbo Co Galway

HOTEL   Tel: 091 592108   Fax: 091 592065

sinnott@iol.ie   www.iol.ie/bizpark/s/sinnott

Like the other Sinnott hotels – Connemera Gateway and the new Brooks Hotel in Dublin – the Connemara Coast is an attractive building which makes the best possible use of the site without intruding on the surroundings. Set on the sea side of the road, in its own extensive grounds, it is hard to credit that Galway city is only a 10 minute drive away. An impressive foyer sets the tone on entering, and both public areas and bedrooms at the hotel are spacious and well-designed throughout. Facilities are particularly good too – a fine bar, two restaurants, a children's playroom and a leisure centre among them – and a range of special breaks is available. • Acc£££ • Closed 25 Dec • Amex, Diners, MasterCard, Visa •

Galway   Ardawn House

31 College Road Galway Co Galway

ACCOMMODATION   Tel: 091 568833   Fax: 091 563454

email: ardawn@iol.ie

Only a few minutes walk from Eyre Square, Mike and Breda Guiloyle's hospitable guesthouse is easily found, just beside the greyhound track. Accommodation is all en-suite and rooms are comfortably furnished, with good amenities. But it's Mike and Breda who make Ardawn House special – they take great pride in every aspect of the business, (including an extensive breakfast) and also help guests to get the very best out of their visit to Galway. • Acc££ • Closed Xmas wk • Amex, MasterCard, Visa •

Galway   Ardilaun House Hotel

Taylor's Hill Galway Co Galway

HOTEL   Tel: 091 521433   Fax: 091 521543

email: ardilaun@iol.ie   www.commerce.ie/ardilaun

Set in extensive wooded grounds, Ardilaun House Hotel is convenient to the city yet retains its original country feeling. Friendly, helpful staff make a good impression on arrival and everything about the hotel – which has recently been extensively renovated, extended and refurbished – confirms the feeling of a well-run establishment. Public areas are spacious, elegantly furnished and some – notably the dining room – overlook gardens at the back. Bedrooms are furnished to a high standard, current in-house leisure facilities include billiards and a new leisure centre is due to open in March 1999. Purpose-built conference facilities offer a wide range of options for large and small groups, with back-up business services. Attractive banqueting facilities are especially suitable for weddings (up to 280 guests). • Acc£££ • Closed Xmas wk • Amex, Diners, MasterCard, Visa •

Galway   Brennan's Yard

Lower Merchants Road Galway Co Galway

HOTEL   Tel: 091 568166   Fax: 091 568262

Located close to Spanish Arch, in a characterful stone building, Brennans Yard first opened in 1992 and a second phase of the development was due to go ahead a couple of years later. It is an interesting hotel – all rooms were individually designed with country pine antiques and Irish craft items, giving the hotel special character. Unfortunately, a delay in finishing the development and poor maintenance have spoilt the effect recently. Work is now proceeding, however, which will add a further 21 rooms to the hotel for the 1999 season, and the original rooms are to be refurbished to the same standard. If all goes according to plan, Brennans Yard will again be among the most desirable hotels in Galway. • Acc££ • Closed 24-26 Dec & 1 Jan • Amex, Diners, MasterCard, Visa •

Galway   Corrib Great Southern Hotel

Dublin Road Galway Co Galway

HOTEL   **Tel: 091 55281   Fax: 091 51390**

This large modern hotel overlooks Galway Bay and has good facilities for business guests and family holidays (ask about their Weekend Specials). Public areas include O'Malleys Pub, which has sea views, and a quieter residents' lounge; in summer evening entertainment and crèche facilities are laid on. Bedrooms vary considerably; the best are spacious and well-planned, with stylish bathrooms. An excellent business/convention centre has facilities for groups from 8 to 800, with banqueting for up to 650. • Acc£££ • Closed 24-26 Dec • Amex, Diners, MasterCard, Visa •

Galway   Galway Ryan Hotel & Leisure Club

Dublin Road Galway City East Co Galway

HOTEL   **Tel: 091 753181   Fax: 091 753187**

Only a mile or so from the city centre, this hotel makes a useful base for business or leisure. En-suite bedrooms (which include four wheelchair-friendly rooms) have bath and showers and are of a good standard throughout. There is desk space for business guests and 24 hour room service. Meeting rooms (for up to 35 people) are available and there is an exceptional leisure centre. Friendly staff and good facilities for children make the Ryan an excellent base for a family holiday. • Acc££-££££ • Closed 24-26 Dec • Amex, Diners, MasterCard, Visa •

Galway   Glenlo Abbey Hotel

Bushypark Galway Co Galway

HOTEL   **Tel: 091 526666   Fax: 091 527800**

email: glenlo@iol.ie   www.glenlo.com

Originally an eighteenth century residence, Glenlo Abbey is just two and a half miles from Galway city yet offers all the advantages of the country – the hotel is on a 138-acre estate, with its own golf course and Pavilion. It enjoys views over Lough Corrib and the surrounding countryside. The scale of the hotel is generous throughout, public rooms are impressive and bedrooms are well-furnished with good amenities and marbled bathrooms. The old Abbey has been restored to provide privacy for meetings and private dining, and there is a fully equipped business service bureau to back up seminars, conferences and presentations. For indoor relaxation there's the Oak Cellar bar (where light food is served) and, in addition to the classical River Room restaurant, the hotel recently acquired an historic Pullman train carriage which now operates as a restaurant in the hotel grounds – it's in beautiful order, has a great atmosphere and, needless to say, makes a meal here a memorable event. • Acc££££ • Open all year • Amex, Diners, MasterCard, Visa •

Galway   Great Southern Hotel

Eyre Square Galway Co Galway

HOTEL   **Tel: 091 564041   Fax: 091 566704**

email: res@galway.gsh.ie   www.gsh.ie

Overlooking Eyre Square right in the heart of Galway, this historic railway hotel was built in 1845 and has retained many of its original features and old-world charm which mixes easily with modern facilities. Public rooms – notably the foyer – are quite grand. There's a rather successful country style bar, O'Flahertys Pub, down in the basement (with access from the Square or the hotel) in addition to a more usual hotel cocktail lounge. Bedrooms, which vary somewhat but are generally spacious and comfortable, are traditionally furnished with dark mahogany and brass light fittings. • Acc££-££££ • Closed 24-26 Dec • Amex, Diners, MasterCard, Visa •

Galway   Jurys Galway Inn

Quay Street Galway Co Galway

HOTEL   **Tel: 091 566444   Fax: 091 568415**

email: tara-flynn@jurys.com

Jurys Galway Inn is magnificently sited to make the most of both the river – which rushes past almost all the bedroom windows – and the great buzz of the Spanish Arch area of the city (just outside the door). Like the other Jurys room-only 'inns', the hotel offers a good standard of basic accommodation without frills. Rooms are large (sleeping up to four people) and well finished, with everything required for comfort and convenience –

ample well-lit work/shelf space, neat en-suite bathroom, TV, phone – but no extras. Beds are generous, with good-quality bedding, and open wardrobes are more than adequate. Neat tea/coffee-making facilities are built into the design, but there is no room service. Public areas include an impressive, well-designed foyer with seating areas, a pubby bar with good atmosphere and self-service cafeteria. • Acc££ • Closed 25 & 26 Dec • Amex, Diners, MasterCard, Visa •

Galway   K C Blakes

10 Quay Street Galway Co Galway

RESTAURANT   Tel: 091 561826   Fax: 091 561829

K C Blakes is named after a stone Tower House, of a type built sometime between 1440 and 1640, which stands as a typical example of the medieval stone architecture of the ancient city of Galway. The Casey's new restaurant, with all its sleek black designer style and contemporary chic could not present a stronger contrast to such a building. The head chef is John Casey, previously the chef at his family restaurant Westwood Bistro – now to become the new Westwood Hotel, under new ownership. True to form, he sources ingredients for K C Blakes with care and cooks with skill to produce dishes ranging from traditional Irish (beef and Guinness stew), new Irish cuisine (black pudding croquettes with pear & cranberry sauce), classical French (sole meunière) to Global cuisine (a huge choice here – let's say chicken fajita). It's a remarkable operation, aimed at a wide market and keenly priced. • L£ Mon-Fri, D££ daily • Closed 25 Dec • Amex, MasterCard, Visa •

Galway   Killeen House

Bushypark Galway Co Galway

COUNTRY HOUSE 🏛   Tel: 091 524179   Fax: 091 528065

Catherine Doyle's delightful house really has the best of both worlds. It's on the Clifden road just on the edge of Galway city yet, with 25 acres of private grounds and gardens reaching down to the shores of Lough Corrib, offers all the advantages of the country, too. The house was built in 1840 and has all the features of a more leisurely era, when space was plentiful – not only in the reception rooms, which include an elegant dining room overlooking the gardens (where delicious breakfasts are served in style), but also the bedrooms. These are luxuriously and individually furnished (1 shower only), each in a different period, eg Regency, Edwardian and (most fun this one) Art Nouveau. • Acc££ • Closed 25 Dec • Amex, Diners, MasterCard, Visa •

Galway   Kirbys of Cross Street

Cross Street Galway Co Galway

RESTAURANT   Tel: 091 569404   Fax: 091 568095

One of a trio of establishments situated on Cross Street, and adjoining Kirwan's Lane (the others are two of Galway's leading pubs, Busker Browne's and The Slate House), this dashingly informal two storey restaurant does a very nice line in contemporary cuisine. Modern Irish Cuisine is what they call it and, unusually, that's really what you get (plus a few influences from further afield). Thus starters like salad of spiced beef with marinated vegetables and grilled black & white seafood pudding on a seafood vegetable salad, a cream of parsnip soup with smoked salmon julienne; and main courses such as fillet of beef in Guinness sauce served with a gratinated oyster and mustard-glazed supreme of chicken with cabbage colcannon. If this all sounds unusually promising for a little restaurant squeezed between two pubs, bear in mind that Stefan Matz of Erriseask House (see entry) helped develop the menu with head chef John Cooney. Busker Browne's bar food is far from ordinary either – their ambitious bar menu even runs to lobster. • L£ & D££ daily • Closed 25 Dec & Good Fri • Amex, MasterCard, Visa •

Galway   Kirwan's Lane Restaurant

Kirwan's Lane Galway Co Galway

RESTAURANT   Tel: 091 568266

Clifden man Michael O'Grady is the chef-proprietor at this classy contemporary restaurant in a laneway just beside the Hotel Spanish Arch. It's been open since 1996, but recently closed for a couple of weeks and re-emerged with double the space. It is a great success and deservedly so – hard work and talent have combined to make Kirwan's Lane the leading restaurant in the city. Menus offer a wide choice of international dishes with a pleasing leaning towards New Irish Cuisine. Evening menus are slightly more formal, but sensibly short à la carte menus apply in both cases and the style is similar.

This is a fine restaurant, with service and surroundings to match the food – don't forget that booking is strongly advised. •L£ & D££ Mon-Sat • Closed Xmas wk • Amex, Diners, MasterCard, Visa •

Galway · The Malt House

Old Malt Shopping Mall High Street Galway Co Galway
RESTAURANT   Tel: 091 567866   Fax: 091 563993
The Cunningham's welcoming old restaurant and bar in a quiet cul-de-sac laneway off High Street has great character and a friendly attitude. There's a cheerful lunchtime bar menu with soups and salads, served with good home-made bread, popular hot seafood dishes – baked garlic mussels, panfried crab claws – steaks and vegetarian dishes; a nice note – they will serve the restaurant menu in the bar if required. Dinner menus are more formal but the emphasis is still on fairly traditional dishes – and none the worse for that. The Malt House has a loyal and well-deserved local following. • L£ & D££ Mon-Sat • Closed Bank Hols • Amex, Diners, MasterCard, Visa •

Galway · McDonagh's Seafood House

22 Quay Street Galway Co Galway
RESTAURANT   Tel: 091 565001   Fax: 091 562246
www.e-maginet.com/mcdonagh
A most unusual restaurant this: McDonagh's is a fish shop during the day – they buy whole catches from local fishermen and have it on sale in the shop within a couple of hours of leaving the boat. Buying the whole catch guarantees the wide variety the shop is famous for. Then, when it comes to the cooking, there's the fish & chips operation – select your variety and see it cooked in front of you. On the other side of the shop is the Seafood bar, a more formal restaurant where an extensive range of dishes is offered. They even do their own smoking on the premises and fish caught by anglers can be brought in and smoked to take home. They do party food, too. The family also owns the dashing Hotel Spanish Arch (091 569600) a couple of doors up the street. • L£ Mon-Sat, D£ daily • Closed Xmas & New Year • Amex, Diners, MasterCard, Visa •

Galway · Nimmo's

Spanish Arch Long Walk Galway Co Galway
RESTAURANT   Tel: 091 563565   Fax: 091 846403
Stephan Zeltner-Healy, chef-proprietor at this extraordinarily old waterside restaurant just through the Spanish Arch, is a very fine chef indeed, as regular visitors to his previous tiny restaurant over Tigh Neachtain pub may remember. Here he is in another tiny restaurant, presenting the same inscrutable menus. Other chefs over-write menus, giving lengthy descriptions for every dish – with Stephan every order is an adventure. It all sounds quite ordinary, so be prepared! Everything is based on carefully sourced seasonal local ingredients – and Stephan's cooking is excellent. • D££ Mon-Sat & Sun Bank Hol wkends • Closed 25 Dec & 1 Jan, Mon low season • Amex, MasterCard, Visa •

Galway · Norman Villa

86 Lower Salthill Galway Co Galway
ACCOMMODATION   Tel: 091 521131   Fax: 091 521131
Dee and Mark Keogh's guesthouse is exquisite. It's a lovely old house, immaculately maintained and imaginatively converted to make the most of every inch, ensuring guest comfort without spoiling the interior proportions. It's dashingly decorated, with lovely rich colours. A great collection of modern paintings looks especially magnificent juxtaposed with antique furniture. Dee and Mark are dedicated hosts, too. But there is a catch – how to get a booking at Norman Villa, especially for an impulse break. The only solution, apart from being lucky enough to pick up a cancellation, seems to be to do what their American guests do – book months in advance. It goes against the grain for many people but is well worth the effort. • Acc££ • Open all year • MasterCard, Visa •

We aim to be as up to date as possible, but changes will inevitably occur after we go to press. We would request that listed establishments inform us as quickly as possible of major changes, eg sale of property or key staff changes, so that our records may be updated through the year. Readers will have access to important changes by visiting our website (www.ireland-guide.com).

Galway   # Tigh Neachtain

Cross Street Galway Co Galway

PUB   **Tel: 091 568820**

Tigh Neachtain is one of Galway's oldest pubs – the origins of the building are medieval – and has been in the same family for a century. Quite unspoilt, it has great charm and a friendly atmosphere – the pint is good and there's bar food. But perhaps the nicest thing of all is the way an impromptu traditional music session can get going at the drop of a hat. • Closed 25 Dec & Good Fri • No credit cards •

Galway   # Westwood House Hotel

Dangan Upper Newcastle Galway Co Galway

HOTEL   **Tel: 091 521442   Fax: 091 521400**

Reaching completion as we go to press, this new hotel will be open for the 1999 season. It is in the same group as the Schoolhouse Hotel in Dublin (see entry) and the Station House Hotel, Clifden (095 21699). This promising establishment is well located, set well back from the Clifden road out of the city, and offers a high standard of accommodation at fairly reasonable prices. • Acc££ • Open all year •

Headford   # Lisdonagh House

Caherlistrane Headford Co Galway

COUNTRY HOUSE   **Tel: 093 31163   Fax: 093 31528**

email: Lisdoonag@iol.ie

Situated about 15 minutes drive north of Galway city in the heart of hunting and fishing country, Lisdonagh house is on an elevated site with beautiful views overlooking Lake Hackett. It is a lovely property, with large well-proportioned reception rooms, a fine staircase and luxurious bedrooms, furnished with antiques and decorated in period style,with marbled bathrooms to match. Dinner, served to residents at 8 pm, was limited to a no-choice 4-course menu on the occasion of our visit. Breakfast, served in the dining room, was good although service was erratic. • Acc££-£££ • D££ • Closed mid Dec–early Feb • Amex, MasterCard, Visa •

Inishbofin   # Day's Hotel

Middle Quarter Inishbofin Island Co Galway

HOTEL   **Tel: 095 45809   Fax: 095 45803**

This modest but hospitable family-run hotel beside the harbour has been first (and last) port of call for many visitors to the island over the years. It has recently changed hands, but only within the family, so there is not too much danger of sudden or dramatic changes taking place just yet. Ferries to the island run regularly from Cleggan, with ticket offices in Clifden (regular buses between Clifden and Cleggan) and also at Kings of Cleggan. Credit card bookings are accepted. For bookings and enquiries, telephone: 095 44642 or 095 21520. Off-season, inquire about the availability of food and drink on the island. • Acc££ • Closed Oct-end Mar •

Kilcolgan   # Moran's Oyster Cottage

The Weir Kilcolgan Co Galway

PUB/RESTAURANT ⭐   **Tel: 091 796113   Fax: 091 796503**

Seafood Pub of the Year

This is just the kind of Irish pub that people everywhere dream about. It's as pretty as a picture, with a well-kept thatched roof and a lovely waterside location (with plenty of seats outside where you can while away the time and watch the swans floating by). It's also brilliantly well-run by the Moran family – and so it should be, after all they've had six generations to practice. They're famed throughout the country for their wonderful local seafood, especially the native oysters (from their own oyster beds) which are in season from September to April. Willie Moran is an ace oyster opener, a regular champion in the famous annual competitions held in the locality. Farmed Gigas oysters are on the menu all year. Then there's chowder and smoked salmon and seafood cocktail and mussels – and, perhaps best of all, delicious crab sandwiches and salads. • Meals£-££ daily • Closed 25 Dec & Good Fri • Amex, MasterCard, Visa •

Kinvara

Merriman Hotel

Main Street Kinvara Co Galway

HOTEL   **Tel: 091 638222   Fax: 091 637686**

Claiming to be the largest thatched building in Ireland, the Merriman Hotel is in the main street of Kinvara and has filled a gap by providing good middle-range accommodation in the area. They are working hard to ensure standards of service and accommodation are as high as possible. Special breaks are sometimes offered- an inquiry is worthwhile. • Acc££ • Closed Jan & Feb • Amex, Diners, MasterCard, Visa •

Kinvara

Tully's

Kinvara Co Galway

PUB   **Tel: 091 637146**

Definitely a spot for traditional music, this is a real local pub in the old tradition, with a little grocery shop at the front and stone-floored bar at the back. Tully's has a fine old stove in the bar for cosy winter sessions, which is always a good sign (They also have a small enclosed garden with a few parasoled tables for fine weather.) Not a food place, although sandwiches, teas and coffees are always available. Normal pub hours. • No credit cards. • Closed 25 Dec & Good Fri •

Kylemore

Kylemore Abbey Restaurant

Kylemore Co Galway

RESTAURANT   **Tel: 095 41146   Fax: 095 41368**

email: enquires@kylemoreabbey.ie

Kylemore Abbey, with its stunning mountain and waterside setting, would make a dramatic location for any enterprise. But what the Benedictine nuns are doing here is truly astonishing. The abbey is not only home for the nuns but is also run as an international girls' boarding school. In addition, the nuns run a farm and garden (walled, recently restored and now open to the public). A short walk further along the wooded shore leads to the Gothic church, a miniature replica of Norwich cathedral. In a neat modern building beside the carpark is one of the country's best craft shops – and an excellent restaurant. Everything at this daytime self-service restaurant is made on the premises, and the range of wholesome offerings includes a good selection of hot and cold savoury dishes, including several vegetarian options – typically black eye bean casserole or vegetarian lasagne. Home baking is a special strength and big bowls of the nuns' renowned home-made jams are set up at the till, for visitors to help themselves. Beside them are neatly labelled jars to buy and take home. • Meals£ all day Mon-Sun • Closed Nov-mid Mar • Amex, Diners, MasterCard, Visa •

Leenane

Delphi Lodge

Leenane Co Galway

COUNTRY HOUSE   **Tel: 095 42211   Fax: 095 42296**

email: delfish@iol.ie   www.ireland.iol.ie/~delfish

One of Ireland's most famous sporting lodges, Delphi Lodge was built in the early 19th-century by the Marquis of Sligo. It is beautifully located in an unspoilt valley, surrounded by the region's highest mountains (with the high rainfall dear to fisherfolk). Owned since 1981 by Peter and Jane Mantle – who have restored and extended the original building in period style – the lodge is large and impressive in an informal, understated way, with antiques, fishing gear and a catholic selection of reading matter creating a stylish yet relaxed atmosphere. The dozen guest rooms are all quite different, but they are en-suite (with proper baths) and very comfortably furnished (with lovely lake and mountain views). Dinner, for residents only, is taken at a long mahogany table. It is cooked by Frank Bennett, who has "a range of dishes that is vast and eclectic – some traditional, some 'nouveau', some oriental – and some Arabic" The famous Delphi Fishery is the main attraction, but people come for other country pursuits, or just peace and quiet. A billiard table, the library and serious wine can get visitors through a lot of wet days. Just across the road, four restored cottages offer self-catering accommodation. • Acc££-£££ • Closed mid-Dec-mid-Jan • Amex, Diners, MasterCard, Visa •

The guide aims to provide comprehensive recommendations of the best places to eat, drink and stay throughout Ireland. We welcome suggestions from readers. If you think an establishment merits assessment , please write or email us.

Leenane Portfinn Lodge Restaurant & Guesthouse

Leenane Co Galway

ACCOMMODATION/RESTAURANT   Tel: 095 42265   Fax: 095 42315

There are few views in Ireland to beat the sight of the sun sinking behind the mountains over Killary harbour. On a good evening that's something you can look forward to at Rory and Brid Daly's seafood restaurant, Portfinn Lodge. The dining area is in a room of the main house and an adjoining conservatory. The lobster tank at the entrance bodes well for a good meal – 90% of the menu will be seafood: prawns, salmon, brill, turbot and many of their cousins make a nightly appearance. There is plenty else to choose from, however, including local lamb in various guises and two vegetarian dishes daily. Good brown bread comes with country butter, which is quite a feature in these parts, and there's always an Irish cheeseboard.

Guesthouse

Modest but comfortable accommodation is offered in eight neat purpose-built en-suite rooms, all sleeping three and one with four beds; one room has wheelchair access. • D£-££ daily • Acc£ • Closed mid-Oct-Apr • Diners, MasterCard, Visa •

Letterfrack Rosleague Manor

Letterfrack Co Galway

COUNTRY HOUSE/RESTAURANT   Tel: 095 41101   Fax: 095 41168

A lovely pink-washed Regency house of gracious proportions and sensitively handled modernisation, Rosleague looks out benevolently over a tidal inlet through gardens planted with rare shrubs and plants. Although the area offers plenty of activity for the energetic, there is a deep sense of peace about the place. It is hard to imagine anywhere better to recharge the soul; or the body, for that matter – breakfast, especially, is a feast of memorable wholesomeness, based on local and home-made speciality produce. Although more sophisticated, dinner – for which non-residents are welcome by reservation – shares the same exceptional respect for home-grown and local ingredients, with specialities including seafood straight from Cleggan harbour and, of course, the famous Connemara lamb. They grow their own basic vegetables, herbs and typical 'cottage garden' fruit like gooseberries and rhubarb, while more sophisticated produce, including Irish farmhouse cheeses, comes from Patrick Perceval's famous old-fashioned van delivery service.• D£££ daily • Acc££-£££ • Closed Nov-late-Mar • Amex, Diners, MasterCard, Visa •

Moyard Garranbaun House

Moyard Co Galway

COUNTRY HOUSE   Tel/Fax: 095 41649

In a spectacular position overlooking Ballynakill Bay, the Finnegans' imposing 19th century Georgian-style manor has wonderful views of the Twelve Bens, Diamond Hill and the Maam Turks – and there is a trout lake, Lough Garraunbaun, attached to the estate. Delia Finnagan is a most hospitable host, keeping her beautifully furnished house immaculate without spoiling the relaxed atmosphere. Books, turf fires and a grand piano say a lot about the things that bring people here – and Delia's cooking, of course. The organic garden, free range chicken and eggs provide an excellent base for her dinners; also wild local lobster, oysters, shrimps, scallops, salmon and Connemara lamb. Cheeses served are all Irish and baking of bread and scones is a daily event. • Acc££ • Open all year •Visa •

Moyard Rose Cottage

Rockfield Moyard Co Galway

FARM STAY   Tel/Fax: 095 41082

email: conamara@indigo.ie

This long-established farmhouse is situated on a working farm in a scenic location surrounded by the Twelve Bens mountains. It has moved into a new generation since Patricia O'Toole took over in 1997. Obviously already well prepared for the job (the family has always helped here), Patricia is full of energy and enthusiasm. Expect simple (but increasingly) comfortable accommodation and good home cooking (especially baking) and you won't be disappointed. There's a sitting room with an open turf fire (and television), a diningroom for guests (separate tables) and eight en-suite bedrooms,(6 shower-only) tea/coffee making trays and hair dryers. Nearby attractions include sandy beaches, scenic walks, fishing, island trips, traditional Irish music, horse riding and golf. • Acc£ • Closed Mar • MasterCard, Visa •

Moycullen

RESTAURANT ★

Irish Food Award Winner

Drimcong House Restaurant

Moycullen Co Galway
Tel: 091 555115 / 555585   Fax: 091 555836
email: drimcong@indigo.ie

Since Gerry and Marie Galvin moved from Kinsale in 1984, this country restaurant just west of Moycullen has become almost a place of pilgrimage for food lovers from all over Ireland (and, indeed, much further afield). It is well-appointed but without pretensions. The restaurant overlooks the garden and is furnished with traditional oak furniture, but any preconception about undue formality will have been banished in the comfortable, book-strewn bar beforehand. Gerry Galvin is one of Ireland's culinary pioneers – indeed he has been described as the father of modern Irish cuisine. Always ahead of his time, Gerry's original approach to food is seen in his early support for Euro-Toques, the European association of chefs dedicated to protecting the integrity of their ingredients, promoting the creation of innovative dishes and encouraging young talent – his entrants in the Euro-Toques Young Chef of the Year Award are invariably exceptionally well tutored. Gerry himself was a worthy first winner of the "New Irish Cuisine" competition in 1996. Many of the ingredients on his menus – for the salads plus the herbs and apples – are grown in his garden at Drimcong. Others are all local. His cooking is inventive, with wide-ranging menus that change weekly (and include a vegetarian menu) as well as a set dinner and à la carte menu. Always keen to encourage the young, Gerry also does a special 3-course menu for "pre-teenage people". A typical spring menu could include grilled oysters with goats' cheese, tomato and olive salsa, a soup (usually making use of whatever is abundant in the garden). Main courses might include the fish of the day and local meats, such as rack of Connemara mutton with garlic and rosemary jus. Desserts tend to be classical – hot rhubarb and amaretto tart, Drimcong ice creams – and there's always an excellent Irish farmhouse cheeseboard, with home-baked biscuits. • D££ Tues-Sat • Closed Xmas-Mar • Amex, Diners, MasterCard, Visa •

Moycullen   Moycullen Country House & Restaurant

Moycullen Co Galway
COUNTRY HOUSE/RESTAURANT   Tel: 091 85566   Fax: 091 85566

Overlooking Lough Corrib, and set peacefully in 30 acres of rhododendrons and azaleas, Moycullen House was built as a sporting lodge in the arts and crafts style at the beginning of the century. Large bedrooms furnished with antiques all have private baths and there's a spacious residents' sitting room with an open log fire . Children welcome; cot/extra bed available; baby-sitting by arrangement.

Casburn Restaurant

Richard and Louise Casburn added a new name to the list of must-visits in Moycullen in 1998 when they opened this very professionally run restaurant. A great deal of thought and work went into getting the changes right, and the effort has paid off handsomely. Louise looks after front-of-house. Richard's menus are ambitious but he offers a sensibly short à la carte with daily extras, eg seafood. The style is modern – dishes like prawn & crab tabouleh salad with chive dressing; roast loin of lamb with a grain mustard crust and lightly minted jus convey the style. Presentation is not overworked and cooking is excellent. It should not take the Casburns long to build up a following.• D££-£££ Wed-Mon • Acc££ • Closed 25 Dec, Good Fri & mid Jan-end Feb • Amex, Diners, MasterCard, Visa •

Moycullen   White Gables Restaurant

Moycullen Village Co Galway
RESTAURANT   Tel: 091 555744   Fax: 091 556004

Kevin and Ann Dunne have been running this attractive cottagey restaurant on the main street of Moycullen since 1991 and it's now on many a regular diner's list of favourites. Open stonework, low lighting and candlelight (even at lunch time) create a soothing away-from-it-all atmosphere. Kevin sources ingredients with care and offers weekly-changing dinner and à la carte menus and a set Sunday lunch (which is enormously popular and has two sittings). Cooking is consistently good and, to indicate the style, expect hearty, wholesome dishes such as black and white pudding with wholegrain mustard sauce, good soups, roast half duckling with orange sauce and a range of seafood including lobster from their own tank. Beef is a speciality – order it for Sunday lunch and you will understand why. Good ices, soft fruit in season; efficient service. • L£ Sun, D££ Mon-Sun • Closed Mons, 24 Dec-14 Feb • Amex, Diners, MasterCard, Visa •

Oranmore — Galway Bay Golf & Country Club Hotel

Renville Oranmore Co Galway

HOTEL   Tel: 091 790500   Fax: 091 790510/792510
email: gbaygolf@iol.ie   www.galwaybay.com

This rather handsome modern hotel, just eight miles from Galway city, looks out over an 18-hole championship golf course (designed by Christy O'Connor Jnr.) towards Galway Bay. It has a wide range of facilities for both business and leisure. Public areas include an impressively spacious lobby, large bar and a well-appointed restaurant with imaginative decor, all views. Generous-sized bedrooms, which include six for wheelchair users and a high proportion of executive suites, are furnished to a high standard with well-designed bathrooms. A number of special packages are offered by the hotel, giving good value on both golf and non-golfing breaks. • Acc£££ • Closed 25 Dec • Amex, Diners, MasterCard, Visa •

Oranmore — Quality Hotel & Leisure Centre

Oranmore Co Galway

HOTEL   Tel: 091 792244   Fax: 091 792246

This large new hotel at a roundabout on the main (N6) road is easy to find (a big plus for business locations) and offers a high standard of accommodation. Excellent leisure facilities – including a 20-metre pool – and, at the time of the guide's visit, a fine meeting room on the top floor was nearing completion. • Acc£££ • Amex, Diners, MasterCard, Visa •

Oughterard — Connemara Gateway Hotel

Oughterard Co Galway

HOTEL   Tel: 091 552328   Fax: 091 552332
email: sinnott@iol.ie   www.iol.ie/bizpark/s/sinnott

An attractive building set well back from the road, this low, neatly designed hotel creates a good impression from the outset. The large foyer has lots of comfortable seating in country-look chintz fabrics. Open turf fires are welcoming and an abundance of fresh and dried flower arrangements bring colour and add interest throughout, as does the work of local artists and sculptors. Bedrooms are variable (reflecting the hotel's origins as a 1960s motel) but all are comfortable, with considerate details (like a little washing line in the bathroom) and some have access to the garden at the back. No rooms designed for wheelchairs, but all are ground floor. There's quite a characterful public bar, used by locals as well as residents, a good leisure centre and a children's games room. • Acc££ • Closed 25 Dec • Amex, Diners, MasterCard, Visa •

Oughterard — Corrib Wave

Portacarron Oughterard Co Galway

ACCOMMODATION   Tel: 091 552147   Fax: 091 552736

A fisherman's dream, Michael and Maria Healy's unpretentious waterside guesthouse offers warm family hospitality, comfortable accommodation (all en-suite), an open turf fire to relax by and real home cooking. All rooms have a double and single bed and some are suitable for families. Best of all at Corrib Wave is the location – utter peace and tranquillity. Golf and horseriding nearby and everything to do with fishing organised for you. • Acc£ • Closed Nov-mid Mar • Diners, MasterCard, Visa •

Oughterard — Currerevagh House

Oughterard Co Galway.

COUNTRY HOUSE   Tel: 091 552312   Fax: 091 552731

Tranquillity, trout and tea in the drawing room – these are the things that draw guests back to the Hodgson family's gracious but not luxurious early Victorian manor overlooking Lough Corrib. Built in 1846, with 150 acres of woodlands and gardens and sporting rights over 5,000 acres, Currerevagh has been open to guests for over half a century. The present owners, Harry and June Hodgson, are founder members of the Irish Country Houses and Restaurants Association (known as the Blue Book). Yet, while the emphasis is on old-fashioned service and hospitality, they are adamant that the atmosphere should be more like a private house party than a hotel, and their restful rituals underline the differences: the day begins with a breakfast worthy of its Edwardian origins, laid out on the sideboard in the dining room; lunch may be one of the renowned picnic hampers required by sporting folk. Then there's afternoon tea, followed by a leisurely dinner. Fishing is the ruling passion, of course – notably brown trout, pike, perch and salmon – but there are plenty of other country pursuits to assist in building up an appetite for June's simple cooking, all based on fresh local produce. • D££ • Acc£££ • Closed Nov-Apr •

Oughterard   Sweeney's Oughterard House

Oughterard Co Galway

HOTEL   Tel: 091 091 552207

The Higgins family have owned and run this attractive creeper-clad old hotel for several generations. Prettily situated opposite the river and surrounded by mature trees (on the Clifden side of the town), it is genuinely old-fashioned with comfortable, cottagey public rooms furnished with antiques. Bedrooms vary considerably – some have four-posters. Fishing is the main attraction, but there are plenty of other outdoor pursuits including the gentle pleasure of taking tea on the lawn. • Acc££-£££ • Closed 22 Dec-mid-Jan •

Portumna   Shannon Oaks Hotel & Country Club

Portumna Co Galway

HOTEL   Tel: 0509 41777   Fax: 0509 41357

sales@shannonoaks.ie   www.shannonoaks.ie

Situated by the shores of Lough Derg, this attractive, privately-owned hotel opened in 1997. The interior is spacious, original and strikingly effective, with decor echoing the themes of river and woodland. A large lobby sets the tone, with polished wooden floor, faux-marble pillaring featuring a winter treescape and ample, well-spaced seating in contemporary style. Public rooms include a warm-toned restaurant, which can be opened up in summer, and a cosy, pub-like bar. Bedrooms are designed and finished to an exceptionally high standard, with air conditioning and fax/modem lines as standard. Thoughtful planning has also gone into the design of the conference and banqueting facilities and there is a fine leisure centre with air-conditioned gymnasium. • Acc££-£££ • Closed 25 Dec • Amex, Diners, MasterCard, Visa •

Recess   Ballynahinch Castle Hotel

Recess Co Galway

HOTEL   Tel: 095 31006   095 31085

bhinch@iol.ie

This crenellated Victorian mansion enjoys a most romantic position in ancient woodland on the banks of the Ballynahinch River. Renowned as a fishing hotel, it is impressive in scale and relaxed in atmosphere. This magic combination, plus a high level of comfort and friendliness (and an invigorating mixture of residents and locals in the bar at night) all combine to bring people back. Renovations and extensions have recently been undertaken, with great attention to period detail, a policy also carried through successfully in furnishing both public areas and bedrooms. Most bedrooms and some reception rooms – notably the dining room – have lovely views over the river. Facilities for small conferences (25). • Acc£££ • Closed Feb & Dec 20-27 & Bank Hols • Amex, Diners, MasterCard, Visa •

Recess   Lough Inagh Lodge Hotel

Recess Connemara Co Galway

HOTEL   Tel: 095 34706   Fax: 095 34708

email: Inagh@iol.ie   www.commerce.ie/inagh

Privately owned by Maire and John O'Connor (previously manager of Ballynahinch Castle), this former sporting lodge on the shores of Lough Inagh is now a small hotel with a country house atmosphere. Completely refurbished by the present owners (and opened as a hotel in 1990), it has large, well-proportioned rooms, interesting period detail and lovely fireplaces with welcoming log fires, plus all the modern comforts. Public areas include two drawing rooms, each with an open fire, a lovely dining room with deep green walls and graceful spoonback Victorian mahogany chairs and a very appealing bar (with a big turf fire and its own back door and tiled floor for wet fishing gear). Bedrooms, some with four-posters, are all well-appointed and unusually spacious, with views of lake and countryside. Walk-in dressing rooms lead to well-planned bathrooms. While it has special appeal to sportsmen, Lough Inagh is only 42 miles from Galway and makes a good base for touring Connemara. Golf and pony trekking nearby. • Acc££-£££ • Closed Dec-Feb • Amex, Diners, MasterCard, Visa •

Roundstone

O'Dowd's

Roundstone Co Galway

PUB   **Tel: 095 35809   Fax: 095 35907**

email: odowds@indigo.ie

The Griffin family have been welcoming visitors to this much-loved pub overlooking the harbour for longer than most people care to remember – and, although there are some new developments from time to time, the old bar is always the same. It's one of those simple places, with the comfort of an open fire and good pint, where people congregate in total relaxation. A reasonably priced bar menu majoring in seafood offers sustenance or, for more formal meals, the restaurant next door does the honours. The Griffins now also have a coffee shop, Espresso Stop, as part of the same building, where they do full Irish breakfast, all day food from the bar menu and speciality teas and coffee with scones, croissants and Danish pastries. • Meals £-££ • Closed 25 Dec, 3-6pm in winter & some Bank Hols • Amex, MasterCard, Visa •

Tuam

Cre na Cille

High Street Tuam Co Galway

RESTAURANT   **Tel/Fax: 093 28232**

Cathal and Sally Reynolds' consistently excellent restaurant in Tuam makes a fine stopping place en-route to Galway city or Connemara but, as it is deservedly popular with the locals both at lunchtime and in the evening, booking is strongly advised. Evenings are a little more formal and the setting softer, but the common link is Euro-Toques chef Cathal Reynolds' confident use of local ingredients in generous food at remarkably keen prices. From wide-ranging menus – set lunch, tea-time special, set dinner and à la carte – offering a wide range of seafood, meats, poultry and game in season come dishes like John Begley's black pudding with apple and onion in a balsamic sauce, followed by grilled darne of wild salmon in a dill and cream sauce or a vegetarian dish of the day – a vegetarian crumble perhaps. A customer-friendly wine list with a special £10 cellar. • L£ Mon-Fri, D££ Mon-Sat • Closed 25 Dec & 1 Jan •

KERRY

What can we say about this splendid place that the Kerrymen (and women) haven't said already? And we can only agree that it's all absolutely true. This magnificent county really is the Kingdom of Kerry. Everything is king size. For not only has Kerry mountains galore – more than anywhere else in Ireland – but the Kingdom also has the highest of all, in Carrantuohill. By international standards, this loftiest peak of MacGillicuddy's Reeks (try pronouncing it "mackil-cuddy") may not seem remarkable at just 1038 m. But when you sense its mysterious heights in the clouds above a countryside of astonishing beauty, its relative elevation is definitely world league. And that beauty of the lower countryside sweeps out into Kerry's fabulous coastline, and up into Kerry's mountains as well. They're beautiful, and remarkably varied with it. So in the upland stakes, Kerry has quantity and quality. Thus it's no surprise to find that, when the enthusiastically visiting Victorians were grading scenery in the early days of tourism, Kerry frequently merited the "sublime" rating. This meant that the county, and particularly the area around Killarney, became a visitors' mecca. At one stage, this was a distinct drawback, with some truth to accusations of tackiness. But in modern times, the entire tourism business in Kerry has put itself through a bootstraps operation, so that by and large they now have – if you'll excuse the expression – a very classy product. And through it all, the Kingdom has a timeless glory which suits man and beast alike. For the folk in Kerry are renowned for their longevity, particularly in the area along the coast from the lovely little town of Kenmare. Down there, along towards Sneem, you'll hear of Big Bertha, the world's longest-lived cow, a great milker, and ancestress in her own lifetime of a veritable herd of progeny. Don't doubt her existence even for a nano-second because, as with everything else in Kerry, it's all absolutely true and then some.

Local Attractions and Information

Beaufort	Hotel Dunloe Castle Gardens 064 44583
Castleisland	Crag Cave 066 41244
Dingle	Oceanworld 066 52111
Glencar	Into the Wilderness Walking Tours (May-Sept) 066-60104
Kenmare	Easter Walking Festival (1st of season) 064 41034
Kenmare	Heritage Centre (lacemaking, history etc) 064 41233
Killarney	Muckross House, Gardens & Traditional Farm 064 31440
Killorglin	Puck Fair (old festival) mid-August 066 62366
Lauragh	Killarney, Derreen Garden 064-83103
Listowel	St John's Art Centre (monthly programme) 068 225662
Listowel	Writers Week (June) 068 21074
Oughterard	Tourist Information 091552808
Tralee	Kerry The Kingdom (3 multi-image, audio-visual attractions) 066 27777
Tralee	Rose of Tralee International Festival (late August) 066 23227
Valentia Island	(near Portmagee), The Skellig Experience 066 76306

Annascaul   The South Pole Inn

Annascaul Co Kerry

PUB   **Tel: 066 57388 /57477**

Annascaul, on the Dingle peninsula, is one of the most-photographed villages in Ireland – mainly because of the brilliantly colourful and humorous frontage painted onto his pub by the late Dan Foley (which appeared on the front cover of at least three international guidebooks last year.) It is still a fine pub, but its theatrical owner is greatly missed since he passed on to the greater stage. Anyway, we have always liked The South Pole, which is down at the lower end of the street – the name becomes clear when you realise there is a connection with the great Irish explorer Sir Ernest Shackleton. As well as being a delightful, well-run pub, The South Pole is full of fascinating Shackleton memorabilia. • Closed 25 Dec & Good Fri •

Ballybunion   The Marine Links Hotel

Sandhill Road Ballybunion Co Kerry

HOTEL   **Tel: 068 27139   Fax: 068 27666**

email: marinelinkshotel@tinet.ie   www.travel-ireland.com/irl/marine.htm

Close to Ballybunion Golf Club, and looking over the mouth of the Shannon River to the Atlantic Ocean, Sandra Williamson and Rosaleen Rafter run as snug and friendly a little hotel as any golfer could wish to find. The growing collection of golf bag tags from around the world in the Hook and Socket Bar is evidence of many an international visitor and a yarn told in this welcoming place. The informally furnished lounge and restaurant have a relaxed holiday atmosphere. Bedrooms, while quite simple, are bright and have all the necessary comforts, with the bonus of sea views across to the cliffs of Clare. Aside from golf, hot seaweed baths, miles of sandy beaches, cliffwalks, horseriding and fishing are all at hand and Kerry's major scenic attractions are only a short drive away. Good value short breaks; discounts at Ballybunion Golf Club except July-September. • Acc££ • Closed Nov-mid Mar • Amex, Diners, MasterCard, Visa •

Caherciveen   Brennan's Restaurant

12 Main Street Caherciveen Co Kerry
RESTAURANT   Tel: 066 72021   Fax: 066 72914
email: brenrest@iol.ie

Conor and Teresa Brennan opened their stylish main street restaurant on a very wet night in July 1993, but the sun seems to have smiled on them ever since. They run a very smooth operation, serving lunch for visitors doing the Ring of Kerry (except Sunday), a deservedly popular early evening menu (main courses under £10, 6-7pm only) and a later wider-ranging à la carte every day. Conor takes pride in using the best of local ingredients and serving them imaginatively but without overdressing: thus "Pure unadulterated Saint Tola goats cheese" comes with a raw tomato dressing and extra virgin olive oil infused with dill, and "roasted tender loin of Kerry mountain lamb" has a sauce of julienne of garlic and restaurant-garden rosemary. Local seafood is a strong feature – a choice of five or six dishes may well include today's 'Harvest of the Sea' Fisherman's Plate, with a variety of the best of the day's catch. A good cheese plate (five farmhouse cheeses, with full details of origin and style, served with water biscuits and grapes) and well-made desserts, notably pastry and ices. As we go to press there are plans to install air conditioning and an application has been made for a full restaurant licence, which will allow a reception/bar offering a full range of drinks. • L£ Mon-Sat, D££ Mon-Sun • Closed Nov & Feb, 25 Dec • Amex, Diners, MasterCard, Visa •

Caherciveen   O'Neills "The Point Bar"

Renard Point Caherciveen Co Kerry
PUB   ⭐   Tel/Fax: 066 72165

In the same family for 150 years, Michael and Bridie O'Neill's pub, The Point Bar, is beside the Valentia Island car ferry. Recently renovated in true character, it's as neat as ninepence. A lovely place to drop into for a quick one while you're waiting for the ferry – but even better to stay awhile and make the most of their super fresh seafood, served during the summer. They do have a menu and it's a good starting point, covering everything from a whole range of salads and open sandwiches on brown bread – fresh and smoked wild salmon, smoked mackerel, crabmeat, crab claws – to hot dishes like deepfried squid and a couple of hake and monkfish dishes with garlic and olive oil. Everything on the menu, bar lobster (market price) is under a tenner. Not very suitable for children. The Valentia Island ferry runs continuously – ie not to a timetable – from April-September inclusive; price at time of going to press £3 single, £4 return. • L£ Mon-Sat, D£-££ daily • Closed mid-Oct-Easter • No credit cards •

Caherdaniel   Derrynane Hotel

Caherdaniel Co Kerry
HOTEL/RESTAURANT   Tel: 066 75136   Fax: 066 75160

If only for its superb location – on the seaward side of the Ring of Kerry road – this unassuming 1960s-style hotel would be well worth a visit, but there is much more to it than the view, or even its waterside position. The accommodation is quite modest but very comfortable, the food is good and, under the excellent management of Mary O'Connor and her well-trained staff, this hospitable, family-friendly place provides a welcome home from home for many a contented guest. Don't leave the area without visiting Daniel O'Connell's beautiful house at Derrynane – or the amazing Ballinskelligs chocolate factory. Well-behaved small dogs with their own beds may stay with their owners.

Restaurant

Beautifully located, overlooking the outdoor swimming pool and the hotel's gardens (which reach down to the shore), the restaurant enjoys stunning sea views on a good day. Head chef Derrick Smith ensures that residents are well looked after – the four-course dinner menu is very fairly priced at £22.50. This is a place to consider planning a lunch stop on the Ring of Kerry. Sunday lunch is served in the restaurant (booking advised) and bar food from 10am-7 pm daily. • Acc££ • Closed Oct-Apr • Amex, Diners, MasterCard, Visa •

Caherdaniel · Iskeroon

Caherdaniel Co Kerry
COUNTRY HOUSE · Tel: 066 75119 · Fax: 066 75488
email: iskeroon@iol.ie · www.homepages.iol.ie/~iskeroon/
Geraldine and David Hare's beautiful old house is in a secluded position overlooking Derrynane Harbour. The effort taken to get there makes it all the more restful once settled in. All three of the comfortable and interestingly decorated bedrooms overlook the harbour – and the islands of Deenish and Scarriff – and each has its own private bathroom just across a corridor. Geraldine enjoys cooking dinner for guests – local seafood is her speciality – and there's a big turf fire in the drawing room to relax beside afterwards. The private pier at the bottom of the garden joins an old Mass Path which, by a happy chance, leads not only to the beach but also to Keatinge's pub (known as Bridie's) where a bit of banter and some good seafood is also to be had in the evenings. • Acc££ • Closed Nov-May • Amex, MasterCard, Visa •

Caherdaniel · The Stepping Stone

Caherdaniel Co Kerry
RESTAURANT · Tel: 066 75444 · Fax: 066 75449
email: thesteppingstone@tinet.ie
The Stepping Stone is a delightful little restaurant, just off the Ring of Kerry and a brisk walk up from the harbour at Derrynane. It's a characterful, cottagey little place, with tables necessarily tightly packed and a cheerful, professional atmosphere. Bear with it if service is slow – the kitchen is also tiny – but food is imaginative, well-cooked and definitely worth waiting for. Joint owner-chefs Stephen McIlroy and Sally Walker present carefully considered eclectic menus which please modern tastes while often retaining classic partnerships – thus, for example, confit of duck with roast spiced pear and home-made fruit preserve jus is contemporary but is based on the traditional duck-with-fruit theme. Shortish à la carte menus offer four or five choices in each course but this may be doubled by daily blackboard specials. Regional Irish cheeses are nicely served with sultana & onion marmalade and sesame & oat biscuits. • D£ daily • Closed Nov-27 Dec, 5 Jan-Good Fri • MasterCard, Visa •

Camp · Barnagh Bridge Guesthouse

Camp Tralee Co Kerry
ACCOMMODATION · Tel: 066 30145 · Fax: 066 30299
Snuggled into the hillside overlooking Tralee Bay, Heather Williams' unusual architect-designed guesthouse is in extensive grounds between the mountains and the sea. Attractive and comfortable, it was purpose-built, with five individually furnished guest bedrooms (decor themed on local wild flowers), all with en-suite shower rooms. In the dining room guests can drink in the view of Tralee Bay while doing justice to Heather's breakfasts – fresh juices, newly baked breads and scones, locally made preserves, and Dingle smoked salmon and scrambled eggs or a traditional fry (in addition to daily specials such as kippers or French toast). The stylishly decorated guest drawing room opens onto a patio overlooking the Maharees islands and their spectacular sunsets. • Acc£ • Closed Nov-Apr • MasterCard, Visa •

Camp · James Ashe

Camp Tralee Co Kerry
PUB · Tel: 066 30133
This fine old pub just off the Tralee-Dingle road has been in the family for 200 years and the present owner, Thomas Ashe, has been keeping things running smoothly since 1978. It's a delightful place, full of genuine character and hospitality. Good home-cooked food is served in the bar (lunchtime, Monday-Saturday and 4-8 on Sunday) and restaurant (à la carte 6-9.15 Monday-Saturday and set 3-course lunch Sunday 12.30-2). • Bar meals daily£ • Closed mid Jan-mid March, 25 Dec & Good Fri • Amex, Diners, MasterCard, Visa •

Caragh Lake

COUNTRY HOUSE/RESTAURANT

Caragh Lodge

Caragh Lake Co Kerry
Tel: 066 69115   Fax: 066 69316
email: caraghl@iol.ie

Less than a mile from the Ring of Kerry, Mary Gaunt's lovely Victorian house and gardens nestling on the shores of the startlingly beautiful Caragh Lake is an idyllic place, with views of Ireland's highest mountains, the McGillicuddy Reeks. The house – which is elegantly furnished with antiques but not too formal – makes a cool, restful retreat. Bedrooms include some recently added garden rooms with wonderful views, their own entrance and sitting room (complete with open log fire), and are all sumptuously furnished with lovely bathrooms. In the elegant dining room overlooking the lake (open to non-residents by reservation), Mary's real love of cooking shines through. Local produce (such as freshly caught seafood, often including wild salmon from Caragh Lake, Kerry lamb and home-grown vegetables) takes pride of place. Baking is a particular strength, not only in delicious home-baked breads, but also baked desserts and treats for afternoon tea that include recipes handed down by her family through the generations. Salmon and trout fishing, boating and swimming are all available at the bottom of the garden. • D£££ daily • Acc££ • Closed mid Oct-May • Amex, Diners, MasterCard, Visa •

Caragh Lake

HOTEL

Hotel Ard-na-Sidhe

Caragh Lake Nr Killorglin Co Kerry
Tel: 066 69105   Fax: 066 69282
email: khl@iol.ie

Set in woodland and among award-winning gardens, this peaceful Victorian retreat is in a beautiful mountain location overlooking Caragh Lake. Decorated throughout in a soothing country house style, very comfortable antique-filled day rooms provide plenty of lounging space for quiet indoor relaxation and a terrace for fine weather – all with wonderful views. Bedrooms – shared between the main house and some with private patios in the garden house – are spacious and elegantly furnished in traditional style, with excellent en-suite bathrooms. This is a sister hotel to the Hotel Europe and Dunloe Castle (see entries), whose leisure facilities are also available to guests of Ard na Sidhe. Dooks golf course is nearby and Waterville, Killeen and Mahony's Point all within easy reach. • Acc££££ • Closed Oct-Apr • Amex, Diners, MasterCard, Visa •

Castlegregory

PUB

Ned Natterjack's

The West End Castlegregory Co Kerry
Tel/Fax: 066 39491

Named after the rare natterjack toad, which makes its residence at nearby Lough Gill, this old-world pub handy to the beach has been run by Vincent and Caroline O'Brien since 1994. It has a youthful, laid-back atmosphere, with traditional Irish music seven nights a week, special live music sessions on Saturday nights in summer and a beer garden where barbecues are held in fine weather. Caroline looks after the food – popular dishes based mainly on local seafood and steaks, plus a children's menu; this is very much a family-friendly place. • Meals£ • MasterCard, Visa •

Castlegregory

RESTAURANT

O'Riordan's Café

Castlegregory Dingle Peninsula Co Kerry
Tel/Fax: 066 39379

Kieran O'Callaghan and Shirley Copeland's smashing little café-restaurant is just the place to take a break on a day out on the Dingle Peninsula, or to have a more serious meal if you're staying nearby. It's cosy and welcoming, everything is spick-and-span and it's the kind of place where children can enjoy finding out more about good grown-up food. Menus change every few days, everything is based on local produce and is home cooked. Brandon Bay seafood, salmon and trout from local rivers feature regularly, as does garden produce in soups, salads and vegetable dishes. Freshly baked breads might include herb and onion, sourdough, rye and tomato and fennel – and there are delicious homely puddings and tarts. Wholesome meat dishes include beef in Guinness and Kerry mountain lamb roasted with rosemary, while vegetarians do very well too – tempura of vegetable with soy and ginger dip or samosas with spiced eggplant, basmati rice and salads are typical choices – and there's always a good selection of interesting farmhouse cheese, such as Lavistown, Cratloe and Ardrahan. Kieran enjoys helping visitors get the best out of a visit to the area – they've even printed their own map, recommending the best places to visit. • Open all day L£ & D££ daily • Closed Oct-May • MasterCard, Visa •

Dingle

ACCOMMODATION

Bambury's Guest House

Mail Road Dingle Co Kerry
Tel: 066 51244   Fax: 066 51786
email: bernieebb@tinet.ie

Just a couple of minutes walk from the centre of Dingle, Jimmy and Bernie Bambury's well-run, purpose-built guesthouse has 12 spacious rooms (including three suitable for disabled guests) all with en-suite shower rooms, tea/coffee trays, phone, satellite TV, hair dryer and complimentary mineral water. Bernie Bambury's breakfasts include griddle cakes with fresh fruit and honey – a house speciality – and vegetarian breakfasts are offered by arrangement. • Acc£ • Open all year, including Xmas • MasterCard, Visa •

Dingle

RESTAURANT

Beginish Restaurant

Green Street Dingle Co Kerry
Tel: 066 51588   Fax: 066 51591
email: patmoore@tinet.ie

Named after one of the nearby Blasket Islands, and conveniently close to the marina, it should come as no surprise that local seafood features strongly on the menu at Pat and John Moore's elegant restaurant. There is a conservatory at the back overlooking the garden – a nice spot for lunch or as a private room for 12 at night, when it is floodlit. The cooking is never too clever or pretentious, but always an experience to relish due to the sheer quality of ingredients and the imaginative but disciplined approach. Decisions can be tough, as the seasonal dinner menu offers around ten individually priced choices on most courses – plus four specials, including a vegetarian option. Lobster can be a bargain, but Kerry mountain lamb is equally attractive and the daily specials are also particularly good – John Dory fillet baked with white (butter) beans and served with anchovy vinaigrette was one such masterpiece on a recent visit. Farmhouse cheeses – a selection of about half a dozen – are served plated, with water biscuits, and there's a choice of freshly brewed coffee, tea or herbal infusions.

Accommodation

Self-catering accommodation is available in several exceptionally well-equipped and comfortably-furnished units for varying numbers. Normally available for a minimum of 1 week, but it is worth inquiring about overnight lettings. • L£-££ & D££ daily • Closed Bank Hols & Dec-mid Mar • Amex, Diners, MasterCard, Visa •

Dingle

RESTAURANT

The Chart House Restaurant

The Mall Dingle Co Kerry
Tel/Fax: 066 52255

Jim McCarthy (previously restaurant manager at The Park Hotel Kenmare) opened this brand new restaurant in Dingle in 1997. Informal in furnishing style and general approach, offering fairly moderately priced seasonal, multi-cultural menus based on local ingredients, the restaurant itself and chef Paul Cosgrove's eclectic cooking style have brought a different element to Dingle's dining scene. Thus Annascaul black pudding and apples may be used in a starter – spiced with ginger, wrapped in filo pastry and served in a bacon jus; similarly, local steamed mussels may be served "Malay style" with chili. Main course roast salmon is cooked "Asian style" and served on a bed of braised cabbage, with herb cream sauce – and grilled supreme of chicken comes on a ratatouille of vegetables with a herb oil. Desserts include some classics -warm pear tart with almond frangipani, sauce anglaise or home-made ice creams – and Irish cheeses are cannily offered, at £7.50, with a glass of vintage port. The wine list is concise, but unhelpful – no country (or even continent) of origin and no tasting notes are given. • D££ daily • Closed 7 Jan-mid Feb • MasterCard, Visa •

Dingle

ACCOMMODATION

Cleevaun

Lady's Cross Milltown Dingle Co Kerry
Tel: 066 51108   Fax: 066 52228
email: cleevaun@iol.ie   www.iol.ie/KerryInsight

A cup of tea or coffee and a slice of home-made porter cake welcomes guests to Charlotte and Sean Cluskey's well-run, recently renovated guesthouse just outside the town. Set in an acre of landscaped gardens overlooking Dingle Bay, it's near enough to Dingle to be handy and far enough away to enjoy the peace that the peninsula promises. Furnishing throughout is in a pleasant country pine style: bedrooms are all non-smoking, have good facilities and are well organised, with quality beds, quilted bedspreads and well-finished en-suite bathrooms (1 shower-only). One bedroom has a separate dressing room. Charlotte's breakfasts – served in a large south-facing dining room overlooking Dingle Bay – are quite a speciality. • Acc££ • Closed mid-Nov-mid-Mar • MasterCard, Visa •

Dingle   Dingle Skellig Hotel

Dingle Co Kerry

HOTEL   **Tel: 066 51144   Fax: 066 51501**
                email: dsk@iol.ie   www.iol.ie/kerry-insight/dingle-skellig

Although modest-looking from the road, this 1960s hotel enjoys a shoreside location on the edge of the town and has won many friends over the years. It is a particularly well-run, family-friendly hotel, with organised entertainment for children and an excellent leisure centre. Roomy public areas are comfortably furnished with a fair degree of style. Good use is made of sea views throughout, especially in the conservatory restaurant which has special anti-glare glass. Bedrooms – ten of which are designated non-smoking – include three suites, one junior suite and two rooms suitable for disabled guests; all are reasonably large, have been recently refurbished and have small but neat bathrooms. On Tuesday nights throughout the summer, from June, the hotel runs a Ceili night of traditional music, song, story-telling and dance, featuring highly accomplished local artists. Although best known as a holiday destination, the Dingle Skellig also has excellent conference and business meeting facilities, with full back-up services including French and German translation. • Acc£££ • Closed 25 Dec & 4 Jan-mid Feb • Amex, Diners, MasterCard, Visa •

Dingle   Doyle's Seafood Restaurant & Townhouse

John Street Dingle Co Kerry

RESTAURANT/ACCOMMODATION   **Tel: 066 51174   Fax: 066 51816**

Established by John and Stella Doyle in 1974, Doyle's Seafood Bar (as it was then known) was Dingle's first serious restaurant – and thus the foundation stone for the town's current culinary reputation. It changed hands in 1998, although to the casual observer there are few clues – the flagstone floors and old furniture still give this restaurant lots of character. It is now in the good hands of Sean Cluskey (previously manager of Dingle Skellig Hotel) and his wife Charlotte (who runs Cleevaun guesthouse), so it is a safe assumption that all will be well. Local seafood is still the main attraction – they have even retained some of Stella Doyle's specialities, including her award-winning starter of hot oysters in Guinness – and lobster, selected from a tank in the bar, is a speciality. There are, however, concessions to non-seafood eaters – chicken, steaks and vegetable paella as well as lamb. Puddings are nice and traditional or there's a plated selection of farmhouse cheeses from the Munster region to finish.

Rooms

High quality accommodation includes a residents' sitting room as well as eight bedrooms. • D££ Mon-Sat • Acc££ • Amex, Diners, MasterCard, Visa •

Dingle   Greenmount House

Gortonora Dingle Co Kerry

ACCOMMODATION   **Tel: 066 51414   Fax: 066 51974**

Just five minutes walk from the centre of Dingle, the Curran family's exceptionally comfortable guesthouse is quietly located on the hillside, with private parking and uninterrupted views across the town and harbour to the mountains across the bay. The well-appointed bedrooms (all of which are non-smoking) fall into two groups – half are in the original house and, although smaller than the newer ones, have recently been refurbished to a very high standard. The others are junior suites with generous seating areas and good amenities, including fridges as well as tea/coffee-making trays, phone and TV (and their own entrance and balcony). There's also a comfortable residents' sitting room and a conservatory overlooking the harbour, where excellent breakfasts are served. • Acc££ • Open all year • MasterCard, Visa •

The guide aims to provide comprehensive recommendations of the best places to eat, drink and stay throughout Ireland. We welcome suggestions from readers. If you think an establishment merits assessment , please write or email us.

Dingle   The Half Door

Mail Road Dingle Co Kerry

RESTAURANT/ACCOMMODATION   Tel: 066 51600/51833   Fax: 066 51883

Since 1991 chef-proprietor Denis O'Connor has been preparing some of the best seafood in the country at the cottagey Dingle restaurant he runs with his wife Teresa. Denis's mainly seafood menus go with the seasons, but whatever is available it is perfectly cooked and generously served without over-presentation. The saucing is excellent and an outstanding speciality of the house is the seafood platter, available hot or cold as either a starter or main course with (depending on availability of individual items) lobster, oysters, Dublin Bay prawns, scallops, crab claws and mussels (attractively presented with garlic or lemon butter). Good puddings or Irish farmhouse cheeses to follow. • L£ & D££ Mon-Sat • Closed 24-26 Dec •

Accommodation

The O'Connors also have accommodation in a separate establishment called the Half Door Waterfront Guesthouse, on the edge of Dingle. Ask at the restaurant or call 066 51883 for details. • Acc££ • Closed 24-26 Dec • Amex, MasterCard, Visa •

Dingle   Lord Baker's

Main Street Dingle Co Kerry

PUB/RESTAURANT   Tel: 066 51277   Fax: 066 52174

Believed to be the oldest pub in Dingle, this business was established in 1890 by a Tom Baker. A very popular businessman in the area, a colourful orator, member of Kerry County Council and a director of the Tralee-Dingle Railway, he was known locally as "Lord Baker" and as such is now immortalised in John Moriarty's excellent pub and restaurant in the centre of Dingle. A welcoming turf fire burns in the front bar, where bar food such as chowder and home-baked bread or crab claws in garlic butter is served. At the back, there's a much more sophisticated dining set-up in the restaurant proper (and, beyond it, a lovely garden). Seafood stars, as it does everywhere in the area, but there's also a good choice of other dishes – local lamb, of course, also beef, chicken and local duckling – all well-cooked and served in an atmosphere of great hospitality. Sunday lunch in the restaurant is a particularly popular event and very well done (booking strongly advised); on other days the lunchtime bar menu, plus one or two daily specials such as a roast, can be taken in the restaurant. The wine list includes a House Selection of ten wines from around the world at £10.50-£13 and an equal choice of half bottles. • L£, D££ daily & bar meals daily • Closed 24-25 Dec • Amex, Diners, MasterCard, Visa •

Dingle   Milltown House

Dingle Co Kerry

ACCOMMODATION   Tel: 066 51372   Fax: 066 51095

email: milltown@indigo.ie   www.indigo.ie/~milltown

This attractive guesthouse on the western side of Dingle, set in immaculate gardens running down to the water's edge, enjoys beautiful views of the harbour and distant mountains. Day rooms include an informal reception room, a comfortably furnished sitting room and a conservatory breakfast room overlooking the garden. The bedrooms – all very comfortable and thoughtfully furnished -include two with private patios. Limited room service is available. Milltown House changed hands late in 1997 but there was little noticeable change on a recent visit. • Acc££ • Closed 23-27 Dec • MasterCard, Visa •

Dingle   Pax Guest House

Upper John Street Dingle Co Kerry

ACCOMMODATION   Tel: 066 51518

email: paxhouse@iol.ie

Just half a mile out of Dingle, this modern house enjoys what may well be the finest view in the area – and, thanks to the exceptional hospitality and high standards of the owners, Joan Brosnan and Ron Wright, is also one of the most comfortable and relaxing places to stay. Rooms are very thoughtfully furnished and decorated in traditional Celtic themes, with well-finished bathrooms (3 shower only). Breakfast is a major event, featuring fresh Dingle Bay seafood as well as an exceptional range of meats and cheeses. Well-behaved dogs are welcome by arrangement. • Acc£ • Closed Nov-Mar • MasterCard, Visa •

Dingle

Tigh Mhaire de Barra

The Pier Head Dingle Co Kerry

PUB   **Tel: 066 51215**

Real hospitality, good food and music are the attractions of Mhaire de Barra and Pat
Leahy's harbourside pub. In unpretentious and comfortable surroundings they serve
good things like home-made soups with freshly-baked bread, local seafood specials,
traditional dishes like boiled bacon and cabbage and Kerry porter cake at lunchtime.
Evening meals include an additional range of hot main courses. Dingle Pies, for which
the pub is famous, are included in the menu off-season, when the rush of the tourist
season has died down. • Meals £ • Closed 25 Dec & Good Fri • No credit cards.•

Fenit

The Tankard

Kilfenora Fenit Co Kerry

RESTAURANT   **Tel: 066 36164**   **Fax: 066 36516**

Easily spotted on the seaward side of the road from Tralee, this bright yellow pub and
restaurant has built up a great reputation, especially for seafood. An imaginative bar
menu is available from lunchtime to late evening, serving the likes of "smokeys" and
boxty, warm chicken salad and vegetarian choices like mushroom & mozzarella salad.
The restaurant is normally open for dinner only (except Sundays), but lunch is available
by arrangement. A phone call is worthwhile to get the best of seafood cooking (which
can be exceptional). Beyond seafood there's quite a wide choice, especially steaks in
various guises, duckling, Kerry lamb and some strong vegetarian options. There's a great
sea view from the restaurant, but not the pub. • D££ daily, L£ Sun & bar meals£ • Amex,
Diners, MasterCard, Visa •

Fenit

West End Bar

Fenit Tralee Co Kerry

Tel: 066 36246

This family-run pub is exactly seven minutes walk from the marina. Good home cooking
is available in the bar and informal restaurant (phone ahead to check times) and there is
simple, inexpensive accommodation too • Meals£ • Acc£ (closed Nov-Apr) • Bar closed
25 Dec & Good Fri only • MasterCard, Visa •

Glencar

The Climbers' Inn

Glencar Killarney Co Kerry

ACCOMMODATION   **Tel: 066 60101**   **Fax: 066 60104**

email: climbers@iol.ie/~climbers

A real inn, The Climbers' is the oldest established walking and climbing inn in Ireland. It
specialises in walking holidays and short breaks, with or without guides, and offers every
comfort for the traveller, whether arriving on foot, on horseback or, more prosaically, by
car. (It may sound less exciting but, whether approaching from Killarney or Sneem, the
drives are spectacular.) Established in 1875 and in family ownership for four generations,
the current owners are Johnny and Anne Walsh, an energetic young couple who have
made big improvements since they took over in 1993. Accommodation comprises
budget (hostel) and bed & breakfast (rooms with en-suite showers) and has all been
recently refurbished. Rooms are simple, functional and spotlessly clean. Home-cooked
dinners are served in the dining area of a bar reminiscent of alpine inns, furnished with
old church furniture. A guest chef is invited from a different country each season, so the
style of cooking varies accordingly. It will, however, be based on local ingredients, often
wild, and will aim to satisfy hearty mountain appetites with big soups, home-baked
brown bread and main courses which include Kerry mountain lamb, wild venison or
salmon (with plenty of wholesome vegetables and a good pudding). Breakfast, which is
served in a separate room (used also for group dining) may be a more pedestrian affair,
with commercial orange juice and cornflakes. Bar food is also available daily from 12
noon – 6 pm in the summer season. "Into the Wilderness" tours are organised from the
inn – details from Johnny Walsh, or any tourist office. • Meals£ • Acc£ • Closed Nov-
Mar • Amex, Diners, MasterCard, Visa •

Kenmare   Bean & Leaf

4 Rock Street Kenmare Co Kerry

CAFE   **Tel: 064 42363   Fax: 064 42196**

email: kburke@mail1.tinet.ie   www.homepage.tinat.ie/~beanandleaf

Up a little side road off the main street (one block up from Quill's) is this surprising little cyber-café. Excellent coffees (with beans to take home), teas and tisanes, scrumptious food (global with South American leanings – tortilla, burrito, chicken taco, guacamole dip) all somehow assembled and/or cooked in a tiny little kitchen in front of your eyes. Lovely pastries and bakes – and art and music too. A one-off. • L£ & D£ daily • Closed 25 Dec, Nov & Feb • MasterCard, Visa •

Kenmare   Café Indigo & The Square Pint

The Square Kenmare Co Kerry

RESTAURANT   **Tel: 064 42356   Fax: 064 42358**

As the name implies, this first floor restaurant has indigo as its primary colour. It is remarkably minimalist, both architecturally and decoratively, for a converted pub in an historic Kerry town. The menu (notable for some modern, minimalist or simply youthful variations on traditional spellings) reflects the trendy surroundings, with modern dishes influenced by many international cuisines – chicken and wild mushroom ravioli with truffle-scented butter sauce or thinly sliced cured fillet of beef with parmesan shavings and pickled sea grass as starters, for example. Main courses could be crispy spring roll of chicken breast and king prawns with a sweet pepper sauce and sun-dried tomato pasta or seared sea scallops with a celeriac purée and mango vanilla bean salsa sauce. Desserts are perhaps easier to visualise: bitter chocolate lemon torte with vanilla sauce or iced honeyed nougatine with coffee sauce. Pancake terrine flavoured with orange blossom and almond served with a passionfruit coulis almost defies description, however. A French bias on the wine list with good house wines. Blinis bar, serving savoury and sweet Russian pancakes from 10.30pm-12.30am. Downstairs, The Square Pint serves a daily-changing lunch menu (spiced lentil soup, Irish stew, seafood pie) and snacky things like mini baguettes or grilled vegetables on toast with tapenade spread. In the evenings there's live music every night. • L£ & D££ daily • Closed 25 Dec & Good Fri • Amex, Diners, MasterCard, Visa •

Kenmare   Ceann Mara

Kenmare Co Kerry

ACCOMMODATION   **Tel: 064 41220   Fax: 064 41220**

In a peaceful location just outside Kenmare, Therese Hayes's pleasing modern house is set in lovely gardens that run down to the water. Interesting, comfortable reception rooms are full of family antiques and mementoes and the four bedrooms are all very different, but thoughtfully furnished. Very good breakfasts are served in a lovely dining room overlooking the garden. • Acc£ • Closed Oct-May •

Kenmare   d'Arcy's

Main Street Kenmare Co Kerry

RESTAURANT ☆⭐   **Tel: 064 41589**

New partners (Pat Gath and Martin Wilde) and new chef James Mulchrone have taken over this former bank – you can still make out where the vault used to be – at the top of the town. The menu is surprisingly modern – definitely less traditional than might be anticipated if you had visited the restaurant previously. Nonetheless, dishes are excellent and well executed – the chef has a sure touch and cooking is spot on. Local ingredients are cleverly used in dishes with overseas influences, mainly oriental and Mediterranean. Thus Kenmare smoked salmon is served with potato pancakes and a sharp red onion salsa, and a bruschetta of goat's cheese comes with tapenade and sun-dried tomato pesto. Roast herb-crusted loin of lamb (a generous portion this) comes with a port and mustard seed sauce; seared scallops are served with fine pasta and a basil pesto broth. Regular patrons will be pleased to see that one of the late Matthew d'Arcy's signature dishes, fillet of beef with mushroom stuffing baked in puff pastry with shallots and a cracked black pepper sauce (an Irish version of beef Wellington?) remains on the menu. For dessert, look no further than a more traditional rhubarb and ginger fool served in a hazelnut tuile, or crème brûlée with lavender honey ice cream. Good wine list, home-made breads, and pleasant service – all in all, a lively and welcoming restaurant with a pleasingly cosmopolitan feel to it.

Accommodation

There are five bedrooms which, it is expected, will be renovated in time for the 1999 season. • D££ daily • Closed mid-Jan-mid-Feb • MasterCard, Visa •

Kenmare   Dromquinna Manor

Blackwater Bridge PO Kenmare Co Kerry

HOTEL   Tel: 064 41657   Fax: 064 41791

email: dromquinna@tinet.ie   www.kenmare.com/dromquinna

Built in 1850 in an idyllic location – the hotel is set in 42 acres of wooded grounds and has three quarters of a mile of sheltered south-facing sea frontage – Dromquinna Manor has a number of unusual features including a romantic tree house (a 2-bedroom suite with four-poster and balcony, 15ft up a tree), a safe little sandy beach (beside the informal Boat House Bistro) and a 34ft Nelson Sport Angler with professional skipper for fishing parties and scenic cruises. The interior of the house features an original oak-panelled Great Hall, a traditional drawing room complete with concert grand piano and an unusual Dragon Bar. The 48 bedrooms include three suites and five junior suites and are all individually decorated to specific themes, with good bathrooms (only two are shower-only). The hotel and surroundings can be very busy at times – they do a barbecue Sunday lunch on the quay with a live band (moving into the Boat House in bad weather) which has become very popular – so reservations are essential. Not surprisingly, weddings are also often catered for, so finding a time when the hotel and grounds are quiet enough to be themselves can sometimes be a matter of luck. • Acc££ • Open all year • Amex, Diners, MasterCard, Visa •

Kenmare   The Horseshoe

3 Main Street Kenmare Co Kerry

RESTAURANT/PUB   Tel: 064 41553   Fax: 064 42502

Chef-proprietor Irma Weeland's nice old-fashioned bar and restaurant is cosy and well-run – and the good home cooking she offers in the informal oil-cloth-tabled restaurant at the back, with its open fire and original cattle stall divisions, is unpretentious and wholesome. Soups, chowders, chicken goujons, burgers and pies will all be home-made, as will the chips (a rare enough event these days). Seafood and steaks are the key players on evening menus, but there's plenty of other dishes to choose from, including strong vegetarian options and local duck (often a good bet in west Cork and Kerry). Classic puddings – crème brûlée, treacle tart – and a short but adequate wine list. • L£ Mon-Sat, D£-££ daily • Closed 25 Dec, Good Fri & closed Feb & Mar • Amex, MasterCard, Visa •

Kenmare   The Lime Tree

Shelburne Street Kenmare Co Kerry

RESTAURANT   Tel: 064 41225/42434   Fax: 064 41839

email: benchmark@iol.ie

Built in 1832, Tony and Alex Daly's restaurant is an attractive cut stone building set well back from the road (next to The Park Hotel). An open log fire, exposed stone walls, original wall panelling and a minstrels' gallery (which is an upper eating area) all give character to the interior. Menus change with the seasons, and there are always daily specials, including several vegetarian options such as goat cheese potato cake or ragout of mushrooms. Local produce – like Sneem black pudding and Kerry lamb (oven-roasted, with thyme honey jus perhaps) – is highly valued, and local seafood appears in delicious dishes such as fruits de mer cassoulet with fettucine, seafood potpourri "en papillotte" and lobster risotto with pesto. Finish, perhaps, with a traditional pudding like warm blackberry and pear fruit crumble. • D££ only • Closed mid-Nov-end Mar • MasterCard, Visa •

Kenmare   Muxnaw Lodge

Castletownbere Road Kenmare Co Kerry

COUNTRY HOUSE   Tel: 064 41252

Within walking distance from town (first right past the double-arched bridge towards Bantry), Mrs Hannah Boland's wonderfully cosy and homely house was built in 1801 and enjoys spectacular views across Kenmare Bay. It is very much a home – relax in the TV lounge or outside in the sloping gardens (you can even play tennis on the all-weather court). Bedrooms are tranquil, all en suite and with cleverly hidden tea/coffee-making facilities, and are individually furnished with free-standing period pieces and pleasant fabrics. Notice is required by noon if guests wish to dine – a typical dinner cooked in and on the Aga comprises carrot soup, oven-baked salmon and apple pie, but guests are always asked beforehand what they like. Two new rooms are planned for 1999. • Acc£ • Closed 25 Dec • No credit cards •

Kenmare   New Delight

18 Henry Street Kenmare Co Kerry

RESTAURANT   Tel: 064 42350

A delightful vegetarian café and restaurant that serves almost wholly organic food. Irish carnivores have traditionally treated such places with deep suspicion, it seems, but happily times have changed and they have embraced this relatively new venture, sampling an array of eclectic dishes (with a more Asian slant in the evening). Typically, you could have a celery soup, warm grilled aubergine with feta cheese and salad, and lemon tart – everything is home-made (bread, scones, carrot cake etc). Enclosed tea garden. • L£ & D£ daily • Closed Dec-mid Mar • No credit cards •

Kenmare   Packie's

Henry Street Kenmare Co Kerry

RESTAURANT   Tel: 064 41508   Fax: 064 42135

Since Tom and Maura Foley opened this buzzy little restaurant in 1992 it has had a special place in the hearts of many who visit Kenmare. It's stylish but unpretentious, with small tables and a big heart. Great local ingredients, especially seafood, mingle with imports from sunnier climes and, in Maura's skilful hands, result in imaginative Ireland-meets-the-Med food that is memorable for its intense flavouring. Although roast pepper salad may come with black olives and pesto, and the impression is somehow of world cuisine, it's not all sun-dried tomatoes and pesto – starters of potato pancakes come with garlic or herb butter and crab cakes with traditional tartare sauce. Red onion and caper salsa may sound like an exotic accompaniment for wild smoked salmon, but it's actually a long-established partnership. Close examination of menus will probably reveal more dishes that have stood the test of time than new ones, but the important factor here is the sheer quality of both food – especially local seafood – and cooking Puddings include good ices and a nice variation on bread and butter pudding – Moriarty's barm brack and butter pudding with rum – or there are Irish farmhouse cheeses to finish. Interesting and well-priced wine list. Private Room. • D££ Tues-Sat only 5.30-10 • Closed Sun and Nov-Easter • MasterCard, Visa •

Kenmare   Park Hotel Kenmare

Kenmare Co Kerry

HOTEL/RESTAURANT   Tel: 064 41200   Fax: 064 41402

email: phkenmare@iol.ie   www.parkkenmare.com

In a lovely location adjoining Kenmare town, with views over sloping gardens to the ever-changing mountains across the bay, this renowned hotel was built in 1897 by the Great Southern and Western Railway Company for passengers travelling to Parknasilla, 17 miles away. The train stopped at Kenmare, where the gentry would stay overnight, before continuing on to Parknasilla. Although sold in the late '70s, 1985 is the key date in the hotel's recent history. It was then that Francis Brennan took over as proprietor and general manager. Since then Park Hotel Kenmare has earned international acclaim for exceptional standards of service, comfort and cuisine – and for Mr Brennan's (growing) collection of antiques. Once inside the granite Victorian building, a warm welcome and the ever-burning fire in the hall begin weaving the Park's special magic: any tendency to formality in the antique furnishings is offset by amusing quirks of taste and despite the constant quest for perfection, it is surprisingly relaxed. Public rooms are not overpoweringly grand and several open onto a verandah overlooking the gardens and Kenmare River. Luxurious accommodation includes nine suites and 31 min-suites; all bedrooms are spacious, with excellent bathrooms (only four are shower-only) and furnished to exceptional standards of comfort with all the amenities expected of top hotels – fresh flowers, robes, mineral water, quality toiletries – and some unexpected, such as the recently introduced hi-fi systems which have been enthusiastically received by guests. • Acc££££ • Closed 4 Jan-Easter • Amex, Diners, MasterCard, Visa •

Restaurant ★

Service in this elegant dining room is unfailingly outstanding and the views from window tables are simply lovely – a fitting setting for very fine food. A stylishly restrained classicism has characterised this distinguished kitchen under several famous head chefs. Currently Bruno Schmidt occupies the role. A wide choice of dishes is available, with seasonal à la carte and set dinner menus (which are changed daily). There is an understandable leaning towards local seafood – two out of three starters or main courses on the dinner menu might be various types of seafood – but the carte offers a wider selection, including Kerry lamb, beef, pork and local duck as well as interesting vegetarian dishes and one or two special seafood dishes, such as lobster. Typically, an early summer menu might start with marinated fillet of salmon with beetroot and wild asparagus, light horseradish and cucumber sauce, then soup such as a light and cold lobster gazpacho – or a witty gin & tonic sorbet. Cannelloni of fresh sole and crab on wild mushrooms with a morel cream sauce is a typical main course. Beautifully presented desserts might include red wine soup with caramelised figs and pistachio ice cream and there's a good choice of local farmhouse cheeses. Excellent service; fine list of 600 wines (House Wine £17.95) A short à la carte lounge menu is available at lunchtime. • D££££, light L in bar • Closed 4 Jan-Easter • Amex, Diners, MasterCard, Visa •

Kenmare   The Purple Heather

Henry Street Kenmare Co Kerry
RESTAURANT/BAR   **Tel: 064 41016**
Daytime sister restaurant to Packie's, this traditional darkwood and burgundy bar gradually develops into an informal restaurant at the rear. Run by the O'Connell family since the mid-1970s, The Purple Heather was among the first to establish a reputation for good food in Kenmare. What they aim for – and achieve, with commendable consistency – is good, simple, home-cooked food. Soups come with home-baked breads, salad is made of organic greens with balsamic dressing. Main courses include a number of seafood salads, vegetarian salads (cold and warm), pâtés – including a delicious smoked salmon pâté– plus a range of omelettes and Irish farmhouse cheeses. The sandwich menu offers every variation – white/brown, closed/open, toasted or otherwise – and there's a good choice of home-made desserts to go with teas, tisanes, coffees, hot chocolate or whatever takes your fancy, including Irish coffee. • Daytime meals£ • Closed 1 wk Xmas • No credit cards •

Kenmare   Riversdale House Hotel

Kenmare Co Kerry
HOTEL   **Tel: 064 41299**
Coming from Killarney, across the double-arched bridge out of town on the N71 road to Bantry; this bright yellowish hotel is just on the left, on the shores of Kenmare Bay. It is set in seven acres of gardens, with car parks to the front and rear. The hotel has a large open-plan lounge with a cluster of chesterfields around an open stone fireplace and a bar, with a long counter, that often provides live Irish entertainment. Best of the bedrooms (those on the ground floor have direct access to the gardens) are obviously those with breathtaking views across the estuary to the hills beyond, and especially worth seeking out are the eaved fifth-floor suites, each with its own patio balcony. But all the rooms are comfortably furnished in contemporary style, providing satellite TV, tea/coffee-making facilities and neat bathrooms. • Acc££ • Closed early Nov-third wk March • Amex, Diners, MasterCard, Visa •

Kenmare   The Rosegarden

Kenmare Co Kerry
ACCOMMODATION   **Tel: 064 42288   Fax: 064 42305**
email: rosegard@iol.ie   www.euroka.com/rosegarden
Peter Ringlever, the former owner of Jugs Restaurant in the 1980s, has returned to Kenmare and, with his wife Ingrid, built and opened this brand new guesthouse out of town at the start of the Ring of Kerry road. Set back from the road, with an immaculate garden and pond at the front, the house has a distinctly continental feel about it (hardly surprising since the couple are Dutch) and is spotlessly clean. The centrally-heated bedrooms, all en suite (possibly the best shower pressure in Ireland!) offer guests satellite TV (including a nightly-changing in-house movie shown at 10pm), tea/coffee-making facilities and biscuits. Dinner (à la carte or nightly-changing table d'hôte) combines local produce with some international touches; witness Kenmare Bay shrimps in a spicy oriental sauce, breaded medallions of pork served with a peppercorn, tomato and basil sauce, finishing with tiramisu. Various breads come with three assorted butters including curry. • Acc£ • D£ • Closed Nov-Mar • Amex, Diners, MasterCard, Visa •

Kenmare

Sallyport House

Kenmare Co Kerry

COUNTRY HOUSE   Tel: 064 42066   Fax: 064 4206

This renovated country house on the edge of Kenmare is in a quiet and convenient location overlooking the harbour, with fine garden and mountain views at the rear. It is spacious throughout, from the large entrance hall (with welcoming fire) to bedrooms that are thoughtfully furnished with a mixture of antique and good quality reproduction furniture, plus orthopaedic beds, TV, phone and (unusual enough to merit mention) lights and mirrors correctly placed for their function. All rooms have practical, fully-tiled bathrooms with powerful over-bath showers and built-in hair dryers. Delicious breakfasts are served in a sunny dining room overlooking the garden. Ample parking. No dogs. Not suitable for children under 12. • Acc££ • Closed Xmas & New Year • No credit cards •

Kenmare

Sheen Falls Lodge

Kenmare Co Kerry

HOTEL/RESTAURANT 🏛 🏛   Tel: 064 41600   Fax: 064 41386
Hotel of the Year   email: sheenfalls@iol.ie   www.iol.ie/sheenfalls

This stunning hotel made an immediate impact from the day it opened in April 1991 and it has continued to develop and mature most impressively since. It has a beautiful waterside location. Welcoming fires always burn in the elegant foyer and in several of the spacious, beautifully furnished reception rooms, including a lounge bar area overlooking the waterfall. Luxurious rooms include one suitable for disabled guests. All have superb amenities, lovely marbled bathrooms and views of the cascading river or Kenmare Bay. Exceptional facilities for business and private guests include state-of-the-art conference facilities, a fine library and an equestrian centre. A recently completed Health Spa includes a pretty indoor swimming pool and, together with an informal bar and bistro ("Oscars", open 6-10 daily), has been so carefully landscaped and integrated with the older building that it feels as if it has always been there. But it is the staff, under the guidance of the exceptionally warm and hospitable General Manager, Adriaan Bartels, who make this luxurious and stylish international hotel the home from home that it quickly becomes for each new guest. Little Hay Cottage, a luxuriously appointed self-contained two-bedroomed thatched cottage in its own garden, is also available to rent.

La Cascade ★

This beautifully appointed restaurant is arranged in tiers to take full advantage of the waterfalls – floodlit at night and providing a dramatic backdrop for Fergus Moore's superb cooking, which is French with modern Irish overtones. Unquestionably one of Ireland's most talented chefs, Fergus has been executive chef since the hotel opened and, with the backing of faultless service under restaurant manager John O'Meara, has earned great praise for consistently high standards. Both a daily table d'hôte (£37.50) and a separate vegetarian menu (£27.50) are offered and will certainly please even the most discerning diner. Menus favour seafood, but the overall choice is balanced with three meat or poultry dishes on a selection of six. Luxurious starters bursting with flavour might typically include fresh lobster with rocket salad, citrus dressing and crisp fried aubergine, terrine of foie gras with freshly toasted brioche and orange and hazelnut dressing, local wild Atlantic salmon (cured and smoked on the premises) or a game consommé with broad beans, tarragon and smoked duck tortellini. Main courses are in a similar vein – fresh scallops might be wrapped in smoked bacon and served with saffron risotto, basil and balsamic dressing, or a filet of beef be served with braised salsify, broad beans and morels. Indulgent desserts include good ices – passion fruit with orange wafer and citrus compote, for example- and classic hot souffles, but the farmhouse cheese selection, with parmesan biscuits, is equally tempting. As to the wine, suffice it to say that the hotel rejoices in having not one, but two superb French sommeliers – Alain Bras and Ronauld Toulon – and that the wine cellar is open for guests to choose their own bottle from nearly 500 wines.(House wines £16-20) Port can also be served in the cellar after dinner. Dinner only, 7.15-9.30 daily. (Light lunches (smoked salmon, club sandwiches etc) are available in the sun lounge, 12-4 daily, followed by afternoon tea, 4-6 pm. • D££££ daily • Acc££££ • Closed early Dec-23 Dec, 4 Jan-6 Feb •

Beside the main building there is also a discreet 3-bedroom apartment, with separate entrance from the grounds, popular for small business conferences, and in the basement an impressive state-of-the-art conference suite, the William Petty Conference Centre, named after the original owner of the land, which has facilities for up to 150, theatre-style. An otherwise well-appointed and luxurious leisure centre is remarkable for having only a post-sauna plunge-pool.• Closed Jan -mid Mar. • Access, Amex, Visa, Diners.•

Kenmare
Shelburne Lodge

Killowen Cork Road Kenmare Co Kerry

ACCOMMODATION 🏛
Tel: 064 41013   Fax: 064 42135

Shelburne Lodge is the oldest house in Kenmare and has all the style and attention to detail that would be expected from Tom and Maura Foley, proprietors of the dashing Kenmare restaurant, Packies. A fine stone house on the edge of the town, the lodge is set back from the road in its own grounds and lovely gardens. Spacious day rooms include an elegant, comfortable drawing room and a large, well appointed dining room where excellent breakfasts are served. Accommodation, in seven rooms individually decorated to a high standard, is extremely comfortable and everything (especially beds and bedding) is of the highest quality; individual decoration extends to the excellent bathrooms – all with full bath except the more informal conversion at the back of the house, which is especially suitable for families and has neat shower rooms. No evening meals are served, but residents are directed to Packies. • Acc££ • Closed early Oct-end Mar • MasterCard, Visa •

Killarney
Aghadoe Heights Hotel

Aghadoe Killarney Co Kerry

HOTEL
Tel: 064 31766   Fax: 064 31345

A few miles out of town and well-signposted off the N22 road (both directions: Tralee and Cork), this low-rise hotel, built in the '60s, enjoys stunning views of the lakes and the mountains beyond. It also overlooks Killarney's two 18-hole championship golf courses. Ownership changed recently, and it is now in the very capable hands of Patrick Curran, a fine hotelier (previously at Castletroy Park, Limerick). It's very luxuriously furnished and decorated, with lots of marble, antiques and good paintings, and the club-like Lake Room with its leather chesterfields and dark wood is particularly relaxing. Less so is the fitness room with its ferocious-looking equipment, part of a magnificent leisure complex that features a superb pool with its own waterfall (there's also an ornamental one at the hotel's entrance), as well as a spa bath, sauna etc. Again, the views from here are sensational. The elegant bedrooms, fitted in a variety of woods and furnished with co-ordinating drapes and fabrics, offer the usual amenities, including mini-bar and satellite TV, while the smartly tiled bathrooms provide robes, slippers and pampering toiletries. Service is exceptional – the head porter has been here over 27 years and there's nothing he doesn't know – including, no doubt, the exact spot for catching salmon and trout on the hotel's own 10-mile stretch of riverbank about six miles away.

Frederick's Restaurant

The restaurant enjoys one of the most dramatic views over the Lakes of Killarney and, like the rest of the hotel, is luxuriously appointed. The change of ownership has not affected the kitchen, where head chef Robin Suter still holds sway. He offers daily changing set menus as lunch and dinner in addition to weekly à la carte menus. The style is formal, imaginative, distinctly French and based on top quality produce, notably Kerry lamb – in roast saddle of Kerry lamb with spinach & ratatouille, perhaps – and seafood, such as sautéed scallops with savoy cabbage in orange butter. Tempting vegetarian choices are always available on the regular menus. Should the weather oblige, there is an outdoor eating area on the pool-side terrace, which has the same wonderful view over lakes and mountains. An interesting wine list includes a section selected for exceptional value, from £16.50 – £25, a collection of 'Wild Geese' wines from Franco-Irish wine families, and a good selection of half bottles. • L££ & D£££ daily • Open all year • Amex, Diners, MasterCard, Visa •

Killarney
Cahernane Hotel

Muckross Road Killarney Co Kerry

HOTEL
Tel: 064 31895   Fax: 064 34340
email: cahernane@tinet.ie   http://homepage.tinet.ie/~cahernane

Formerly the residence of the Earls of Pembroke, this beautifully situated hotel is set in parkland with wonderful views of Killarney's lakes and mountains. A welcoming fire burns in a large entrance hall (that has probably seen little change since the original house was built in 1877) and, although a large modern wing has added a new dimension, it is the character of the old building that holds the spirit of the hotel. Rooms vary from traditional master bedrooms in the manor house, which are furnished with antiques, to the simpler but spacious and well-appointed rooms with good bathrooms in the new wing. Reduced green fees are available for residents playing the local championship courses; tee-off times can be booked through the hotel. Flying lessons can also be arranged. Well behaved pets are allowed by arrangement. • Acc£££ • Closed Nov-Mar • Amex, Diners, MasterCard, Visa •

Killarney   Celtic Cauldron

27 Plunkett Street Killarney Co Kerry

RESTAURANT   **Tel: 064 36821**

Ireland's first and reputedly only traditional restaurant offering authentic fare from the Celtic nations, based on original recipes and medieval cooking methods. The dining-room is reminiscent of a farmhouse kitchen, with lots of bric-a-brac scattered around, ranging from old box cameras to medical dictionaries! Wherever possible produce is organic and local: shellfish in mead sauce, a combination of Irish cockles, mussels and prawns, cooked in a cream and mead sauce with herbs and served with potato cakes; Glamorgan sausage, a Welsh vegetarian dish made from cheese, wholemeal breadcrumbs, leeks and herbs; Scottish pheasant and port pâté. Main courses might include braised venison in port and juniper berries, pheasant breasts stuffed with apple and nuts, wrapped in bacon and served with plum and cardamom sauce, or braised beef in a rich ale gravy. For lunch, a wholesome Irish stew will suffice: lean lamb and fresh seasonal vegetables, cooked in a rich dark gravy flavoured with Guinness and served with a crusty farle of bread and a chunk of cheese. Desserts are traditional too; perhaps apple pie or bread and butter pudding. This is an unusual restaurant and deserves to succeed. • L£ & D££ daily • Closed 25 Dec & 1 Jan • MasterCard, Visa •

Killarney   Fuchsia House

Muckross Road Killarney Co Kerry

ACCOMMODATION   **Tel: 064 33743   Fax: 064 36588**

A short walk from the town centre, on the N71 road to Kenmare, this is a purpose-built and very affordable guesthouse. It is set well back from the road, with a well-maintained rear garden and ample car parking in the front. On arrival in the afternoon you'll be served tea and home-made cake in the drawing room, a prelude to an outstanding breakfast the next morning, with many fresh goodies on show. Spacious bedrooms, very luxuriously furnished with smart co-ordinating fabrics and quality bedding (the beds are especially firm and comfortable), offer facilities more usually associated with expensive hotels, from remote-control satellite TV and direct-dial telephone to a professional hairdryer and power shower in the well-equipped bathrooms. Hosts Tom and Mary Treacy are part of a family of well-known and dedicated Killarney hoteliers (Killarney Lodge, Killarney Park and Ross Hotels), ensuring the house is immaculately run and maintained. •Acc££ • Closed mid Dec-end Feb • Diners, MasterCard, Visa •

Killarney   Gaby's

27 High Street Killarney Co Kerry

RESTAURANT   **Tel: 064 32519   Fax: 064 32747**

One of Ireland's longest established seafood restaurants, Gaby's has a cosy little bar beside an open fire just inside the door, then several steps lead up to the main dining area, which is cleverly broken up into several sections and has a nice informal atmosphere. Chef-proprietor Gert Maes offers well designed seasonal à la carte menus in classic French style – and in three languages. Absolute freshness is clearly the priority – a note on the menu reminds that availability depends on daily landings – but there's always plenty else to choose from, with steaks and local lamb as back-up. Start with a cassoulet of prawns and monkfish perhaps – Dublin Bay prawns and monkfish in a lightly gingered sauce – or Gaby's "Famous Smoked Salmon Pâté", served in a little pot with a salad garnish and crisp hot toast. Main course choices may include oak-smoked fillets of trout (smoked while you wait), brill fillets in a tomato and Pernod cream sauce and classics like sole meunière. Lovely desserts – a striped light and dark chocolate mousse, served on a cool crème anglaise, perhaps, or a trio of home-made ices in a crisp tuile basket with blackcurrant coulis – and freshly brewed coffee to finish. • D££ Mon-Sat • Closed mid Feb-mid Mar • Amex, Diners, MasterCard, Visa •

We aim to be as up to date as possible, but changes will inevitably occur after we go to press. We would request that listed establishments inform us as quickly as possible of major changes, eg sale of property or key staff changes, so that our records may be updated through the year. Readers will have access to important changes by visiting our website (www.ireland-guide.com).

Killarney

Hotel Dunloe Castle

Beaufort Killarney Co Kerry

HOTEL   Tel: 064 44111   Fax: 064 44583

email: khl@iol.ie   www.iol.ie/khl

Sister hotel to the Hotel Europe (Fossa) and Ard-na-Sidhe (Caragh Lake), Dunloe Castle has many features in common with the larger Europe: the style of the building is similar, the same priorities apply – generous space is allowed for all areas throughout, the quality of furnishing is exceptionally high and both maintenance and housekeeping are superb. The original castle is still part of the development, but the hotel is mainly modern and, like the Europe, the atmosphere is distinctly continental. But Dunloe Castle has some special features of its own, including the park around the hotel, which is internationally renowned for its unique botanical collection, and an equestrian centre. • D£££ • Acc£££ • Closed Oct-April • Amex, Diners, MasterCard, Visa •

Killarney

Hotel Europe

Fossa Killarney Co Kerry

HOTEL   Tel: 064 31900   Fax: 064 32118

email: khl@iol.ie   www.iol.ie/khl

Surrounded by spectacular countryside, Killarney's most luxurious hotel overlooks the Lakes of Killarney. Although now around thirty years old, the Europe was exceptionally well built and has been so immaculately maintained through the years that it still outshines many a new top level hotel. Public areas are very large and impressive, furnished to the highest standards and make full use of the hotel's wonderful location. The leisure facilities – which include a 25 metre swimming pool and seaweed bath, all dating back to the time of the hotel's construction – are also a credit to the vision and wisdom of the original developers. Bedrooms follow a similar pattern, with lots of space, best quality furnishings, beautiful views and balconies all along the lake side of the hotel. Given the high standards and facilities offered, rates are very reasonable, and it is also worth inquiring about special breaks. The hotel's continental connections show clearly in the style throughout but especially, perhaps, when it comes to food -breakfast, for example, is a hot and cold buffet. Excellent conference and meeting facilities include a 450 seat auditorium with built-in microphones and translation system. • L££ daily, D£££ daily • Acc£££ • Closed Nov-Mar • Amex, Diners, MasterCard, Visa •

Killarney

Kathleen's Country House

Madam's Height Tralee Road Killarney Cp Kerry

ACCOMMODATION   Tel: 064 32810

Long before the current rash of purpose-built guesthouses, Kathleen O'Regan Sheppard was offering hotel standard accommodation at guesthouse prices, and this family-run business continues to offer good value, hospitality and comfort in a quiet location – in gardens just a mile from the town centre. All of the individually decorated rooms are non-smoking and furnished to a high standard, with orthopaedic beds, phone, TV, tea/coffee-making facilities and fully tiled bathrooms with full bath and shower. Spacious public areas provide plenty of room for relaxing and include a pleasant dining room where good breakfasts are served overlooking the garden. Not suitable for very young children. Special rates are offered off-season. • Acc££ • Closed mid Nov-early Mar • Amex, MasterCard, Visa •

Killarney

Killarney Great Southern Hotel

Killarney Co Kerry

HOTEL   Tel: 064 31262   Fax: 064 31642

email: res@killarney.gsh.ie   www.gsh.ie

This classic railway hotel was established in 1854 and its pillared entrance and ivy-clad facade still create a sense of occasion. Recent refurbishment has been done with due respect for the age and history of the building, and the spacious foyer, especially, has retained a high level of grandeur. Belying its central position, the hotel is set in 36 acres of landscaped gardens, providing peace and relaxation on the premises. Facilities which have been added over the years include two tennis courts, an indoor heated swimming pool and a leisure centre. Regularly refurbished bedrooms include one suitable for disabled guests, three suites, two junior suites and – unusually these days – 12 single rooms. Almost all rooms have bath and shower. The hotel makes a good venue for conferences, with facilities for up to 1,000 delegates and back-up services. • Acc££££ • Open all year • Amex, Diners, MasterCard, Visa •

Killarney

ACCOMMODATION

Killarney Lodge

Countess Road Killarney Co Kerry
Tel: 064 36499   Fax: 064 31070
email: kylodge@iol.ie

This purpose-built guesthouse is set in private walled gardens just a two minute walk from the town centre. Owner-run by Catherine Treacy, this is a place that offers hotel standards at guesthouse prices: private parking, large en-suite air-conditioned bedrooms with all the amenities expected of a hotel room, wheelchair facilities (one bedroom designed for disabled guests) and large public rooms to relax in. • Acc£-££ • Closed 15-28 Dec • Amex, Diners, MasterCard, Visa •

Killarney

HOTEL/RESTAURANT

Killarney Park Hotel

Kenmare Place Killarney Co Kerry
Tel: 064 35555   Fax: 064 35266

Situated in its own grounds, a short stroll from the town centre, this luxurious, well run and deceptively modern hotel has already undergone a recent transformation, with the refurbishment of all public areas and the leisure centre, and the addition of several new superior bedrooms (incorporating entrance halls) and a conference suite (capacity 150). The library has been extended, a new drawing room added and the bar renovated, creating an elegant Victorian feel, enhanced by the sweeping staircase that leads to the bedrooms. Many of these have been refurbished in a contemporary country house style, with soft fabrics, warm colours, large beds and splendid bathrooms Sister hotel to the much older Ross Hotel nearby..

Restaurant

A large and opulent room with an ornate ceiling, heavy drapes and grand paintings, with a pianist playing the usual favourites throughout dinner. Note the attractive open – but no doubt closed after hours! – walk-in cellar next to him. A lengthy à la carte menu is available in high season, otherwise a fixed-price menu with several choices is offered. The cooking is competent, without reaching great heights, but commendable nonetheless for a dining-room that has to accommodate large groups as well as individual hotel guests and outsiders. • Acc££££ • L£ Sun & D£££ daily • Closed 24-26 Dec • Amex, Diners, MasterCard, Visa •

Killarney

HOTEL

The Killarney Ryan Hotel

Killarney Co Kerry
Tel: 064 31555   Fax: 064 32438

This modern hotel on the edge of Killarney is set in 20 acres of grounds and has earned an exceptional reputation for family holidays. In the summer holidays, especially, but also on holiday weekends and special breaks, the facilities and activities available for children from tiny tots to teenagers are outstanding – a supervised crèche, children's entertainment (including a 'club' for older children), indoor and outdoor supervised sports and special menus and meal times. All rooms are comfortably furnished with good facilities including TV, phone, hair-dryer and trouser press, and (except for family rooms which do not have them for safety reasons) also have tea/coffee-making facilities. In addition to on-site activities, golf, pitch & putt, riding and fishing are all available nearby. • Acc£££ • Closed Dec & Jan • Amex, Diners, MasterCard, Visa •

Killarney

HOTEL

Killeen House Hotel

Aghadoe Killarney Co Kerry
Tel: 064 31711   Fax: 064 31811
email: charhing@indigo.ie

Recognising its potential as "a charming little hotel" Michael and Geraldine Rosney bought this early nineteenth century rectory in 1992. Just 10 minutes drive from Killarney town centre and 5 minutes from Killeen and Mahoney's Point golf courses, the hotel makes a homely base for business or leisure. There's a warm, welcoming atmosphere that is especially noticeable in the pubby little bar, which is popular with locals as well as residents (run as an "honour" bar with golf balls accepted as local tender!) Rooms vary in size but include eight executive rooms; all have full bathrooms en-suite (one with jacuzzi) and are freshly-decorated, with phone and satellite TV. There's a traditional drawing room for guests, furnished with a mixture of antiques and newer furniture, and an open fire. Dogs permitted by arrangement. • Acc££-£££ • Closed Nov-Apr • Amex, Diners, MasterCard, Visa •

Killarney   Lake Hotel

Muckross Road Killarney Co Kerry

HOTEL   **Tel: 064 31035   Fax: 064 31902**

lakehotel@tinet.ie   www.homepage.tinet.ie/~lakehotel

Coming into town from Kenmare on the N71, the hotel is set well back from the road on the lake shore, with the ruins of McCarthy Mor Castle within the grounds. The hotel was built in 1820 and visited by Queen Victoria when she came to Ireland in 1861 (the hotel still has the original horse-drawn carriage in which she travelled). In the late spring of 1998 a lift was being installed and several new suites, with a four-poster bed, spa bath and their own balcony overlooking the lakes, were being constructed. The other existing en-suite bedrooms are smartly decorated and furnished and have the usual modern amenities. Don't be alarmed if you see deer frolicking about – they quite often venture out of the woods to see who's playing tennis on the court in front of the hotel! Own fishing.• Acc££ • Closed early Dec-mid Feb • Amex, Diners, MasterCard, Visa •

Killarney   Muckross Park Hotel

Muckross Village Killarney Co Kerry

HOTEL   **Tel: 064 31938   Fax: 064 31965**

Just across the road from Muckross House and Garden, Muckross Abbey and the Muckross Traditional Farms, this hotel has retained a real "country house" feeling – despite its close proximity to "Molly's", the hotel's large traditional-style pub/restaurant (which is accessible through an independent entrance from the car park).The proportions of the building contribute to the country house feel. There's a spacious, elegant reception area and well-proportioned day rooms include a residents' sitting room and a restaurant (the "Bluepool", named after the nearby Cloghreen Blue Pool Nature Trail) overlooking gardens towards the river. There's also a dining room suitable for private dinner parties and small conferences (30). Generous bedrooms have large double and single beds, quality furnishings and well-planned bathrooms. Rear rooms overlook the garden and front ones, although not as quiet, look over the woodland in Muckross Park. Two unusual suites are on a separate staircase – one has a gallery sleeping area and the other a bathroom with original stone walling and a corner bath. In addition to rooms in the main building, the Muckross Suites offer 48 two-bedroom apartments in a new block just behind the hotel. No dogs. Banqueting for 150. • Acc£££ • Closed Nov-Mar • Amex, Diners, MasterCard, Visa •

Killarney   Randles Court Hotel

Muckross Road Killarney Co Kerry

HOTEL   **Tel: 064 35333   Fax: 064 35206**

email: randles@iol.ie

Within easy walking distance of the town centre, but also convenient to attractions such as Muckross House and Killarney National Park, this attractive house was originally built in 1906 as a family residence and underwent extensive refurbishment before Kay Randles opened it as an hotel in 1991. Although it has grown a little since then (and now has 50 bedrooms) it has retained the domesticity and warmth of the family home. Period features, including fireplaces and stained glass windows, have been retained. Comfortably furnished public rooms include a small bar, a large drawing room with log fire, tapestries and antiques and an elegant restaurant opening onto a sheltered patio. Spacious bedrooms include three rooms suitable for disabled guests, two suites, 12 executive rooms and 10 no-smoking rooms; all are furnished to a high standard, with direct dial telephones, satellite television, radio, hair dryers and well-appointed bathrooms. 24 hour room service. Laundry and dry cleaning are all available. • Acc£££-££££ • Closed Xmas wk & early Jan-mid Mar • Amex, Diners, MasterCard, Visa •

Killarney   Torc Great Southern

Park Road Killarney Co Kerry

HOTEL   **Tel: 064 31611   Fax: 064 31824**

email: res@torc.gsh.ie

On the main Cork road, this modern hotel set in gardens is just 5 minutes walk from the town centre. Well-run, with views of the Kerry mountains, it makes a good base for a holiday in the area. Accommodation includes one room suitable for disabled guests, 10 single rooms and 18 non-smoking rooms. Very handy for Killarney's championship golf courses (closed mid Oct- mid April) – special breaks available. • Acc££ • Closed Xmas & New Year • Amex, Diners, MasterCard, Visa •

Killorglin

Nick's Restaurant
Lower Bridge Street Killorglin Co Kerry

RESTAURANT   Tel: 066 61219/61936   Fax: 066 61233

Nick and Anne Foley have been running this popular restaurant in the centre of Killorglin since 1978 . During that time Nick's cooking – a mixture of traditional Irish and classic French – has earned a particular reputation for his way with local seafood, although there are always other choices, notably prime Kerry beef and lamb. Moules marinière or provençale, lobster thermidor, shellfish mornay and peppered steak in brandy cream sauce are all typical of his classic style. Vegetarians aren't forgotten either – there's a choice of three dishes on the regular menu. Dessert choices are changed daily and there's a good cheeseboard. Aside from providing excellent food, Nick's is also renowned for its great atmosphere. • L£ Sun & D£££ Mon-Sun • Closed Nov & 25 Dec • Amex, Diners, MasterCard, Visa •

Listowel

Allo's Bar & Bistro
41 Church Street Listowel Co Kerry

RESTAURANT   Tel: 068 22880

Named after the previous owner ("Alphonsus, aka Allo") Armel Whyte and Helen Mullane's cafe-bar seems much older than it is – they have reconstructed the whole interior with salvaged materials (the flooring was once in the London Stock Exchange). It is convincingly done with the long, narrow bar divided up in the traditional way. Likewise Armel's cooking – a lively combination of traditional and new Irish cooking with some international influences – is based on all the best local ingredients. Main courses – which change daily – could include pan-fried lamb cutlets in a mushroom, onion and smoked bacon sauce and poached fillet of Atlantic salmon with oriental vegetables in a fish glaze. These could be followed by classic desserts: tangy lemon tart or bakewell tart with home-made custard. Evening menus, which include many of the daytime dishes in a more formal menu structure, broaden the choice to include dishes like grilled fillet of turbot with brown sage butter and chargrilled fillet of Irish beef with a hot pepper and mushroom glaze. Finish with an irresistible pudding – strawberry shortbread or Helen's home-made ice cream selection – or a platter of Irish cheeses with a glass of port. • Meals£-££ • Closed 25 Dec & Good Fri • Amex, MasterCard, Visa •

Parknasilla

Great Southern Hotel
Parknasilla Sneem Co Kerry

HOTEL   Tel: 064 45122   Fax: 064 45323

email: es@parknasilla.gsh.ie

Overlooking Kenmare Bay, set in 300 acres of sub-tropical parkland, this classic Victorian hotel is blessed with one of the most beautiful locations in Ireland. The spacious foyer with its antiques and fresh flowers sets a tone of quiet luxury. Whether activity or relaxation is required there are excellent amenities at hand – including an outdoor swimming pool and Canadian hot tub, horseriding, archery, clay pigeon shooting and snooker for the restless – and an abundance of comfortable places (including a no-smoking drawing room) for a quiet read or afternoon tea. Public rooms include an impressive restaurant and a library (added in 1995 for the hotel's centenary and available for the use of all guests, although also ideal for meetings and small conferences). Bedrooms vary in size and outlook but include one full suite, nine junior suites and one suitable for disabled guests; all have en-suite bathrooms with bath and shower, direct-dial telephone, radio, TV with in-house movie channel, trouser press and hair dryer. Most also have tea/coffee making facilities. Children are welcome, but not under 10 years old after 7 pm. • Acc££££ • Open all year • Amex, Diners, MasterCard, Visa •

Portmagee

Fisherman's Bar
Portmagee Co Kerry

PUB   Tel: 066 77103

Whether for a cup of coffee – very enjoyable taken at an outside table beside the sea on a fine day – or something more substantial from the all-day bar menu, this comfortable, well-run pub just beside the Valentia Island bridge is always a delightful place to take a break. Local seafood stars – a bowl of chowder, perhaps, or hot crab claws with garlic butter, both served with home-made brown bread – and main dishes include seafood platters and Irish stew. There's also an attractive evening restaurant beside the bar, which is especially highly regarded by sailing folk. Bar food should be available all day in high season; a call to check times is advised. • Closed 25 Dec & Good Fri • MasterCard, Visa •

Sneem

The Blue Bull

South Square Sneem Co Kerry

PUB Tel: 064 45382   Fax: 064 45382

This characterful pub in one of Ireland's neatest villages has become something of a legend. Many is the holidaymaker who has fallen for chef-proprietor Katie O'Carroll's wholesome cooking. A wide range of food and dishes is offered, but the emphasis is on local ingredients – Sneem black pudding for example, and other local meats from the village butcher – and the style is mainly traditional: Irish stew, bacon and cabbage, and shepherd's pie are regulars, alongside local seafood in salads, open sandwiches and hot dishes (such as steamed mussels). Vegetarian options such as vegetable stir-fry and pasta dishes are regularly included on the menu. • L£ & D£ daily • Closed 25 Dec & Good Fri • Amex, Diners, MasterCard, Visa •

Tahilla

Tahilla Cove Country House

Tahilla Sneem Co Kerry

COUNTRY HOUSE Tel: 064 45204   Fax: 064 45104

This family-run guesthouse feels more like a small hotel – it has a proper bar, for example, with its own entrance (which is used by locals as well as residents). This is a low-key place, with an old country house in there somewhere (which has been much added to) and there is a blocky annexe in the garden. It has two very special features, however: the location, which is genuinely waterside, is really lovely and away-from-it-all, and the owners, James and Deirdre Waterhouse. Tahilla has been in the family since 1948, and run since 1987 by James and Deirdre – who have the wisdom to understand why their many regulars love it just the way it is. Comfort and relaxation are the priorities. All the public rooms have sea views, including the dining room and a large sitting room, with plenty of armchairs and sofas, which opens onto a terrace (where there are patio tables and chairs overlooking the garden and the cove with its little stone jetty). Accommodation is divided between the main house and another close by; rooms vary considerably but all except two have sea views, many have private balconies and all are en-suite, with bathrooms of varying sizes and appointments (only one single is shower-only). All rooms have phone, TV, hair-dryer and individually controlled heating.. Food is prepared personally by the proprietors and, although the dining room is mainly intended for residents, others are welcome when there is room – simple 4-course country house style menus change daily – and bar food is available from noon to 7 pm. Pets are allowed by arrangement. • Acc££ • Closed Nov-Easter • Amex, Diners, MasterCard, Visa •

Tralee

Abbey Gate Hotel

Maine Street Tralee Co Kerry

HOTEL Tel: 066 29888   Fax: 066 29821

Situated in a relatively quiet corner in the centre of Tralee, this large and rather stylish modern hotel has become one of the area's leading hotels since opening in 1994. A large marble-floored foyer has ample seating space and other public areas include the main Vineyard Restaurant and its own bar. There's also an enormous traditional-style Market Place pub, where bar food is served all day. Bedrooms include four equipped for disabled guests and are of good size, comfortably furnished in a modern style with usual amenities including phone, satellite TV, tea/coffee-making facilities and well-finished en-suite bathrooms (all with bath and shower except the disabled rooms). Children are welcome – there's an outdoor playground, informal meals at the Market Place buffet and Tralee's famous Aquadome is nearby. •Acc£££ • Closed 25 Dec • Amex, Diners, MasterCard, Visa •

Tralee

The Brandon Hotel

Princes Street Tralee Co Kerry

HOTEL Tel: 066 23333   Fax: 066 25019

Overlooking a park and the famous Siamsa Tire folk theatre, and close to the Aquadome, Tralee's largest hotel is at the heart of activities throughout the area. Spacious public areas are quite impressive, and while some bedrooms are on the small side, all have been recently refurbished and have direct-dial phone, radio and TV (no tea/coffee-making facilities) and tiled bathrooms. There's a well-equipped leisure centre and good banqueting/conference facilities. The recently opened Brandon Court Hotel (066 29666), an interesting smaller establishment in a very central position, is a sister hotel. • Acc££-£££££ • Closed 24-28 Dec • Amex, Diners, MasterCard, Visa •

Waterville

Butler Arms Hotel

Waterville Co Kerry

HOTEL   Tel: 066 74144   Fax: 066 74520

One of Ireland's best-known hotels – it is one of several to have strong links with Charlie Chaplin – Peter and Mary Huggards' Butler Arms Hotel dominates the seafront at Waterville. Like many hotels which have been owner-run for several generations it has established a special reputation for its homely atmosphere and good service. Improvements are constantly being made and public areas, including two sitting rooms, a sun lounge and a cocktail bar, are spacious and comfortably furnished, while the beamed Fishermen's Bar (which also has a separate entrance from the street) provides a livelier atmosphere. Bedrooms vary from distinctly non-standard rooms in the old part of the hotel (which many regular guests request) to smartly decorated, spacious rooms with neat en-suite bathrooms and uninterrupted sea views in a wing constructed in the early '90s. • Acc£££ • Closed mid-Oct-early Apr • Amex, MasterCard, Visa •

Waterville

The Huntsman

Waterville Co Kerry

RESTAURANT   Tel: 066 74124   Fax: 066 74560

Raymond and Deirdre Hunt's landmark restaurant has been providing a warm and restoring stop on the Ring of Kerry since 1978. There's always a welcoming turf fire in the bar and tables are set up in both bar and restaurant to maximise some of Kerry's finest sea and mountain views. Raymond specialises in classic French seafood cookery. The full à la carte menu is also available for bar meals. The bar menu is quite extensive and includes popular dishes such as deep-fried fish and fries, Irish stew, omelettes and pasta, as well as classics – grilled black sole and shellfish in garlic butter. Mixing choices from the two menus is allowed. Accommodation is available in a luxurious development alongside the restaurant – ask Ray about overnight stays and The Huntsman Club, which is a time-share operation of special interest to golfers.

• L£ & D££ daily • Closed 3 days Xmas • Amex, Diners, MasterCard, Visa •

Waterville

The Smuggler's Inn

Waterville Co Kerry

ACCOMMODATION/RESTAURANT   Tel: 066 74330   Fax: 066 74422

Harry and Lucille Hunt's famous clifftop pub enjoys a remarkable location right beside the world famous championship Waterville Golf Course (and overlooking a mile of sandy beach to the sea and mountain views beyond). Pleasantly decorated, quite spacious rooms vary in size, outlook and facilities (and price – one has a balcony) but all offer comfortable en-suite accommodation (the less expensive rooms are shower-only). There's a first-floor residents' sitting room with sofas and armchairs, books, television – and magnificent sea views. Local ingredients provide the base for Harry's mainly traditional cooking, with seafood (including lobster from their own tank) being the speciality. Non seafood-lovers have plenty of other choices, including Kerry lamb and beef, of course, and there's a separate vegetarian menu available. A fine place to take a break from the Ring of Kerry on a good day – bar food is available from 11am-10pm daily (snack menu only 3-6 pm), both lunch and dinner are served in the restaurant daily and there are garden tables overlooking the beach for fine summer days. • L£, D££ daily & bar meals£ • Acc££ • Closed Dec-Feb • Amex, Diners, MasterCard, Visa •

KILDARE

The horse is so central and natural a part of Irish life that you'll find significant stud farms in a surprisingly large number of counties, but it is in Kildare that they reach their greatest concentration in the ultimate equine county. Thus it's ironic that, a mere 400 million years ago, Kildare was just a salty ocean where the only creatures remotely equine were the extremely primitive ancestors of sea horses. However, things have been looking up for the horse in County Kildare ever since, and today the lush pastures of the gently sloping Liffey and Barrow valleys provide ideal country for nurturing champions. Apart from many famous private farms, the Irish National Stud in Kildare town, just beyond the legendary gallops of The Curragh, is open for visitors, and it also includes a remarkable Japanese garden, reckoned the best Japanese rock garden in Europe, as well as the Museum of the Horse. Once you get away from the busy main roads, Kildare is full of surprises, and in the northwest of the county you enter the awe-inspiring Bog of Allen, the largest in Ireland, across whose wide open spaces the early engineers struggled to progress the Grand Canal on its route from the east coast towards the Shannon. Inevitably, Kildare is feeling an element of commuter pressure from Dublin, and the fact that it is on the main route from the capital to the south and southwest means that it has more miles of motorway per square mile of county than anywhere else. Yet the underlying quality of the land is such that only the shortest diversion from the arterial roads is required to find total rural peace.

Local Attractions and Information

Kill	Goffs Bloodstock Sales (frequent) 045 886600
Straffan	Steam Museum 01 627 3155
Celbridge	Castletown House 01 628 8252
Tully	Irish National Stud 045 21617
Tully	Japanese gardens 045 21251
Kilcock	Larchill Arcadian Gardens (follies) 01 6287354
Naas	Furness (Palladian House) 045 866815
Straffan	Lodge Park Walled Garden (beside Steam Museum) 01 6288412

Athy

Tonlegee House & Restaurant

Athy Co Kildare

COUNTRY HOUSE/RESTAURANT

Tel/Fax: 0507 31473

email: tonlegeehouse@tinet.ie

Mark and Marjorie Molloy's elegant country house just outside Athy was built in 1790 and now combines modern comfort with an element of old-fashioned style. The nine individually furnished en-suite bedrooms include a junior suite and one single room and all are comfortably furnished to a high standard with phones, TV and complimentary mineral water. Well-finished bathrooms all have bath and shower except one, which is shower only. Well-behaved dogs allowed by arrangement.

Restaurant

Mark's seasonal menus are in a modern European style and based firmly on local produce – including some from their own garden. Four-course dinner menus offer a choice of five starters and main courses – typical dishes include quail in pastry with wild mushroom sauce, or steamed mussels with tomato, saffron and chorizo. Main courses offer a well-balanced choice, with local Kildare lamb an especially strong option – in an imaginative dish of noisettes with peppered lamb sausage, puy lentils and tarragon jus. Finish with good, uncomplicated desserts like thin apple tart with cinnamon cream (cooked to order) or home made ice creams – or make the most of a good Irish farmhouse cheeseboard, then tea or coffee and petits fours. • D£££ Tues-Sat (Mon & Sun residents only) • Closed Xmas, New Year, Good Fri & Bank Hols • Amex, MasterCard, Visa •

Ballymore Eustace

Ballymore Inn

Ballymore Eustace Co Kildare

PUB ⭐

Tel: 045 864585

Vegetarian Dish of the Year

The O'Sullivan family's pub, the Ballymore Inn, looks simple enough from the outside. Inside, there's interesting furniture in unusual colours, but the fresh flowers are the biggest giveaway – huge vases of lovely big, generous lilies, perhaps, on the mantelpiece, on the bar and even, when you get through that far, in the Ladies. But it's for the food that people come – of the kind that's so good they're reluctant to let their friends into the secret. But word about the food has definitely got out and people are coming from all over to get a taste of the wonderful things this country kitchen has to offer. There's lots to choose from, such as delicious soups, Caesar salad with crispy bacon, excellent steaks, pasta dishes – with chicken, tomato and goat's cheese perhaps – and stir fries. One of the best things they've done recently is install a really good pizza oven, though this is not a pizza restaurant. There's a separate pizza menu – and what pizzas they are. Not only are the bases wonderfully light, thin and crisply cooked, but every ingredient is in tip-top condition and the range includes some wonderful combinations, most of which happen to be vegetarian. No ordinary pizzas these, you can choose from the likes of Pepperoni, Tomato, Chilli & Mozzarella or Grilled Peppers with Olives and Pesto, or dither between Spinach, Oyster Mushroom and Goat's Cheese and Anchovy, Black Olives, Capers, Red Onion and Cooleeney Cheese. They're all wonderful but best of all, we think, is the Grilled Fennel, Roasted Peppers, Basil and Ardrahan Cheese, winner of our Vegetarian Dish of the Year 1999. • L£ & D£-££ Mon-Sat • Closed 25 Dec & Good Fri • Amex, MasterCard, Visa •

Castledermot

Kilkea Castle & Golf Club

Kilkea Castledermot Co Kildare
HOTEL/RESTAURANT   Tel: 0503 45156   Fax: 0503 45187
email: kilkea@iol.ie

The oldest inhabited castle in Ireland, Kilkea dates back to the twelfth century and has been sensitively renovated and converted into a hotel without loss of elegance and grandeur. Rooms, many with lovely views over the formal gardens and surrounding countryside, are splendidly furnished to incorporate modern comforts. Public areas include a hall complete with knights in armour and two pleasant ground floor bars – a cosy back one and a larger one that opens onto a terrace overlooking gardens and golf course. Some of the bedrooms in the main castle are very romantic – as indeed is the whole setting – making it understandably popular for weddings. The adjoining leisure centre, architecturally discreet, offers state-of-the-art facilities: indoor swimming pool, saunas, jacuzzi, steamroom, well-equipped exercise room and sunbed. Outdoor sports include clay pigeon shooting, archery, tennis and fishing. An 18-hole championship golf course, which has views of the castle from every fairway, opened in 1994, using the river Greese flowing through the grounds as a natural hazard and adding a couple of extra lakes to increase the challenge still further; informal meals are served in the golf club. Special weekend breaks at the castle are good value.

De Lacy's Restaurant

Named after Hugh de Lacy, who built Kilkea Castle in 1180, this beautiful first-floor restaurant has a real "castle" atmosphere and magnificent views over the countryside. It also overlooks the delightful formal kitchen garden (source of much that appears on the table in summer) and has a bright, airy atmosphere. Scottish chef George Smith has a distinctive style seen in a uniquely decorative approach to presentation in some dishes. The quality of ingredients shines through, with good contrast in flavour and, in specialities such as the roast of the day, there are excellent simpler alternatives available (and certainly no lack of generosity). On a recent visit, for example, Roast Rack of Kildare Lamb was coated with herbed breadcrumbs and served with garlic and rosemary flavoured sauce – delicious and perfectly cooked; and there were no less than eight dainty chops on the rack. Grilled Fillet of Cod, also perfectly cooked and (more moderately) generous was served on a tasty bed of lightly spiced stir-fry style root vegetables. Guests can take coffee on the terrace in summer and wander around to see the old fruit trees, vegetables and herbs. • L££ & D££-£££ daily • Acc£££ • Closed 23-27 Dec • Amex, Diners, MasterCard, Visa •

The Curragh

Martinstown House

The Curragh Co Kildare
COUNTRY HOUSE   Tel: 045 441269   Fax: 045 441208

Just on the edge of the Curragh, near Punchestown, Naas and The Curragh race courses, this delightful 200 year old 'Strawberry Hill' gothic style house is on a farm, set in 170 acres of beautifully wooded land. It also has a lovely walled garden that provides vegetables, fruit and flowers for the house in season. There are also free range hens, sheep, cattle and horses. Meryl Long welcomes guests to this idyllic setting, aiming to offer them "a way of life which I knew as a child (but with better bathrooms!) a warm welcome, real fires and good food." It is a lovely family house, with very nicely proportioned rooms – gracious but not too grand – and bedrooms that are all different, very comfortably furnished with fresh flowers and with their own special character. A stay here is sure to be enjoyable, with the help of a truly hospitable hostess who believes that holidays should be fun, full of interest and with an easy-going atmosphere. • Acc££ • Closed Easter • Amex, MasterCard, Visa •

Kilcullen

PUB

Berneys Bar & Restaurant

Kilcullen Co Kildare
Tel: 045 481260   Fax: 045 481877
email: berneys@indigo.ie

Paul and Freda Mullen have been running this welcoming bar on the main street since 1989 – it's a real local, with its own character, a beer garden for summer and a log fire that makes a welcome sight on cold days. Freda's cooking is a mixture of Irish and country French, and in addition to a good choice of sandwiches and salads and one or two regulars she offers a short bar menu of 2-3 soups, hot dishes and puddings, changed daily. Evening meals are served in the restaurant, a large L-shaped room beside the bar with warm red walls and interesting pictures. The restaurant menu moves up a few gears and offers a much wider choice and more elaborate dishes. There's always a good choice of seafood and vegetarian dishes as well as popular fare like steaks (various ways), roast venison and duck – although limited bar food such as sandwiches and salads is available until 11 pm. • L£ & D££ daily • Closed 25 Dec & Good Fri • Amex, Diners, MasterCard, Visa •

Leixlip

HOTEL/RESTAURANT

Leixlip House Hotel

Captain's Hill Leixlip Co Kildare
Tel: 01 624 2268   Fax: 01 624 4177

Up on a hill overlooking Leixlip village, this lovely Georgian house is just eight miles from Dublin city centre. Having undergone extensive renovation (it was furnished and decorated to a very high standard in period style) it opened as an hotel in 1996. Gleaming antique furniture and gilt-framed mirrors enhance thick carpeted public rooms in soft country colours, all creating an atmosphere of discreet opulence. Bedrooms include two suites furnished with traditional mahogany furniture. The strong, simple decor particularly pleases the many business guests who stay here. Attention to detail is good throughout although it is surprising that, while all are en-suite, nine of the fifteen bedrooms have shower-only. The hotel's conference centre has facilities for up to 120 people, can be adapted to suit a wide range of uses and has back-up business services. Hotel guests have complimentary use of a nearby gym. Special dinner and overnight rates are available at certain times; details from Reservations.

The Bradaun Restaurant

The commitment to quality evident in the hotel as a whole is continued in the restaurant, a bright, high-ceilinged, formally appointed dining room. Head chef Declan Raggett, who has been with the hotel since it opened, offers modern Irish cooking in lunch and dinner menus that change twice weekly. Menus are imaginative, wide ranging, based on fresh seasonal produce and well-executed. Main courses offer a balanced choice, usually with two fish dishes and often including Kildare lamb – loin with glazed shallots and a thyme & garlic sauce perhaps. Desserts are equally good – fresh fruit terrine and a caramelised confit was especially enjoyed on a recent visit, for example, – and all the details are right including good coffee and petits fours. Service, in our experience, was mixed, with younger staff willing and friendly but insufficiently trained to do justice to the high standard of food. • D£££ daily & L£ Sun • Acc£££ • Closed 25 Dec • Amex, Diners, MasterCard, Visa •

Maynooth

HOTEL

Glenroyal Hotel, Leisure Club & Conference Centre

Straffan Road Maynooth Co Kildare
Tel: 01 629 0909   Fax: 01 6290919
email: manager@glenroyal-hotel.ie   www.indigo.ie/glenroyal

Situated on the outskirts of the university town of Maynooth, and only 20 minutes from Dublin city centre, this large hotel was in the process of growing even larger at the time of our visit but the dust will no doubt have settled by the time this guide appears. It serves the needs of a large area requiring facilities for a wide range of events, notably conferences, corporate events and weddings. Demand is high. It also has extensive leisure facilities. These include a dramatically designed 20 metre pool (with underwater loungers, whirlpool and children's splashpool), a gymnasium and much else besides. Bedrooms, which include one room suitable for disabled guests and 10 executive rooms, are all comfortably furnished – mostly in contemporary style – with all the amenities expected of this kind of hotel and neat en-suite bathrooms (7 shower only). • Acc£££ • Closed 25 Dec & Good Fri • Amex, Diners, MasterCard, Visa •

Maynooth   Moyglare Manor

🏛

Maynooth Co Kildare

COUNTRY HOUSE/RESTAURANT   Tel: 01 628 6351   Fax: 01 628 5405

Wine List of the Year   email: moyglare@iol.ie   www.iol.ie/moyglaremanor

Country hedges and workaday farmland give way to neatly manicured hedging, rolling parkland and, eventually, beautifully tended gardens as one approaches this imposing classical Georgian manor – and it comes as no surprise to find that the owner, Norah Devlin, lavishes her love of beautiful things on the place, with a passion for antiques that has become legendary. Gilt-framed mirrors and portraits are everywhere, shown to advantage against deep-shaded damask walls. The remarkable abundance of chairs and sofas of every pedigree ensures comfortable seating, even when the restaurant is fully booked with large parties milling around before and after dining. First-time visitors sometimes describe it as "like being in an antique shop", but after recovering from the stunning effect of its contents guests invariably reflect on the immaculate maintenance and comfort of the place under the careful stewardship of long-time manager Shay Curran. Spacious bedrooms are also lavishly furnished in period style, some with four-posters or half testers, and include a ground-floor suite; all have well-appointed bathrooms with quality appointments and good attention to detail. Television is only available in rooms on request, as peacefulness is the aim at Moyglare.

Restaurant

Hotel manager Shay Curran personally supervises the formally-appointed restaurant, which is in several interconnecting rooms; the middle ones nice and cosy for winter, those overlooking the garden and countryside pleasant in fine weather. Grand and romantic, it's just the place for a special occasion. Jim Cullinane, who has been head chef since 1983, presents lunch (£21.95) and dinner (£29.50) in menus that change daily (plus an à la carte at dinner). He is known for his nicely balanced combination of traditional favourites and sophisticated fare, attractively presented, with a vegetarian option always available. There is an emphasis on seafood and game in season – roast pheasant, perhaps, hung long enough to give it a gamey flavour, perfectly cooked and served off the bone accompanied by a nice little serving of green-flecked champ as well as game chips and Cumberland sauce. Lunch menus offer less choice than dinner, but are nevertheless quite formal and convey a sense of occasion. Fine meals are complemented by an exceptional wine list of special interest to the connoisseur – which is why Moyglare Manor is the winner of our 1999 Wine List of the Year Award. • L££ & D£££ daily • Acc£££-££££ • Closed 24-26 Dec & 1 Jan • Amex, Diners, MasterCard, Visa •

Moone   Moone High Cross Inn

Bolton Hill Moone Co Kildare

PUB   Tel: 0507 24210

The Clynch family has been running this characterful country pub since 1978, although it dates back to the 1870s when it was a pub and grocery shop. It's a warm, welcoming place with open fires in both the bars. The larger one is well set up with rustic tables (including old school desks) for the comfortable service of bar food, where traditional dishes like Irish stew, bacon and cabbage (and often a fresh fish of the day) are served between 11 am and 9 pm.

Accommodation

Upstairs there are eight simple en-suite letting bedrooms, which are very popular for overflow from weddings at nearby Kilkea Castle as well as normal holiday business. • Meals£ • Acc££ • Closed 25 Dec & Good Fri • MasterCard, Visa •

Naas   Fletcher's

Commercial House Naas Co Kildare

PUB   Tel: 045 897328

This great old pub goes back well into the 1800s and has been in the Fletcher family since Tom Fletcher's father ran it in the 1930s. It's the kind of place that puts Irish theme pubs to shame, with its simple wooden floor and long, plain mahogany bar broken up in the traditional way with mahogany dividers and stained glass panels. They did up the back lounge recently, but there's no need to worry – it shouldn't need work for another couple of hundred years. • Closed 25 Dec, Good Fri & Bank Hols •

Naas   Manor Inn

Main Street Naas Co Kildare

PUB   **Tel: 045 897471   Fax: 045 897139**

Dennis and Margaret Curry have run this thriving traditional pub since 1972. It always used to be a great stopping place for Dubliners heading to Cork, until the new roads by-passed the town. The lack of this particular passing trade has not done any harm, however, as it's handy to the Curragh (racing crowds and army base) and Mondello Park (note the racing helmet clock in the back bar). The chef, Anthony Hogan, has been in situ since 1979, which probably explains the commendable consistency of cooking standards. The menu is quite long – usually a bad sign, but the kitchen seems to be on top of it here – and includes a Junior Menu, lots of good Irish steaks, a range of house specials (including beef in Guinness) and a wide selection of popular bar dishes. But the best bet is often one of the daily specials – usually including fish – so don't forget to check the blackboard menu. Nice new toilets were noted on a recent visit – something more pubs could invest in with benefit. • L£ & D£-££ daily • Closed 25 Dec & Good Fri • Amex, Diners, MasterCard, Visa •

Newbridge   Hotel Keadeen

Curragh Road Newbridge Co Kildare

HOTEL   **Tel: 045 431666   Fax: 045 434402**

email: keadeen@iol.ie

Centrally located and easily accessible off the M7 motorway, this family-owned hotel is set in eight acres of fine landscaped garden just south of the town (and quite near the Curragh racecourse). The 55 bedrooms and suites are generously sized and furnished to a high standard. A fine romanesque Health & Fitness Club was opened in 1996 with an 18-metre swimming pool and scented aromatherapy room among its attractions, plus a staffed gymnasium with specialist equipment imported from America. Extensive conference and banqueting facilities cater for anything from 15 to 800 people. • Acc££-£££ • Open all year • Amex, Diners, MasterCard, Visa •

Newbridge   The Red House Inn

Newbridge Co Kildare

RESTAURANT   **Tel: 045 431657   Fax: 045 431934**

Proprietor-manager Brian Fallon runs a tidy ship at this cosy inn just off the Naas dual carriageway. It has a very relaxed atmosphere, especially in the characterful bar and the restful conservatory and garden at the back. The dining room is well-appointed in a classic, elegant style, very suitable for the mainly traditional home-cooked food for which The Red House is famous. Local meats – prime beef and Kildare lamb – usually star, but vegetarian options are always given too. • D£££ Tues-Sat, L£ Sun only • Amex, Diners, MasterCard, Visa •

Straffan   Barberstown Castle

Straffan Co Kildare

COUNTRY HOUSE/RESTAURANT   **Tel: 01 628 8157   Fax: 01 627 7027**

email: castleir@iol.ie

Barberstown Castle is fascinating; steeped in history through three very different historical periods, it's one of the few houses in the area to have been occupied continuously for over 400 years. The oldest part is very much a real castle – the original keep in the middle section of the building, which includes the atmospheric cellar restaurant, was built by Nicholas Barby in the early 13th century. This was followed by a more domestic Elizabethan house, added in the second half of the 16th century. Hugh Barton (also associated with nearby Straffan House, now the Kildare Hotel & Country Club, with whom it shares golf and leisure facilities) built the 'new' Victorian wing in the 1830s. Most recently, in the current ownership of Kenneth Healy, the property has been thoroughly renovated and appropriately refurbished, in keeping with its age and style, to offer a high standard of modern comfort throughout. Very comfortable accommodation is provided in well-appointed, individually decorated en-suite rooms – some are in the oldest section, the Castle Keep, others are more recent, but all have great style. Public areas, including two drawing rooms and an elegant bar, have been renovated with the same care, and there are big log fires everywhere. A separate function room in converted stables has banqueting facilities for 160 and there are conference facilities for 50.

The Castle Restaurant

The restaurant is in a series of whitewashed rooms in the semi-basement of the old Castle Keep, which gives it great atmosphere, heightened by fires and candles in alcoves. The present head chef Thomas Haughton joined the castle in 1997 and is continuing the longstanding policy of using as much local produce as possible in stylish country house cuisine. He presents menus – set lunch (£17.50) and dinner (£32.50) – which change weekly and always include some vegetarian dishes, typically torte of wild mushroom and goat's cheese or poached egg with a confit of leek and truffle dressing. Seafood dishes tend to be luxurious – lobster, scallops. Local lamb and beef also feature and there's a good selection of Irish farmhouse cheeses. Home baked breads include speciality breads as well as traditional brown soda. • Acc£££ • L££ & D£££ • Closed 24-27 Dec • Amex, Diners, MasterCard, Visa •

Straffan   Kildare Hotel & Country Club

Straffan Co Kildare

COUNTRY HOUSE/RESTAURANT 🏛 🏛   Tel: 01 601 7200   Fax: 01 601 7299

Golf Hotel of the Year   email: hotel@kclub.ie

The origins of Straffan House go back a long way – the history is known as far back as 550 AD – but it was the arrival of the Barton wine family in 1831 that established the tone of today's magnificent building, by giving it a distinctively French elegance. It was bought by the Smurfit Group in 1988 and, after extensive renovations, opened as an hotel in 1991. Set in lush countryside, and overlooking its own golf course, the hotel boasts unrivalled opulence. Under the guidance of Ray Carroll, who has been general manager from the outset, it is run with apparently effortless perfection. The interior is magnificent, with superb furnishings and a wonderful collection of original paintings by well-known artists, including William Orpen, Louis le Brocqy, Sir John Lavery and Jack B. Yeats, who has a room devoted to his work. All bedrooms and bathrooms are individually designed in the grand style, with superb amenities and great attention to detail. Equally sumptuous accommodation is available in the self-contained Courtyard Suites, which have one or two bedrooms and private entrances into a living/dining room. Outstanding facilities at the hotel include an indoor sports centre for the seriously active, a health and leisure club with everything from a fine swimming pool to massage and hairdressing, and a fine range of outdoor sports including private fishing, horseriding, clay target shooting and, of course, golf. The 18 hole golf course and facilities at the K Club are exceptional, making it a very worthy winner of our Golf Hotel of the Year Award. The course, which was designed by Arnold Palmer, has a par of 72 and covers 220 acres; featuring 11 lakes and the River Liffey, it gives a demanding game to even the best of players. The K Club is home to the Smurfit European Open, which was first played here in 1995, and has a magnificent clubhouse. Overlooking the 18th green, players can relax in style in the elegantly appointed Legends Bar and Restaurant and there is also a private dining room, The Arnold Palmer Room, available for private functions. Catering at the clubhouse is overseen by Michel Flamme, executive chef at the hotel.

The Byerley Turk   ★

Dramatically draped tall windows, boldly striped in deep terracotta, cream and green, marble columns, paintings of racehorses, tables laden with crested china, monogrammed white linen, gleaming modern crystal and silver – these all create an impressive background for the hotel's fine food. Executive chef Michel Flamme, who has been with the hotel since it opened, bases his cooking on classical French cuisine with some traditional Irish influences – in, for example, a starter of pan-fried Clonakilty black and white pudding, colcannon potato and parsley jus. He presents a seasonal à la carte, a daily changing set dinner menu (£45) and a special "Dining Experience" for complete parties (£80); all the menus are very luxurious and notable for a growing number of specialities. These include braised ox cheeks with puréed root vegetables and flatleaf parsley served with a rich claret sauce, poached Galway Bay lobster surrounded by a chilled vegetable salad with parsley oil and mesclun and, to finish, a range of hot speciality souffles. Given the intermingled history of Straffan House and the Barton family, it is appropriate that Bordeaux Reserve from Barton and Guestier should be the label chosen for the hotel's house wine (£16.95). • Acc£££ • L££ & D££££ • Open all year • Amex, Diners, MasterCard, Visa •

KILKENNY

Kilkenny is a land of achingly beautiful valleys where elegant rivers weave their way through a rich countryside spiced by handsome hills. Rivers are the key to the county. Almost the entire eastern border is marked by the Barrow, which becomes ever more spectacularly lovely as it thrusts towards the sea at the tiny river port of St Mullins. The southern border is marked by the broad tidal sweep of the Suir, and this fine county is divided diagonally by the meandering of the most beautiful river of all, the Nore. Invaders inevitably progressed up its tree-lined course towards the ancient site of Kilkenny city itself. They quickly became Kilkenny folk in the process, for this is a land to call home. The monastic and later medieval city lent itself so naturally to being an administrative centre that at times it appeared set to become the capital of Ireland. Today, it seems odd at first that this miniature city doesn't have its own university. But after you've enjoyed Kilkenny's time-hallowed streets and old buildings, you'll soon realise that, with a plethora of festivals featuring artistic, theatrical and comedy themes, Kilkenny has its own individual buzz of creativity and energy which many an arid modern university campus might well envy.

Local Attractions and Information

Kilkenny	Cat Laughs Comedy Festival (May) 056 63416
Kilkenny	Rothe House (16th century house, exhibitions) 056 22893
Kilkenny	City Tourist Information 056 51500
Thomastown	Kilfane Glen & Waterfall 056 24558
Thomastown	Mount Juliet (parkland surrounding hotel) 056 24455

Bennettsbridge

RESTAURANT

Mosse's Mill Café

Bennettsbridge Co Kilkenny
Tel: 056 27644   Fax: 056 27491
www.NicholasMosse.com

One of the best reasons to go just outside Kilkenny city to Bennettsbridge is to visit the Nicholas Mosse Pottery, where you can see the full range – including acres of his famous spongeware – in the factory shop (and buy seconds at a price that will allow you to spend the change at the family-owned Mill Café, which is just next door). The restaurant is very informal, in an attractive setting overlooking a garden with pond and millstone. It has been designed to show off Irish table dressing (they also do linen now) as well as the good food on it. Lunch and afternoon tea is served in the garden in fine weather. Menus offer a range of light, modern dishes including some Irish influences – smoked salmon slices on potato cakes of dill and salmon or 'The Irish Ploughman' (farmhouse cheeses with home-made chutneys) as well as lots of pasta dishes, enchiladas and much else besides. There will always be about six dishes for vegetarians. Although mainly a daytime place, the café opens for dinner on Saturday. • Meals £-££ • Closed 2 wks mid-Oct & 2 wks at Xmas • Amex, Diners, MasterCard, Visa •

Inistioge

COUNTRY HOUSE

Berryhill

Inistioge Co Kilkenny
Tel/Fax: 056 58434

George and Belinda Dyer's delightful country house was built by George's family in 1780 – it has been immaculately maintained by successive generations and stands high above a valley, on the family's 250 acre farm, proudly overlooking the River Nore. Handsomely covered with virginia creeper, it is comfortably big rather than grand, with a homely hall and well-proportioned reception rooms full of lovely old family things. Bedrooms are very spacious – junior suites really, with a dressing/sitting area and room to make tea and coffee – and each has an animal theme. Good home cooking (with some international influences) is the aim for residents' dinner and local produce will be much in evidence – notably Berryhill trout and salmon from their own private stretch of the Nore – and home-produced lamb as well as local cheeses. Breakfast is a speciality – fresh fruits, Nore smoked salmon & scrambled egg and "anything the heart desires" taken at the dining room table in front of a log fire. • Acc££ • Closed mid Nov-mid Apr • MasterCard, Visa •

Inistioge

The Motte

Plas Newydd Lodge Inistioge Co Kilkenny

RESTAURANT
Tel: 056 58655

On the edge of the picturesque village of Inistioge, with views of extensive parklands and the River Nore, The Motte is situated in a classically proportioned hunting lodge called Plas Newydd Lodge, named in honour of the ladies of Llangollen, who eloped from Inistioge in the late 18th century. Although small in size, this unique country restaurant is big on personality – of the host, the irrepressible Tom Reade Duncan, and of the chef, Alan Walton, as conveyed through his imaginative menus and distinctive style of cooking. The pair of them combine a special blend of classical style and wacky artistic inspiration. Menus are sensibly limited to six choices on each course – starters such as classic Duck Liver Terrine or a witty Cold Curried Chicken Salad (a clever tall dish of miniature poppodums layered up with a light curried chicken breast mixture, served with mango sauce on the side). Main courses range from the unconventional – Kangaroo rump steak for example – to the locally popular, as in a perfect sirloin steak with a classic burgundy butter sauce. World flavours may crop up – in couscous, sauced with lively middle eastern flavours of cumin, lemon and mint, for example, to accompany a pork dish. Side vegetables are always imaginative and perfectly cooked. Desserts on a recent visit were a chocoholics dream, but short on simple, refreshing options. Great service; interesting, moderately priced, wine list. • D££ Tues-Sat (& Sun of Bank Hol w/ends) • Closed 1 wk Xmas, 2 wks Oct • MasterCard, Visa •

Kilkenny

Butler House

Patrick Street Kilkenny Co Kilkenny
056 65707 / 22828   **056 65626**

ACCOMMODATION   email: rer@butler.ie

Located close to Kilkenny Castle, this elegant Georgian townhouse was restored by the Irish State Design Agency in the 1970s.The resulting combination of what was at the time contemporary design and period architecture leads to some interesting discussions. However, the accommodation is all en-suite (although all but one of the 13 bedrooms are shower-only) and very adequate, with all the amenities now expected of good accommodation. There are also conference facilities, for up to 120 delegates and two meeting rooms, for up to 40. • Acc££-£££ • Closed 24-29 Dec • Amex, Diners, MasterCard, Visa •

Kilkenny

Café Sol

William Street Kilkenny Co Kilkenny

RESTAURANT
Tel: 056 64987

Eavan Kenny and Gail Johnson came to Kilkenny via Ballymaloe, Co Cork and made their reputation at The Millstone Café in Bennettsbridge before moving into the centre of Kilkenny. They opened this fun café-restaurant just off the High Street in 1995. Although they do open for dinner on Fridays and Saturdays – when they soften the ambience with the generous use of candles – it is for their good home-cooked all-day food that they are best known: big home-made soups with freshly baked scones, imaginative sandwiches, great vegetarian dishes like warm salad of goats cheese with walnuts and beetroot, light fish dishes like potato cakes with smoked salmon and sour cream, gorgeous salads like Lavistown sausages with mashed potato, mustard mayonnaise and salad. Lots of nice bakes, too – and a good range of teas, coffees and other drinks such as homemade lemonade to wash them down. Evening menus are more formal, but the same sound principles apply. • L£ daily, D££ Mon-Sat • Closed 5 days Xmas & Good Fri • MasterCard, Visa •

Kilkenny

Lacken House

Dublin Road Kilkenny Co Kilkenny

RESTAURANT/ACCOMMODATION   **Tel: 056 61085   Fax: 056 62435**
Sommelier if the Year – Breda McSweeney   email: lackenhs@indigo.ie

Eugene and Breda McSweeney bought this period house on the edge of Kilkenny city in 1983, setting up an establishment that they were to develop into the leading restaurant in the area. Now guests come from far and wide to sample their fare. Eugene takes pride in using the best of local produce in a fine 4-course table-d'hôte menu as well as a wide-ranging à la carte. This features many of the specialities which have won awards and become essential to the repertoire – starters like baked crab gateau and grilled goat's cheese on beetroot bread, and main courses such as roast crispy duckling, served off the bone with a port and Grand Marnier sauce, black sole with fresh Dublin Bay prawns, or superb local fillet steak on a bed of bubble and squeak, with a pepper and brandy sauce. Fresh lobster attracts a small supplement (£2.50). Menus reflect the seasons, with game available in winter, and always include something interesting for vegetarians, based on whatever's best in the market. Desserts are always good – or there are Irish farmhouse cheeses from the trolley, served with home-made biscuits. Needless to say, as Breda McSweeney receives our 1999 Sommelier of the Year Award, the wine list merits a special look – and is made even more interesting by a word or two of well-informed advice. Small conferences by arrangement for up to 12 people. • D££-£££ Tues-Sat • Amex, Diners, MasterCard, Visa •

Rooms

Nine en-suite guest bedrooms are available, all with phone TV, tea/coffee-making trays. Rooms vary in size and outlook, but are due to be upgraded for the 1999 season. Excellent breakfasts. • Acc££ • Closed 1 wk Xmas & 1 wk Jan • Amex, Diners, MasterCard, Visa •

Kilkenny   Newpark Hotel

Kilkenny Co Kilkenny

HOTEL   Tel: 056 22122   Fax: 056 61111

Very much at the heart of local activities, this 1960's hotel on the N77 boasts major conference and banqueting facilities, a good leisure centre and has a family-friendly attitude. • Acc££-£££ • Open all year • Amex, Diners, MasterCard, Visa •

Maddoxtown   Blanchville House

Dunbell Maddoxtown Co Kilkenny

COUNTRY HOUSE   Tel: 056 27197   Fax: 056 27636

email: blanchville@indigo.ie

Tim and Monica Phelan's elegant Georgian house is just 5 miles out of Kilkenny city, surrounded by its own farmland and gardens. It's easy to spot – there's a folly in its grounds. This lovely house has undergone painstaking renovations – thereby providing modern comforts with old-fashioned style – and has the advantage of being close to the city yet in a very peaceful rural setting. The house has an airy atmosphere, with matching well-proportioned dining and drawing rooms on either side of the hall. The six pleasant, comfortably furnished bedrooms in period style overlook attractive countryside (five are en-suite, one has a private bathroom; two have shower only) Dinner is available to residents (bookings required before noon) and, like the next morning's excellent breakfast, is taken at the communal mahogany dining table. No wine licence but guests are welcome to bring their own. Well-behaved dogs are permitted by arrangement. • Acc£££ • Closed Nov-Feb • Amex, MasterCard, Visa •

Thomastown   Mount Juliet Estate

Thomastown Co Kilkenny

HOTEL/RESTAURANT 🏛 🏛   Tel: 056 73000   Fax: 056 73009

email: info@mountjuliet.ie

Built over 200 years ago by the Earl of Carrick, and named in honour of his wife, Mount Juliet House is one of Ireland's finest Georgian houses. Lying amidst 1500 acres of unspoilt woodland, pasture and formal gardens beside the River Nore, it is one of Europe's greatest country estates, with world class sporting amenities and conference facilities. It retains an aura of eighteenth century grandeur. The original elegance has been painstakingly preserved, so that the hand-carved Adam fireplaces, walls and ceilings decorated with intricate stucco work and many other original features can still be enjoyed today. The 32 bedrooms have period decor with all the comfort of modern facilities. Additional bedrooms on the estate are in the Hunters yard and the Rose Garden two-bedroom lodges. The Jack Nicklaus-designed golf course on the estate went straight into the list of top-ranking courses when it opened in 1991; it hosted the Irish Open for three years consecutively (from 1993 to 1995). Informal dining is available at Hunters Yard, Presidents Bar.

Lady Helen Dining Room

Although grand, this graceful high-ceilinged room, softly decorated in pastel shades and with sweeping views over the grounds, is not forbidding and has a pleasant atmosphere. To match these beautiful surroundings, executive chef Stan Power presents a classic daily dinner menu based on local ingredients, including wild salmon from the River Nore, vegetables and herbs from the Mount Juliet garden and regional Irish farmhouse cheese. Service is efficient and friendly. • Acc££££ • D£££ daily, L££ Sun only • Amex, Diners, MasterCard, Visa •

LAOIS

With its territory bisected by the rail and road links between Dublin and Cork, Laois is often glimpsed only fleetingly by inter-city travellers. But as with any Irish county, it is a wonderfully rewarding place to visit as soon as you move off the main roads. and a salutary place to visit as well. For, in the eastern part between Stradbally and Portlaoise, there's the Rock of Dunamase, that fabulous natural fortress which many occupiers inevitably assumed to be impregnable. Dunamase's remarkably long history of fortifications, defences, sieges and eventual captures has a relevance and a resonance for all times and all peoples and all places. But there's much more to Laois than mournful musings on the ultimate vanity of human ambitions. With its border shared with Carlow along the River Barrow, eastern Laois comfortably reflects Carlow's quiet beauty. To the northwest, we find that Offaly bids strongly to have the Slieve Bloom Mountains thought of as an Offaly hill range, but in fact there's more of the Slieve Blooms in Laois than Offaly. And though the River Nore may be thought of as quintessential Kilkenny, long before it gets anywhere near Kilkenny it is quietly building as it meanders across much of Laois, gathering strength from the weirdly-named Delour, Tonet, Gully, Erskina and Goul rivers on the way. The Erskina and Goul rivers become one in Laois's own Curragh, a mysterious place of wide open spaces and marshy territory northwest of Durrow which, in marked contrast, was created as a planned estate town by the Duke of Ormond.

Local Attractions and Information

Ballinakill
Emo Court

Heywood (Sir Edwin Lutyens gardens) 0502 33563
(James Gandon) & Gardens 056 21450

Abbeyleix   Morrissey's

Main Street Abbeyleix Co Laois

PUB   Tel: 0502 31233/31281   Fax: 0502 31357

One of Ireland's finest and best-loved pubs, Morrissey's is a fine building on the wide main street of this attractive little town. It's a great place to lift the spirits while taking a break between Dublin and Cork – food is not its strength but a quick cup of coffee and enjoyment of the atmosphere is sometimes all that's needed. Morrissey''s has been in the same family since it first opened as a grocery in 1775, when it started life as a thatched one-storey house. In 1880 it was rebuilt as the lofty two-storey premises we see today, with high shelf-lined walls and a pot belly stove to gather round on cold days. The present owner, Patrick Mulhall, is rightly proud of this special place, which is unique in so many ways. They have a list of people who have served their time at Morrissey's since 1850 – and, true to the old tradition, television, cards and singing are not allowed. • Closed 25 Dec & Good Fri •

Abbeyleix   Preston House

Main Street Abbeyleix Co Laois

RESTAURANT/ACCOMMODATION   Tel/Fax: 0502 31432

While Morrissey's pub is a must, if you fancy a bite to eat just walk down the hill a few doors to Michael and Allison Dowling's attractive creeper-clad house, where a sign on the pavement welcomes people to their friendly and informal country-style restaurant. Allison's good home cooking starts off with delicious scones, served with coffee and home-made preserves before lunch, at which time the choice widens to a short but tempting à la carte – typically including starters like smoked haddock chowder with freshly-baked brown bread or grilled goat's cheese and side salad. Vegetarians can look forward to colourful, zesty dishes such as ratatouille or spinach crèpe with salad. Delicious desserts range from the simple – apple crumble and cream – to sophisticated classics like crème brûlée. Dinner menus are also à la carte and, although more formal and offering a wider choice, the same philosophy applies. A first-floor ballroom running across the whole width of this substantial building was in the final stages of renovation on a recent visit, and with a library area up a few stairs at one end providing comfortable seating for non-participants and a minstrels' gallery at the other, it makes a superb venue for local events.

Rooms

Accommodation is available in four large bedrooms, all no-smoking and interestingly furnished with antiques. Unusual en-suite facilities have been cleverly incorporated without spoiling the proportions of these fine rooms – by hiding them in what appears to be a long wardrobe but which opens up to reveal a row of individual facilities – shower, WC etc. Children over 5 are welcome. • Acc£ • Meals£ all day Tues-Sat, L£ Sun • Closed Bank Hols, Xmas, 2 wks Jan • MasterCard, Visa •

Mountrath

COUNTRY HOUSE

Roundwood House

Mountrath Co Laois
Tel: 0502 32120   Fax: 0502 32711
email: roundwood@tinet.ie

Just a couple of miles off the main Dublin-Limerick road, Frank and Rosemarie Kennan's unspoilt early Georgian house lies secluded in mature woods of lime, beech and chestnut. A sense of history and an appreciation of genuine hospitality are all that is needed to make the most of a stay here – forget about co-ordinated decor and immaculate maintenance, just relax and share the immense pleasure and satisfaction that Frank and Rosemarie derive from the years of renovation work they have put into this wonderful property. Although unconventional in some ways, the house is extremely comfortable and well-heated (with central heating as well as log fires) and all the bathrooms are being renovated as we go to press (all have full bath). The Kennans have also been taking on the outbuildings of late and now have several beautifully converted rooms at the back. Their latest venture is two-fold; conversion of further outbuildings for self-catering accommodation and the renovation of an extraordinary (and historically unique) barn. This enterprise – which was at an early stage on a recent visit – defies description, but don't leave Roundwood without seeing it. Children, who always love the unusual animals and their young in the back yard, are very welcome and Rosemarie does a separate tea for them.

Restaurant

Rosemarie Kennan's food suits the house perfectly – good interesting cooking without unnecessary frills – and Frank is an excellent host. Sunday lunch is especially good value. • Acc£££ • Closed 25 Dec & Jan • Amex, Diners, MasterCard, Visa •

LEITRIM

Of all Ireland's counties, it is Leitrim which has to try hardest. That's official. Because, according to government data, it is Leitrim which has the doubtful distinction of having the poorest soil in the entire country. It's a covering of such low fertility, so we're told, that it is barely capable in some places of growing even the scrubbiest trees. Yet the very fact that Leitrim is thus categorised in the official statistics shows that such general overviews can easily become blunt instruments of analysis. For there are pockets of fertility in Leitrim of such good quality that, for instance, one of Ireland's leading organic horticulture firms is able to grow superb produce in the north of the county. And as for Leitrim lacking in glamorous tourist attractions other than the obvious one of the magnificent inland waterways, well, even that is largely a matter of perception. For Leitrim shares the shores of Lough Gill with Sligo, so much so that Yeat's Lake Isle of Innisfree is within an ace of being in Leitrim rather than Sligo of Yeatsian fame. To the northward, we find that more than half of lovely Glencar, popularly perceived as being one of Sligo's finest jewels, is in fact in Leitrim. As for the notion of Leitrim being the ultimate inland and rural county – not so. Leitrim has an Atlantic coastline, albeit of only four kilometres, around Tullaghan. It's said this administrative quirk is a throwback to the time when the all-powerful bishops of the early church aspired to have ways of travelling to Rome without having to cross the territory of neighbouring clerics. Whatever the reason, it's one of Leitrim's many surprises, which are such that it often happens that when you're touring in the area and find yourself in a beautiful bit of country, a reference to the map produces the unexpected information that you're in Leitrim. So forget about those gloomy soil facts – this is a county of hidden quality which deserves to be better known. And for anyone who seeks the essential Ireland, it's worth noting that the ancient Irish system of bar licences resulted in Leitrim having more pubs per head of population than any other county -148 souls per licence, which barely stands comparison with the Dublin figure of 1,119. This means the Leitrim pubs, like the county itself, have to try harder with all sorts of quaint ancillary trades, and they're all the better for that.

Local Attractions and Information

Carrick-On-Shannon
Rossinver

Tourism Information (May-September) 078 20170
Eden Plants & The Organic Centre 072 54122

Carrick-on-Shannon   Hollywell

Carrick-on-Shannon Co Leitrim

COUNTRY HOUSE   Tel: **078 21124**

After many years as hoteliers in the town (and a family tradition of inn-keeping that goes back 200 years), Tom and Rosaleen Maher moved to this delightful period house on a rise over the bridge, with beautiful views over the Shannon and its own river frontage (so guests may fish without leaving the property). It's a lovely, graciously proportioned house, furnished to a high standard but not overdone and with a relaxed family atmosphere. Tom and Rosaleen have an easy hospitality (not surprisingly, perhaps, as their name derives from the Gaelic "Meachar" meaning hospitable), making guests feel at home very quickly and this, as much as the comfort of the house and its tranquil surroundings, is what makes "Hollywell" special. Bedrooms are all individually furnished in period style and have en-suite bathrooms (1 shower only). It's worth getting up in good time for delicious breakfasts, with freshly-baked bread and home-made preserves. No evening meals, but Tom and Rosaleen advise guests on the best local choices and there's a comfortable guests' sitting room with an open fire to gather around on their return. Not suitable for children under 12. • Acc££ • Closed 10 days Xmas • MasterCard, Visa •

Glencar   Glencar Lodge

Glencar Co Leitrim (via Sligo)

CAFÉ   Tel/Fax: **071 45475**
email: glencar@tinet.ie

The drive down the Glencar valley towards Sligo is one of the most beautiful in Ireland and – apart from the well-documented attractions of the lake and waterfalls – there is now another good reason to stop along the way. At Glencar Lodge, which was the hunting lodge of Lissadell House and is set in beautiful gardens, Frank Slevin and Helen Crowley have established a delightful little café/restaurant and craft shop. They serve home-made soups, salads made from locally grown organic vegetables, quiches, open and toasted sandwiches, delicious Illy coffee and all sorts of irresistible home-made cakes, gateaux and tarts – or you can have a glass of wine with some Irish farmhouse cheeses if you like. During the winter they are also doing private parties and corporate functions, serving modern Irish cuisine. They may later develop the café to become a full restaurant. Open daily in summer. Meals £ weekends only in winter • Closed April/May & Oct • MasterCard, Visa •

Keshcarrigan   Canal View House & Restaurant

Keshcarrigan nr Carrick-on-Shannon Co Leitrim

RESTAURANT/ACCOMMODATION   Tel: 078 42056   Fax: 078 42404

A fireside cup of tea and home-baked scones or biscuits in the comfortable residents' lounge (with views of the cruisers passing) welcomes guests on arrival at Jeanette Conefry's immaculate guesthouse and restaurant overlooking the Shannon-Erne Waterway. Bedrooms – some with water views, all with a pleasant outlook – are individually furnished to a high standard. Direct-dial telephones have recently been installed and all have neat en-suite shower rooms. Peace and quiet are an attraction here, but television is available in bedrooms on request. Families are welcome and well looked after.

Restaurant

Gerard and Jeanette Conefry opened the restaurant to coincide with the opening of the waterway in 1992, and it has been a great success. Since 1995 they've been ably assisted in the kitchen by Rita Duggan, and at the time of going to press they propose building private mooring facilities so that restaurant guests can stay there on boats overnight. Table d'hôte and à la carte menus are based on the best ingredients, including locally grown organic vegetables and home-grown herbs, plus carefully sourced produce such as Keshcarrigan venison, fish from Killybegs, veal and steak from local farms. There is a generous sprinkling of vegetarian dishes, marked with a leaf symbol. The dessert menu offers a choice of five or six, including home-made ice creams with butterscotch sauce. Farmhouses cheeses are also available. • Acc££ • D££ daily L£ Sun only • Closed 25 Dec • MasterCard, Visa •

LIMERICK

The story of Limerick city and county is to a large extent the story of the Shannon Estuary, for in times past it was the total access and ready availability of the transport provided by Ireland's largest estuary which dictated the development of life along its southern shore and into the River Shannon itself. But as we move inland from the river, the very richness of the countryside soon begins to develop its own dynamic. After all, eastern Limerick is verging into Tipperary's Golden Vale, and the eastern county's Slieve Felim hills, rising to Cullaun at 462m, reflect the nearby style of Tipperary's Silvermine Mountains. Southwest of Limerick city, the splendid hunting country and utterly rural atmosphere of the area around the beautiful village of Adare makes it a real effort of imagination to visualise the muddy salt waters of the Shannon Estuary just a few miles away down the meandering River Maigue, yet the Estuary is there nevertheless. Equally, although the port of Foynes and the nearby jetty at Aughinish may be expanding to accommodate the most modern large ships, just a few miles inland we find ourselves in areas totally remote from the sea, in countryside which lent itself so well to mixed farming that the price of pigs in Dromcolliher (a.k.a. Drumcolligher) on the edge of the Mullaghareirk Mountains used to set the price of pigs throughout Ireland. Limerick city may have come to international attention in the late 1990s through the popular success of Frank McCourt's moving book Angela's Ashes, but by the time it appeared the picture it conveyed was long since out of date. Nobody would deny that Limerick can be a gritty place with its own spin on life, but in recent years the growth of the computer industry in concert with the rapid expansion of the remarkably vibrant university has given Limerick a completely new place in Irish life, and the city's energy and urban renewal makes it an entertaining place to visit. The eclectic collection on stunning display in the unique Hunt Museum sets a style which other areas of Limerick life are keen to match. That said, Limerick still keeps its feet firmly on the ground, and connoisseurs are firmly of the opinion that the best pint of Guinness in all Ireland is to be had in this no-nonsense city, where they insist on being able to choose the temperature of their drink, and refuse to have any truck with modern fads which would attempt to chill the rich multi-flavoured black pint into a state of near-freezing tastelessness aimed at immature palates.

Local Attractions and Information

Adare	May Fair 061 396894
Glin Castle	Pleasure Grounds & Walled Garden 068 34364
Limerick City	Hunt Museum , Customs House, Rutland Street 061 312833
Limerick City	King John's Castle 061 411201
Lough Gur	Interpretative Centre (3000BC to present day) 061 360788

Adare   Adare Manor

Adare Co Limerick

HOTEL/RESTAURANT 🏛 🏛   **Tel: 061 396566   Fax: 061 396124**

email: reservations@adaremanor.com   www.adaremanor.ie

The former home of the Earls of Dunraven, this magnificent neo-Gothic mansion is set in 900 acres on the banks of the river Maigue. Its splendid chandeliered drawing room and the glazed cloister of the dining room look over formal box-hedged gardens towards the Robert Trent Jones golf course. Other grand public areas include the gallery, named after the Palace of Versailles, with its unique 15th century choir stalls and fine stained glass windows. Luxurious bedrooms have individual hand carved fireplaces, fine locally-made mahogany furniture, cut-glass table lamps and impressive marble bathrooms with strong showers over huge bathtubs. Additional bedrooms are planned for 1999 and also a new Clubhouse. Banqueting for 200.

Gallery Restaurant

Gerard Costelloe has been Chef de Cuisine since 1993. Local produce, including vegetables from the estate's own gardens, is included on menus, and although based on classical cuisine, the style includes some modern Irish food, as in roast lamb cutlets on colcannon, for example. Seasonal menus, augmented by daily changes, are presented as an à la carte, with the proviso that the minimum price per head is £35. The minimum meal in the Gallery is three courses, and there is a 15% service charge. House wine, £19 + 15 %. Alteratively, bar food is available from May-September inclusive, 12-9 daily. • Acc££££ • L££ & D£££ daily • Open all year • Amex, Diners, MasterCard, Visa •

Adare

Carrabawn Guesthouse
Adare Co Limerick

ACCOMMODATION   Tel: 061 396067   Fax: 061 396925

In an area known for high standards, with prices to match, this immaculate owner-run establishment provides a good alternative to the local luxury accommodation. Bernard and Bridget Lohan have been welcoming guests here since 1984 – and many of them return on an annual basis because of the high level of comfort and friendly service provided. Bedrooms (all shower-only and all non-smoking) seemed a little dated in decor on a recent visit, but are very well-maintained with all the amenities required. In addition to seeing guests off with a good Irish breakfast, light evening meals can be provided by arrangement. • Acc££ • Closed 23-28 Dec • MasterCard, Visa •

Adare

Dunraven Arms Hotel
Adare Co Limerick

HOTEL/RESTAURANT   Tel: 061 396633   Fax: 061 396541
email: dunraven@iol.ie   www.iol.ie/hotels

Established in 1792, and set in one of Ireland's most picturesque villages, the Dunraven Arms has seen many changes over the last few years and is now a large hotel. It has been developed with commendable discretion and, under the personal management of Bryan and Louis Murphy, somehow manages to retain the comfortable ambience of a country inn. A very luxurious inn nevertheless – the 76 rooms are all furnished to the highest of standards: there are six suites and 14 junior suites and all the remaining accommodation is in executive rooms. There is also an unusually high proportion of rooms (20) suitable for disabled guests. The furnishing standard is superb throughout, with antiques, private dressing rooms and luxurious bathrooms, plus excellent amenities for private and business guests, all complemented by an outstanding standard of housekeeping. It's an excellent base for sporting activities – equestrian holidays are a speciality and both golf and fishing are available nearby – and also extremely popular for both conferences and private functions, which are held beside the main hotel (with separate catering facilities). A leisure centre has also been recently completed.

Maigue Restaurant

Named after the River Maigue, which flows through the village of Adare, the restaurant is delightfully old fashioned – more akin to eating in a large country house than in an hotel. Mark Phelan, who has been head chef since 1996, takes pride in using the best of local produce in meals that combine the traditions of the area with influences from around the world. Mark is also responsible for food served in the bar. Across the road, in one of the traditional thatched cottages, head chef Sandra Earl cooks for an informal restaurant, The Inn Between, which is in common ownership with the Dunraven Arms; details of opening times are available at the hotel. • Acc£££ • L£ & D££ daily • Closed 25 Dec • Amex, Diners, MasterCard, Visa •

Adare

The Wild Geese Restaurant
Rose Cottage Adare Co Limerick

RESTAURANT   Tel/Fax: 061 396451
email: wldgeese@iol.ie

In one of the prettiest cottages in the prettiest village in Ireland, Conleth Roche and Serge Soustrain's restaurant has great charm that is matched only by the service they provide. Serge presents mainly French menus based on the best local produce – all transformed into something very special by his highly skilled cooking. Semi à la carte dinner menus are priced by the course, with one or two supplements (Liscannor bay lobster, Clare oysters). Main courses, offered with a choice of vegetables or salad, are imaginative and well-judged; thus, from three meat choices, roast saddle of rabbit with panfried polenta and crispy pancetta in a wild mushrooms and Guinness sauce and, from four seafood options, panfried fillet of John Dory with new potatoes, wild mussels and pearl vegetables in a bouillabaisse sauce. Delicious desserts tend to be classic – a good crème brûlée perhaps (served with home-made biscuits) – or you can round off with Irish cheeses. Not suitable for children under 12. A short à la carte menu is offered at lunchtime and served informally.• L£ & D£££ Tues-Sat • Closed first 3 wks Jan • Amex, Diners, MasterCard, Visa •

Visit our web site (www.ireland-guide.com) for new recommendations, news and other relevant travel and dining information.

Adare

Woodlands House Hotel

Knockanes Adare Co Limerick

HOTEL   Tel: 061 396118   Fax: 061 396073

email: woodlands\hotel@iol.ie   www.woodlands\hotel

Just outside Adare, the Fitzgerald family's hotel has grown quite dramatically since it opened in 1983 and management has now moved into the next generation. The whole hotel has been systematically upgraded and developed over the years – the low, grey-tiled building is set in well-kept gardens and presents a very neat and welcoming appearance from the road. It has always been a popular venue for weddings and is particularly well suited to large gatherings, with spacious public areas throughout, including two bars, and a restaurant and banqueting suite overlooking gardens and countryside. Bedrooms include two suitable for disabled guests and four mini suites, and most have a pleasant outlook. A number of new bedrooms have recently been added, but older ones have also been upgraded – all are en-suite and 16 have whirlpool baths, although ten rooms have a shower only. Further developments announced just as we were going to press include another 33 bedrooms and a leisure centre, jacuzzi, sauna, steamroom and gym, all expected to be up and running for the 1999 season. • Acc££ • Closed 24-25 Dec • Amex, Diners, MasterCard, Visa •

Ballingarry

The Mustard Seed at Echo Lodge

Ballingarry Co Limerick

COUNTRY HOUSE/RESTAURANT   🏛   Tel: 069 68508   Fax: 069 68511

One of the country's prettiest and most characterful restaurants, Dan Mullane's famous Mustard Seed started life in Adare in 1985. Having celebrated its first decade it began the next one by moving just ten minutes drive away to Echo Lodge, a spacious Victorian country residence set on seven acres, with mature trees, shrubberies, kitchen garden and orchard. The Mustard Seed's new home offers luxurious accommodation, allowing Dan to provide the thorough-going hospitality that comes so naturally to him. Elegance, comfort and generosity are the key features – seen through decor and furnishings which bear the mark of a seasoned traveller whose eye has found much to delight in while wandering the world.

Restaurant 🍴

While the accommodation offered at Echo Lodge is exceptional , the main emphasis of the establishment is on food and hospitality, with admirable attention to detail. Drinks, served in the Library, come with a tasty amuse-bouche, fresh flowers are carefully selected to suit the decor in the dining room. Head chef David Norris takes great pride in sourcing his ingredients from the best local producers and suppliers; much of the food carefully prepared in his kitchen is organic and the herbs and vegetables come from their own gardens. David's cooking is country house style, based on the disciplines of classical French cooking, with modern Irish and global influences. He presents wide-ranging menus that might include dishes such as a starter of crisp-skinned confit of duck on a bed of oriental vegetables; a soup course influenced by garden produce, eg creamy leek; an imaginative main course, perhaps of lamb – pink loin served with a skewer of liver and kidney on a rosemary jus and garlic cream. A good plated Irish cheese selection or gorgeous puddings are followed by coffee and irresistible home-made petits fours, served at the table or in the Library. •D£££ daily except Sun & Mon, residents only low season. • Acc£££-££££ • Closed 25 Dec & mid-Jan-early Mar • Amex, MasterCard, Visa •

Castleconnell

Castle Oaks House Hotel

Castleconnell Co Limerick

HOTEL   Tel: 061 377666   Fax: 061 377717

Set quietly in 26 acres of wooded countryside on the banks of the Shannon, this attractive hotel is in an idyllic location on the edge of the picturesque village of Castleconnel, just a few miles on the Dublin side of Limerick. The old part of the hotel is a Georgian mansion, with the gracious proportions and elegance that that implies, although a new wing provides extra accommodation which makes up in comfort and convenience for what it might lack in character. Rooms include two executive rooms with whirlpool baths (and a romantic bridal suite) and are all en-suite with full bathrooms (bath and shower) . One room was specially designed for asthmatics, with hard surfaces and specially chosen fabrics. Private fishing is a particular attraction, and the hotel also offers an unusual venue for conferences and weddings in a converted chapel, which accommodates up to 300 people. Nice, helpful staff and a family-friendly attitude make this a pleasant hotel. There's a well equipped leisure centre in the large wooded grounds (15-metre pool), and also 24 self-catering holiday houses – but no dogs. • Acc££ • Closed 24-26 Dec • Amex, Diners, MasterCard, Visa •

Croom   Croom Mills

Croom Co Limerick

RESTAURANT/VISITOR CENTRE   Tel: 061 397130   Fax: 061 397199

One of the most imaginatively handled restorations of its type, a visit to Croom Mills shows the whole traditional corn milling process from beginning to end – including a sample of freshly baked bread hot from the oven. Many other exhibits illustrate related operations and crafts – the blacksmith, for instance, in his 19th century forge – and several primary power sources are to be seen in action, including the giant 16 foot cast iron waterwheel, built in Cork in 1852. The tour takes about an hour – but there are other attractions here too, notably one of the country's best craft and gift shops and the Mill Race Restaurant. Major improvements were in progress on a recent visit, but building work had no adverse effect on the food, which has been exemplary from the start. Starting from early morning there's a full breakfast menu available, then a full lunch menu (plus a light lunch menu available for groups) and a great range of home-cooked goodies on display all day for lighter bites. Vegetarians are well looked after, there's an outdoor eating area overlooking the millrace and they also do "Irish Nights At The Mill" (phone for details). This is good home cooking served in very pleasing surroundings – Mary Hayes and her team deserve great credit. • Open all day meals£ • Closed 25 Dec-2 Jan & Good Fri • Amex, MasterCard, Visa •

Glin   Glin Castle

Glin Co Limerick

COUNTRY HOUSE 🏛   Tel: 068 34112/34173   Fax: 068 34364

email: knight@iol.ie

The Fitzgeralds, hereditary Knights of Glin, have lived in Glin Castle for 700 years and it's now the home of the 29th Knight and his wife Madame Fitzgerald. The interior is stunning, with beautiful interiors enhanced by decorative plasterwork and collections of Irish furniture and paintings. Guests are magnificently looked after by manager Bob Duff. Accommodation was originally all in suites – huge and luxurious, but not at all intimidating because of the lived-in atmosphere that characterises the whole castle – but we are informed that additional rooms – "small, friendly, with a family atmosphere" – will be available for the 1999 season. No doubt they will have all the wonderful details for which the castle is renowned, such as a torch beside the bed. Excellent dinners, prepared by Bob Duff's wife Rachel Collins, who has been chef since 1997, are served communally in the beautiful dining room and are very good value at £25 for five courses, although choice is limited. (House wine £11.50) When the Knight is at home he will take visitors on a tour of the house and show them all his pictures and old furniture. Not to be missed while in Glin is O'Shaughnessy's pub, just outside the castle walls; one of the finest pubs in Ireland it is now in its sixth generation of family ownership and precious little has changed in the last hundred years. The garden and house open to the public at certain times. Non-residents are welcome to dine by reservation. • L£ & D££ • Acc££££ • Closed Dec & Jan • Diners, MasterCard, Visa •

Limerick   Castletroy Park Hotel

Dublin Road Limerick Co Limerick

HOTEL   Tel: 061 335566   Fax: 061 331117

sales@castletroy-park.ie   www.castletroy-park.ie

Although far from enticing from the road, this blocky redbrick hotel has a warm and welcoming atmosphere in all the public areas and, while not individually decorated, the rooms are thoughtfully furnished with special attention to the needs of the business traveller (good desk space, second phone, fax and computer points). Rooms include two suites, five junior suites and 25 executive rooms. There is one room especially equipped for disabled guests and 25 rooms are designated non-smoking. It is much sought after as a conference venue; the purpose-built conference centre is designed to cope equally well with a small board meeting or conference for 400. After work, The Merry Pedlar pub offers a change of scene. • L£ & D££ daily • Acc££££ • Amex, Diners, MasterCard, Visa •

Limerick DuCartes at the Hunt Museum

Hunt Museum Old Custom House Rutland Street Limerick Co Limerick

RESTAURANT/MUSEUM   **Tel: 061 312662   Fax: 061 417929**

This delightful modern café/restaurant is at the back of the museum, overlooking the river, with tables outside on the terrace in fine weather. As well as providing an appropriately elegant space to restore visitors to the museum, it is a popular lunchtime venue for locals. Attractively presented and healthy home-cooked food in the modern idiom should not disappoint. • Meals£ daily (Sun from 2pm) • MasterCard, Visa •

Limerick Green Onion Caffé

Ellen Street Limerick Co Limerick

RESTAURANT/CAFE   **Tel: 061 400710**

If you took a straw poll of Limerick people this is the place they're most likely to nominate as their favourite eating place. The rather gloomy decor probably won't impress and it's pot luck if you happen to like the style of music – but you'll never hear a bad word about Diarmuid O'Callaghan's food. Daytime menus are heavy on sandwiches (eg crab and dill mayonnaise, brie and sundried tomato or roast sirloin and horseradish mayonnaise), all made to order on homemade brown bread or bap and served with a seasonal salad garnish, herbs and cherry tomatoes. Or there are salads – Greek, chicken caesar, cheese filo parcel (goat's cheese topped with apple and walnuts, wrapped in filo and baked) and a couple of pasta dishes available as starter or main course portions. There's a fine drinks menu to go with the food too, ranging from Illy coffees through numerous mineral waters and fresh juices to hot chocolate. Evening menus see a change of pace, with a well-balanced and imaginative à la carte offering serious starters like Clonakilty black pudding, onion jam and colcannon or smoked Irish Gubbeen cheese and spinach tartlet, followed perhaps by pork fillet coated in pistachio nuts, with herb butter or darne of salmon with basil beurre blanc. Puddings tend towards the classics – crêpes with orange caramel sauce, chocolate and hazelnut cheesecake – and there's an interesting moderately priced wine list with good tasting notes. • L£ & D££ Mon-Sat • Closed Xmas, New Year & Bank Hols • Amex, Diners, MasterCard, Visa •

Limerick Greenhills Hotel

Ennis Road Limerick Co Limerick

HOTEL   **Tel: 061 453033   Fax: 061 453307**

Owner-managed by the Greene family since 1969, this friendly hotel is conveniently located just 5 minutes from the city and 20 minutes from Shannon airport. As well as providing a convenient base for touring the west, the hotel makes a useful business location and offers good conference facilities for up to 400 delegates (with back-up business services including French and German translation). Bedrooms include 11 executive rooms, 15 for non-smokers and ten rooms suitable for disabled guests – an unusually high proportion. Bedrooms are comfortably furnished in contemporary style and have full en-suite bathrooms (bath and shower). Excellent health and leisure facilities are a major attraction. • Acc££ • Closed 25 Dec • Amex, Diners, MasterCard, Visa •

Limerick Jurys Hotel

Ennis Road Limerick Co Limerick

HOTEL   **Tel: 061 327777   Fax: 061 326400**
email: margaret-holian@jurys.com

Set in a garden site on the banks of the Shannon, the hotel is just two minutes walk from the city centre and 15 minutes from Shannon airport. Good-sized rooms are decorated to a high standard with plenty of work space for business guests and neat, well-lit bathrooms. Unusually for a city centre hotel, Jurys has a good leisure centre and also an outdoor tennis court. • Acc£££ • Closed 24 & 25 Dec • Amex, Diners, MasterCard, Visa •

Limerick Jurys Inn Limerick

Lower Mallow Street Limerick Co Limerick

HOTEL   **Tel: 061 207000   Fax: 061 400966**
email: ronan_mcauley@jurys.com

Like other Jurys Inns, this budget hotel enjoys a prime city centre location and has carparking available in an adjoining multi-storey carpark (with direct access to the hotel). Rooms are large, comfortable and furnished to a high standard, especially considering the moderate cost. Bathrooms are fairly basic but have everything required including a proper (if budget-sized) bath as well as overbath shower. Don't expect high levels of service – that's what keeps the costs down – but there is a restaurant and pub-like bar as part of the development. • Acc££ • Closed 25 Dec • Amex, Diners, MasterCard, Visa •

Limerick   Limerick Inn

Ennis Road Limerick Co Limerick

HOTEL   **Tel: 061 326666   Fax: 061 326281**

email: limerick-inn@limerick-inn.ie   www.commerce.ie/cl/limerick-inn.ie

This large low-rise modern hotel a few miles out of town on the Shannon Airport road is owner-run by the Ryan family. Although well-placed as a base for touring, its main strength is as a conference venue – the largest of five conference rooms can accommodate 600 delegates and there are smaller meeting rooms for groups of up to 30; backup secretarial services are available. Bedrooms, all of which have full en-suite bathrooms (bath and shower), include four suites and 30 executive rooms, and there is a fine health and leisure centre. • Acc££ • Closed 24 & 25 Dec • Amex, Diners, MasterCard, Visa •

Limerick   Limerick Ryan Hotel

Ardhu House Ennis Road Limerick Co Limerick

HOTEL   **Tel: 061 453922   Fax: 061 326333**

Situated on the outskirts of Limerick city, this hotel is built around an attractive old house dating from 1780. The original building is still gracious and has some elegantly proportioned rooms, including a peaceful drawing room. Unfortunately the new wing – effectively a completely separate block reached by a corridor – was added at a time when modern architecture did not always blend in well with the past. However, it does provide a large number of convenient modern bedrooms (with voicemail phones), and two suites. Conference and business facilities – located in the old house – comprise 11 meeting or private dining rooms catering for anything from two to 250 people, and back-up services are provided by a 24 hour business centre. No leisure facilities on site, but residents have complimentary use of a nearby fitness centre. • Acc££-£££ • Open all year •

Limerick   Mortell's Delicatessen & Seafood Restaurant

49 Roches Street Limerick Co Limerick

RESTAURANT   **Tel: 061 415457   Fax: 061 318458**

Behind their shop the Mortell family run an unpretentious, inexpensive daytime restaurant where chef Brian Mortell cooks good simple food based on the freshest of ingredients, especially fish. The day starts with a big traditional breakfast. If seafood is not your thing, the steaks and roasts that are an additional lunchtime feature should please – and there are always salads and extras from the deli counter in the shop and their own home-baked bread – followed by homely desserts such as apple, rhubarb or lemon meringue pie. • Meals£ all day Mon-Sat • Closed Xmas Day, New Year & Bank Hols • Amex, Diners, MasterCard, Visa •

Limerick   Quenelles

Unit 4 Steamboat Quay Dock Road Limerick Co Limerick

RESTAURANT   **Tel: 061 411111   Fax: 061 400111**

Having made a major impact on the Limerick dining scene in their previous restaurant, Kieran and Sindy Pollard moved down to the new development on Steamboat Quay in 1998. They set up their new restaurant in a very upbeat contemporary style, with lots of Mediterranean colour in strong blocks – mismatched single-colour chairs for example – both in the reception area downstairs and in the first floor restaurant. Lunch was particularly popular in their previous, smaller premises but the new restaurant is open for dinner only. A recent visit was made too soon after opening for a fair judgment, but the following examples should indicate the style and format. Menus are organised as semi-à la carte, with each course priced separately plus some supplements. (including an extraordinary £4 extra for a main course of breast of barbary duck on top of the standard £15.95 course price). Soup of the day comes with home-baked breads; a choice of six starters might include terrine of Irish breakfast (all the traditional ingredients, finished with a poached egg and green tomato marmalade) or half a dozen oysters with lemon or Kilpatrick with a topping of Tabasco and bacon (£2 supplement on £5.50 course price). Eight main courses (£15.95) could include "This tender Cut of Sirloin Steak is pan fried how you like it with bitter chocolate sunken souffle". And so on. We suspect Kieran Pollard is trying too hard to be different – but we know he can cook confidently in an adventurous style and predict that the kitchen will settle down to its previous high standard. • D££-£££ Mon-Sat • Closed 25 Dec •

Limerick — South Court Business & Leisure Hotel

Raheen Roundabout Limerick Co Limerick

HOTEL

Tel: 061 487487   Fax: 061 487499

email: cro@lynchotel.com   www.lynchotels.com

Ideally located for Shannon Airport and the Raheen Industrial Estate, the South Court Hotel presents a somewhat daunting exterior, but once inside visitors soon discover that it caters especially well for business guests, both on and off-duty. In addition to excellent conference and meeting facilities, the bedrooms are comfortable, impressively spacious and well-equipped, with generous desk areas and the latest technology – including fax/modem/ISDN points – in every room. Executive bedrooms even have a separate work area providing a "mini-office" with a leather desk chair and private fax machine. Local, as well as hotel, residents will value having access to the hotel's excellent leisure facilities and the informal bar and café/restaurant which are an important part of the development. • Acc££ • Amex, Diners, MasterCard, Visa

LONGFORD

The good people of Longford have become so accustomed to seeing their county dismissed as "the least interesting in all Ireland" in "speed-through" travel guides that they've adopted a sensibly wry attitude to the whole business. Thus they get on with life in a style appropriate to a quietly prosperous and unpretentious county which nevertheless can spring some surprises. These are not, however, to be found in the scenery, for Longford is either gently undulating farming country, or bogland. The higher ground in the north of the county up towards the intricate Lough Gowna rises to no more than 276 m in an eminence which romantics might call Carn Clonhugh, but usually it's prosaically known as Corn Hill. Over to the east, where there's more high ground, there's even less pulling of the punches in the name of the little market town in its midst, for Granard – which sounds rather elegant – can actually be translated as "Ugly Height". Yet this suggests a pleasure in words for their own sake, which is appropriate as Longford produced novelist Maria Edgeworth of Edgeworthstown, and down towards that fine place Ballymahon and the south of its territory on the Westmeath border, Longford takes in part of the Goldsmith country. Goldsmith himself would be charmed to know that, six kilometres south of the road between Longford and Edgeworthstown, there's the tiny village of Ardagh, a place of just 75 citizens which is so immaculately maintained that it has been the winner of the Tidiest Village in the Tidy Towns awards three times during the past ten years. On the most recent occasion, in 1998, it won the top award as well, the neatest place in all Ireland in every sense of the word. Over to the west, the scenery becomes more varied as Longford has a lengthy shoreline along the northeast part of Lough Ree. It also has pretty Richmond Harbour west of Longford town at Cloondara, where the Royal Canal – gradually being restored along its meandering track from Dublin – finally gets to the Shannon. And as for Longford town itself, they're working on it, and some day the rest of Ireland will wake up to find that there's life a-plenty going on there, if you just know where to look for it.

Local Attractions and Information

Longford	Tourist Information (seasonal) 043 46566
Longford	Carriglass Manor (James Gandon stableyard, lace museum) 043 41026

Granard   Toberphelim House

Granard Co Longford

FARM STAY   **Tel/Fax: 043 86568**

email: tober@tinet.ie   www.Ireland.travel.ie

Dan and Mary Smyth's Georgian farmhouse is about half a mile off the road, on a rise that provides a lovely view of the surrounding countryside. Very much a working farm – cows, beef cattle and sheep plus an assortment of domestic animals and hens – it is a very hospitable place. Guests are welcome to wander around and walk the fields.("Rubber boots are a must"). There's a guests' sitting room with television and three bedrooms: two en-suite (shower) with a single and double bed in each and one twin room with a separate private bathroom. All are comfortably furnished, but don't expect amenities like phones and TV in the rooms. Families are welcome – there's a family room and children's playground – and dinner, light meals and snacks can be arranged as long as notice is given before 12 noon. Cooking is traditional farmhouse fare – no wine licence but guests are welcome to bring their own – and meals are taken around a big mahogany dining table. • Acc£ • Closed Oct-Apr • MasterCard, Visa •

Longford   Longford Arms Hotel

Main Street Longford Co Longford

HOTEL   **Tel: 043 46296   Fax: 043 46244**

email: longfordarms@tinet.ie

Located right in the heart of the midlands, this comfortable family-run hotel has recently been renovated to a high standard. Public areas give a good impression on arrival. Bedrooms are comfortably furnished and particularly convenient for business guests as they have adequate desk space and the amenities required for this type of travel (including trouser presses and irons). Bedrooms include 18 executive rooms, all with good bathrooms (with both bath and shower) and nearly half are designated non-smoking. Good conference facilities (900). The coffee shop provides good casual daytime food and they do all their baking in-house – a good place to take a break. (Bar/coffee shop food is available from 8 am-8 pm). • Acc££ • Closed 25 Dec • Amex, Diners, MasterCard, Visa •

LOUTH

Louth may be Ireland's smallest county at only 317 square miles, but it still manages to be two or even three counties in one. Much of it is fine farmland, which is at its best in the area west of the extensive wildfowl paradise of Dundalk Bay. But as well there are the distinctive uplands in the southwest, whose name of Oriel recalls an ancient princedom. And in the north of the county, the Cooley Mountains sweep upwards in a style which well matches their better-known neighbours, the Mountains of Mourne, which lie across the handsome inlet of Carlingford Lough. As its name suggests, this is one of Ireland's few genuine fjords, and on its Louth shore the ancient little port of Carlingford town used to be one of the country's best-kept secrets, a quiet little place imbued with history. Today, it is happily prospering both as a recreational harbour for the Dundalk and Newry area, and as a bustling visitor attraction in its own right. The county's three main townships of Ardee, Dundalk and Drogheda each have their own distinctive style, and all three have been coming vibrantly to life in recent years. The historic borough of Drogheda is the main commercial port, while the evocatively-named Port Oriel at Clogher Head is an active little fishing harbour. Inevitably, Louth's location plumb on the main east coast corridor between Belfast and Dublin hampered its image in times past, for the trunk road battered its way mercilessly through towns and villages. But now that the M1 is developing to remove the weight of through traffic and speed access throughout the county, Louth is re-discovering its own identity, and it's an attractive one at that.

Local Attractions and Information

Dundalk
Dunleer

Tourist Information 042 35484
White River Mill 041 51141

Ardee   Red House

Ardee Co Louth
COUNTRY HOUSE   Tel/Fax: 041 53523
Although it is just off a busy road, Red House is set in parkland that has been well maintained for 200 years. The trees surrounding this lovely Georgian house insulate it so well that it seems in a world apart. It is a beautiful and interesting house, with lovely reception rooms and a mahogany panelled library. The three spacious bedrooms are elegantly proportioned and furnished with antiques, and while one has an en-suite bathroom the others are private but (in true country house style) along a corridor. Linda Connolly runs the house with warmth and efficiency and cooks very acceptable dinners for residents (by arrangement). There is a floodlit tennis court and (in summer) indoor heated swimming pool and sauna. • Acc££ • Closed mid-Dec-mid-Jan • Amex, MasterCard, Visa •

Blackrock   Brake Tavern

Main Street Blackrock Co Louth
PUB   Tel: 042 21393   Fax: 042 22568
Although it may not look especially inviting from the outside, first-time visitors are always amazed by the warmth and country charm of the Brake once they get in the door – all old pine and rural bric-a-brac, it has open fires and friendly staff. It's a great place to stop even for a cup of tea, but even better if you're hungry – it has a well-deserved reputation for good bar meals, with a wide range offered – not just the usual pub staples, but seafood such as smoked mussels, jumbo prawns and even lobster. There are lots of meat dishes, too, especially steaks with a range of sauces and creamy dishes that come with rice, such as prawns provençal, beef stroganoff and pork a la crème. Salads and accompaniments are particularly good, all arranged buffet style. Beware of the unusual opening hours though – this is a late afternoon into evening place. • Meals£-££ • Closed 25 Dec & Good Fri •

Carlingford   Ghan House

Carlingford Co Louth
COUNTRY HOUSE   Tel/Fax: 042 73682
This 18th century house is an attractive location in its own walled grounds on the edge of Carlingford village. It is of interest both for its accommodation and, more unusually, because the Carroll family run a cookery school on the premises. The accommodation is in four very different country rooms, each with sea or mountain views and three of which

have well-finished en-suite bathrooms. Needless to say dinner is something of a priority – the style is country house, there is a licence and non-residents are welcome (bookings advised). In addition to the cookery school (contact Paul Carroll for the 1999 programme), Ghan House is also a good venue for small conferences and meetings; details of services and rates available on request. At the time of going to press an extra eight en-suite bedrooms were under construction. • L£ & D££ • Acc££ • Closed Xmas & New Year • MasterCard, Visa •

Carlingford Jordan's Town House & Restaurant

Newry Street Carlingford Co Louth
TOWNHOUSE/RESTAURANT Tel: 042 73223 Fax: 042 73827
email: jordans@iol.ie

Since Harry and Marian Jordan opened their restaurant in the centre of Carlingford in 1984 the village has seen great changes – not least in the number and variety of eating places visitors can now choose from. But Jordan's has not stood still either: not only have Harry and Marian moved with the times and kept their serious interest in food alive (unusually they take turn-about in the kitchen and front-of-house), but they have also added a very high quality accommodation element to the business – they are effectively running a country house, although it operates as a leading restaurant with separate accommodation. The rooms are in a converted row of stone fisherman's cottages – very attractive, exceptionally spacious and well-furnished, with lovely bathrooms (bath and shower in all rooms). The restaurant has a little traditional bar area at the front, a reception area with comfortable seating in the middle and a dining room up a few stairs at the end. Fresh local produce provides the basis for everything served – especially seafood, but Carlingford lamb and local beef are not forgotten. Bread is made daily from flour milled by a stone watermill at nearby Dunleer. The style is essentially hearty country house with occasional international influences: expect dishes like caper-baked hake, braised shank of lamb and vegetarian choices such as vegetarian moussaka or wok-fried vegetable hotpot. This is good food and Louth is renowned for large portions, so make sure of a good appetite. • D££ daily, L£ Sun only • Acc££ • Closed Xmas, Good Fri & last 3 wks Jan • Amex, MasterCard, Visa •

Carlingford Magee's Bistro

Tholsel Street Carlingford Co Louth
RESTAURANT Tel/Fax: 042 73751

Hugh Finegan and Sheila Keiros built up a great reputation for their tiny, tightly packed restaurant in the D'Arcy Magee centre. As we go to press they are about to open up in new premises around the corner (just along from PJs /The Anchor Bar) so Sheila's wholesome home cooking will once more be available to the many who have suffered withdrawal symptoms during the unexpectedly long changeover. The new place is much bigger and stylish; it's in two sections, with a 'cheap'n'cheerful' café/pizza side which can be used on its own in low season, and a slightly more formal restaurant alongside. Expect her new open kitchen to produce lots of snappy, zappy new wave food with heaps of flavour – and Hugh will be out front making sure there's lots of fun. • Meals£-££ daily in summer – check times of season • Closed Jan • MasterCard, Visa •

Carlingford O'Hares

Carlingford Co Louth
PUB Tel: 042 73106

Paul McPartland took over this renowned pub a couple of years ago; thankfully, there has been little noticeable change. It's one of those lovely places with a grocery at the front and an unspoilt hard-floored pub with an open fire at the back. Loos (always clean) are in the yard and the food is simple but good. You can have soup and sandwiches if you like, but the speciality is Carlingford oysters – with a pint of stout of course. •Closed 25 Dec & Good Fri •

Carlingford The Oystercatcher Lodge & Bistro

Market Square Carlingford Co Louth
RESTAURANT/ACCOMMODATION Tel: 042 73922 Fax: 042 73987

Brian and Denise McKevitt's little restaurant with rooms opened on the square in Carlingford village in summer 1998. The restaurant has an hospitable atmosphere – there's always someone on hand to greet anyone who pops their head around the door. Seafood is the main offering – Carlingford oysters, of course (several ways), crab puffs and Carlingford Lough mussels with a leek, saffron and wine sauce are all typical first courses. There are half a dozen seafood main courses to match, but carnivores do well too, with local lamb, steaks, duck and pork done in various ways. There are also a couple of vegetarian pastas although, in our experience, vegetarians would do better to take a selection from the excellent range of salads and vegetables which are laid out for self-service with the main course. Prices can add up rather quickly to £20+ per head for 3 courses, which might seem a bit much for the café-style atmosphere but the cooking, especially of seafood, is good.

Rooms

There are seven guest rooms available, all bright, spacious and very clean although a little spartan, with hard floors and only showers in the en-suite facilities. • D£-££ daily • Acc££ • Closed Xmas • MasterCard, Visa •

Collon   Forge Gallery Restaurant

Collon Co Louth

RESTAURANT   Tel: 041 26272   Fax: 041 26584

email: forgrgallery@intel.ie

For the best part of fifteen years Des Carroll and Conor Phelan's charming two-storey restaurant has been providing consistently excellent food, hospitality and service. They've earned a great reputation and a devoted following along the way. It's a most attractive place – the building itself is unusual and has been furnished and decorated with flair, providing a fine setting for food that never disappoints. Des offers weekly menus that combine country French and New Irish styles, with a few other influences along the way – notably Thai. Everything is based on the best possible seasonal produce, much of it local – seafood, game in season, vegetables, fruit – and great home-made breads -white yeast bread, scones or brown bread with thyme perhaps. Typical main courses include a special vegetarian dish such as pillows of filo with leeks and roquefort as well as local meat, such as rack of tender Cooley lamb, and seafood such as prawns and scallops in wine and garlic sauce. But the really good news is that accommodation and private dining facilities are planned "in the coming year". • D££ Mon-Sat • Closed 25 Dec & 2 wks Jan • Amex, Diners, MasterCard, Visa •

Drogheda   Black Bull Inn

Dublin Road Drogheda Co Louth

PUB   Tel: 041 37139

This attractive roadside pub is on the left of the hill, just as you leave Drogheda in the Dublin direction. It has built up a considerable reputation for bar food over the years and now has an interesting food shop/delicatessen next door. • Closed 25 Dec & Good Fri •

Drogheda   Boyne Valley Hotel & Country Club

Drogheda Co Louth

HOTEL   Tel: 041 37737   Fax: 041 39188

At the heart of this substantial hotel, set in large gardens just on the Dublin side of Drogheda town, lies an 18th century mansion. It is not as obvious as it used to be since recent developments created a completely new entrance, but it is still there and provides some unspoilt, graciously proportioned rooms that contrast well with the later additions. Owner-run by Michael and Rosemary McNamara since 1992, it has the personal touch unique to hands-on personal management and is very popular with locals, for both business and pleasure, as well visitors using it as a base for touring the famous historic sites of the area. Bedrooms include eight suitable for disabled guests. While rooms in the old building have more character, the new ones are finished to a very high standard. Conference and business facilities are also good (back up services available) and there is an exceptionally fine leisure centre in the grounds. Well-behaved pets are allowed by arrangement. • L£ & D£-££ daily • Acc££ • Open all year • Amex, MasterCard, Visa •

Dundalk   Ballymascanlon House Hotel

Ballymascanlon Dundalk Co Louth

HOTEL   Tel: 042 71124   Fax: 042 71598

Set in 130 acres of parkland this hotel just north of Dundalk has developed around a large Victorian house. Although it has been in the same family ownership since 1948, major improvements have been made over the last couple of years (since it was decided to demolish an old squash court and use the space to build a new leisure centre and extra accommodation). This has been done with great style, and lifted the hotel into a completely different class. Corporate facilities include three versatile meeting rooms (max 275 in largest room) and there are back-up business services available. The new leisure facilities, which include 20 metre deck level pool and tennis courts, are very impressive. The hotel also has its own 18-hole golf course. • Acc££-£££ • Closed 24-26 Dec • Amex, Diners, MasterCard, Visa •

Dundalk   Quaglino's
Quaglino's Restaurant Dundalk Co Louth

RESTAURANT   Tel: 042 38567   Fax: 042 28598

Quaglino's is a long-established and highly regarded restaurant in Dundalk. Here owner-chef Pat Kerley takes great pride in the active promotion of Irish cuisine and uses as much local produce as possible. He operates no less than three menus at this popular restaurant – not just a table d'hôte and an à la carte, but an Italian one too. They all feature local specialities, notably oysters from the beautiful Carlingford Lough and organic vegetables – typically in a tradition-inspired dish like pot-roasted beef with Deerpark organic vegetables. An experienced and successful competition cook, Pat – who has been a finalist in the New Irish Cuisine competition run by the Restaurants Association of Ireland and Bord Bia – is rightly proud of the growing popularity of Irish cuisine in recent years and does all he can to encourage it. The restaurant is run on traditional lines, with good service a priority. As in most Louth restaurants, generosity is the keynote. • D££-£££ Mon-Sat • Closed Xmas & New Year • Amex, Diners, MasterCard, Visa •

Termonfeckin   Triple House Restaurant
Termonfeckin Co Louth

RESTAURANT   Tel/Fax: 041 22616

The pretty village of Termonfeckin provides a fine setting for Pat Fox's attractive restaurant, which is in a 200-year-old converted farmhouse in landscaped gardens surrounded by mature trees. On cold evenings a log fire in the reception area (an alternative to the conservatory used for aperitifs in summer) is very welcome. Pat presents a number of menus, including an early evening one that is especially good value (£12.50), a wide-ranging dinner menu, an à la carte and also blackboard seafood extras from nearby Clogherhead. What they all have in common is a commitment to using the best of local produce – particularly seafood – fresh Clogherhead prawns, Annagassan crab, and a dish he entitles, intriguingly, Port Oriel Pot-Pourri. But locally-reared meats feature too, in rack of local lamb with a herb crust, for example. Vegetarians do well, too, with vegetable filled crêpes – perhaps with a colourful light tomato sauce and cheese topping or fettucine pesto. Finish, perhaps, with a speciality dessert, a dacquoise that varies with the season's fruits or a plated selection of farmhouse cheeses such as Cashel Blue, Cooleeney and Wexford Cheddar. The wine list reflects Pat's particular interests and special evenings are sometimes held for enthusiasts off-season. • D££ daily, L£ Sun only • Closed 25-28 Dec & Mon Sept-May • Amex, Diners, MasterCard, Visa •

MAYO

Mayo is magnificent. All Ireland's counties have their devotees, but enthusiasts for Mayo have a devotion which is passionate. In their heart of hearts, they feel that this austerely majestic Atlantic-battered territory is somehow more truly Irish than anywhere else, and who could argue with them after experiencing the glories of scenery, sea and sky which this western rampart of Ireland puts on ever-changing display? Yet among Mayo's many splendid mountain ranges we find pockets of fertile land, through which there tumble fish-filled streams and rivers. And in the west of the county, the rolling hills of the drumlin country, which run in a virtually continuous band right across Ireland from Strangford Lough, meet the sea again in the island studded wonder of Clew Bay. At its head is the delightful town of Westport, one of the most attractive small towns in all Ireland, a cosmopolitan jewel of civilisation set in dramatic country with the holy mountain of Croagh Patrick (762 m) soaring above the bay. Along Mayo's rugged north coast, turf cutting at Ceide Fields near Ballycastle has revealed the oldest intact field and farm system in existence, preserved through being covered in blanket bog 5,000 years ago. An award-winning interpretive centre has been created at the site, and even the most jaded visitor will find fascination and inspiration in the clear view which it provides into Ireland's distant past.

Local Attractions and Information

Ballina	Street Festival/Arts Week (July) 056 70905
Ceide Fields	Visitor Centre 0996 43325
Foxford	Woollen Mills Visitor Centre 094 56756
Wesport	House & Children's Zoo 098 25430 / 27766
Westport	Tourist Information 098 25711

Ballina   Mount Falcon Castle

Foxford Road Ballina Co Mayo

COUNTRY HOUSE/RESTAURANT   **Tel: 096 21172   Fax: 096 71517**

email: mfsalmon@iol.ie

Not really a castle at all, Mount Falcon is a substantial neo-Gothic house, built around 1876. Mrs Constance Aldridge has personally made guests welcome at her home for over half a century. Connie, as she is affectionately known, is a most entertaining hostess, a personality perfectly suited to the house, with its dramatic entrance hall (complete with piano for impromptu late-night sessions), comfortable chintzy drawing room with huge fire fed by logs from the estate, genuinely old-fashioned bedrooms and, perhaps most of all, the dining room where she reigns supreme each evening, "dispensing wine and wit in equal measure" as a visiting writer once summed it up. Country pursuits really are at the heart of Mount Falcon and her kitchen uses only the best local produce, mostly from the estate farm and walled kitchen gardens. This is wholesome, no-nonsense cooking: salmon is straight from the River Moy and great joints of Aga-roasted local meat take pride of place on the sideboard. Even the butter is home-made. Non-residents are welcome to dinner by reservation. • L££ & D££ daily • Acc£££ • Closed Xmas wk & Feb & Mar •

Clare Island   Clare Island Lighthouse

Clare Island Co Mayo

LIGHTHOUSE   **Tel: 098 45120**

Should you happen to visit this wondrous place on a fine day it will undoubtedly remain in your heart for ever – and even if the weather gods are less generous, you will be sure of shelter, comfort, good food and companionship which will all add up to a unique experience. Perched 387 feet above the Atlantic, above a sheer cliff, this sturdy lighthouse was in use until 1965 and then lay unused until Robert and Monica Timmerman took on its restoration in 1991. It now makes a wonderful place for a break, and the Timmermans are also promoting it for small seminars, workshops and special groups. If the usual ferry service is too time-consuming they can arrange a water-taxi or helicopter transfer from the mainland. Best of all, perhaps, they recommend slowing down and taking the scenic route – by train to Westport, where they can arrange collection at the station. The six (non-smoking) bedrooms are all different but comfortably furnished in an appropriate country style and all have en-suite facilities, while living areas are spacious, with polished wooden floors, oriental rugs, leather furniture and turf fires. [Details of ferry services are available from Chris O'Grady (098 26397) and Charles O'Malley (098 25045); in high season, June-August, there is a regular service, at other times it is essential to check.] • D££ • Acc££ •

Cong   Ashford Castle

Cong Co Mayo

HOTEL/RESTAURANT 🏨🏨   **Tel: 092 46003   Fax: 092 46260**
email: ashford@ashford.ie   www.ashford.ie

Ireland's grandest castle hotel, with a history going back to the early 13th century, Ashford is set in 350 acres of beautiful parkland. Grandeur, formality and tranquillity are the essential characteristics, first seen in the approach through well manicured lawns, in the entrance and formal gardens and, once inside, in a succession of impressive public rooms that illustrate a long and proud history – panelled walls, oil paintings, balustrades, suits of armour and magnificent fireplaces. Public rooms include two famous dining rooms – the grand George V Dining Room and even grander Connaught Room – but, although they are open to non-residents, would-be diners would be well advised to arrange a visit off-season: when the castle is full, which often happens in summer, dining is reserved exclusively for residents. Accommodation at the castle varies considerably due to the size and age of the building, and each room in some way reflects the special qualities of this unique hotel. The best bedrooms and the luxurious suites at the top of the castle are elegantly furnished with period furniture, some with enormous and beautifully appointed bathrooms, others with remarkable architectural features, such as a panelled wooden ceiling recently discovered behind plasterwork in one of the suites (and now fully restored). Many of the rooms also have magnificent views of Lough Corrib, the River Cong and wooded parkland, but some smaller ones overlook the car park and lack the sense of grandeur expected of a castle. In addition to the more obvious outdoor activities (which include an equestrian centre) the castle has what might be described as a bijou health centre, incorporating computerised exercise equipment, steam room, sauna and whirlpool, all beautifully designed in neo-classical style. Impressive conference facilities, for up to 110 delegates, are backed up by a specialist team. The hotel general manager, Rory Murphy, brings his own natural and easy charm to the job of making guests feel comfortable and relaxed in what are admittedly rather awesome surroundings, while at the same time managing to ensure that the appropriate standards are continually maintained at what is one of the great hotels of the world.

The Connaught Room ⭐

The Connaught Room is the jewel in Ashford Castle's culinary crown and one of Ireland's most impressive restaurants. This lovely, classically furnished evening dining room has heavy gold drapes framing views of the grounds. Tables are beautifully appointed, with fine china and crystal providing a fitting setting for fine food. Denis Lenihan, who has been Executive Chef at the castle since 1978, oversees the cooking for both this and the George V Dining Room. Always a strong supporter of regional produce and local suppliers, he presents a seasonal à la carte menu and also a tasting menu (£46), which is available to a whole table or a minimum of two persons. The style is classical French using the best of Irish ingredients – Atlantic prawns, Galway Bay sole, Cleggan lobster, Connemara lamb – in sophisticated dishes that will please the most discerning diner. Irish farmhouse cheeses and warm souffles are among the tempting endings for luxurious meals, which are greatly enhanced by a meticulous attention to detail. Service, under the direction of Peter Cullen, will invariably be discreet and extremely professional. An extensive wine list is enhanced by the inclusion of a special selection of Wines of the Month, of varying styles and from several regions, at friendly prices.

George V Dining Room

Lunch and dinner are served in this much larger but almost equally opulent dining room, and an all-day snack menu is also available. A five-course dinner menu is offered (£37), and although the standard of cooking and service equals that of The Connaught Room, there is a more down to earth tone about the menus, which are in English, with a choice of about eight on the first and middle courses. Cleggan mussels baked on the half shell under a provençale crust with a little shaved fennel salad, sauté of river salmon on a julienne of red cabbage, cider and ginger are typical of menus that major in seafood but have plenty of other options to choose from. A separate vegetarian menu (£36 plus service) has less choice but is more modern and includes some tempting suggestions. Lunch (£23 for the full lunch, £18 for two courses) offers a shortened and somewhat simplified version of the dinner menu. A 15% service charge is added to all prices. • L££ & D£££-££££ daily • Acc££££ • Amex, Diners, MasterCard, Visa •

Crossmolina

Enniscoe House

Ballina Nr Crossmolina Co Mayo

COUNTRY HOUSE/RESTAURANT   Tel: 096 31112   Fax: 096 31773

email: enniscoe@indigo.ie   www.indigo.ie/~enniscoe

In parkland and mature woods on the shores of Lough Conn, Enniscoe is stern and gaunt, as Georgian mansions in the north-west of Ireland tend to be, but any intimidating impressions of "the last great house of North Mayo" are quickly dispelled once inside this fascinating old place. Built by ancestors of the present owner, Susan Kellett, (they settled here in the 1660s), Enniscoe attracts anglers and visitors with a natural empathy for the untamed wildness of this little known area. The house itself has great charm and makes a lovely place to come back to after a day in the rugged countryside. Family portraits, antique furniture and crackling log fires all complement Susan's warm hospitality and wholesome dinners, which non-residents are welcome to share by reservation. It is the activities in the old farm buildings that have attracted special interest since 1992, when the local Historical Society opened a genealogy centre, The Mayo North Family History Research Centre (096 31809) that researches names and families of Mayo origin. Also – and an especially appropriate development for this remote rural area – there's a little agricultural museum that houses a display of old farm machinery. Well-behaved dogs are welcome by arrangement. • D££ • Acc£££ • Closed mid Oct-Mar • Amex, MasterCard, Visa •

Dugort

Gray's Guest House

Dugort Achill Island Co Mayo

ACCOMMODATION   Tel: 098 43224/43315

Vi McDowell has been running this legendary guesthouse in the attractive village of Dugort since 1979, and nobody understands better the qualities of peace, quiet and gentle hospitality that have been bringing guests here for the last hundred years. It is an unusual establishment, occupying a series of houses, and each area has a slightly different appeal. There's a large, traditionally furnished sitting room with an open fire and several conservatories for quiet reading. Bedrooms and bathrooms vary considerably due to the age and nature of the premises, but the emphasis is on old-fashioned comfort; they all have tea & coffee-making trays and there are extra shared bathrooms in addition to en-suite facilities. Children are welcome (under 10s 50%) and there's an indoor play room and safe outdoor play area plus pool and table tennis for older children. Dogs are allowed by arrangement. It's a nice place to drop into for coffee, light lunch or afternoon tea (which is served in the garden in fine weather) and the dining room is open to non-residents for evening meals by arrangement (7pm). •D££ • Acc£-££ • No credit cards (personal cheques accepted) •

Keel

The Beehive

Keel Achill Island Co Mayo

CAFÉ   Tel: 098 43134/43240   Fax: 098 43018

At their informal restaurant and attractive craft shop in Keel, husband and wife team Patricia and Michael Joyce take pride in the careful preparation and presentation of the best of Achill produce, especially local seafood such as fresh and smoked salmon, mussels, oysters and crab. Since opening in 1991, they have extended the menu each year and now offer an all-day menu from 10.30 am to 6 pm daily. Everything is homemade, and they specialise in home-made soups such as seafood chowder, leek and mussel, tomato and basil and carrot and coriander, all served with homemade brown scones. Baking is a speciality, so there's always a tempting selection of cakes, bracks, teabreads, fruit tarts, baked desserts and scones with home-made preserves or you can simply have a toasted sandwich, or an Irish farmhouse cheese plate (with a glass of wine perhaps). For fine weather there are tables on a raised patio, overlooking Keel beach. • Daytime meals£ • Closed Nov-Easter • MasterCard, Visa •

Newport

Newport House

Newport Co Mayo

COUNTRY HOUSE/RESTAURANT   Tel: 098 41222   Fax: 098 41613

Country House of the Year

To its many visitors, a stay at Newport House symbolises all that is best about the Irish country house. Currently in the capable and caring hands of Kieran and Thelma Thompson, Newport has been especially close to the hearts of fishing people for many years. But although an interest in fishing is certainly an advantage, the comfort and warm hospitality of this wonderful house is accessible to all its guests – not least in shared enjoyment of the club-fender cosiness of the little back bar. The house has a beautiful central hall, sweeping staircase and gracious drawing room, while bedrooms, like the rest of the house, are furnished in style with antiques and fine paintings. Bathrooms, which can be eccentric, work well. The day's catch is weighed and displayed in the hall and a cosy fisherman's bar provides the perfect venue for a reconstruction of the day's sport.

Restaurant

Kieran and Thelma Thompson dine in their high-ceilinged dining room overlooking the gardens most evenings, which is a good recommendation. John Gavin, who has been head chef since 1983, presents interesting five courses menus which, at £32, are good value for the quality and range offered. Not surprisingly, perhaps, fresh fish is a speciality – not only freshwater fish caught on local lakes and rivers, but also a wide variety of sea fish from nearby Achill. An outstanding wine list includes a great collection of classic French wines – 170 clarets from 1961-1990 vintages, a great collection of white and red burgundies, excellent Rhones – and a good New World collection too. • Acc££££ •D£££ daily • Closed early Oct-mid-Mar • Amex, Diners, MasterCard, Visa •

Pontoon   Healy's Hotel

Pontoon Co Mayo

HOTEL   Tel: 094 56443   Fax: 094 56572

email: healyspontoon@tinet.ie

This famous old hotel, loved by fisherfolk, landscape artists and many others who seek peace and tranquillity, changed hands in 1998, and on our most recent visit there was much evidence of bustle as renovations were under way both inside and out. As far as could be ascertained, the improvements were not so dramatic as to spoil the old-fashioned qualities that have earned this hotel its special reputation: a good bit of painting and decorating had been done, some overdue refurbishment in the bar and a general tidy up around the front. Major work was going on at the back, clearing overgrowth to re-establish old gardens, but also development of a beer garden and construction of a helipad. We look forward to next year's visit with interest. • Acc££ • Amex, Diners, MasterCard, Visa •

Rosturk   Rosturk Woods

Rosturk Mulranny Westport Co Mayo

ACCOMMODATION   Tel/Fax: 098 36264

stoney@iol.ie

Beautifully located in secluded mature woodland, with direct access to the sandy seashore of Clew Bay, Louisa and Alan Stone's delightful family home is between Westport and Achill Island, with fishing, swimming, sailing, walking, riding and golf all nearby. It is a lovely, informal house; the three guest bedrooms are all en-suite and very comfortably furnished (one is suitable for disabled guests). Louisa Stoney enjoys cooking for guests, but please book dinner 24 hours in advance. There is also self-catering accommodation available. •D££ • Acc££ • Closed Dec-Mar •

Westport   Hotel Westport

The Demesne Newport Road Co Mayo

HOTEL   Tel: 098 25122   Fax: 098 26739

email: sales@hotelwestport.ie

Set in its own grounds on the edge of Westport town centre – which is just a short stroll away – this large modern hotel has recently completed a major expansion. It has excellent facilities to offer the business and leisure guest. With 127 bedrooms (including six suites) it is the largest hotel in the area and also the only one in Westport with a swimming pool and leisure centre. The conference and business centre can cater for anything from two to 550, with excellent back-up business services – and the leisure facilities that conference delegates also value highly. The whole hotel is wheelchair-friendly, with no steps or obstacles, and seven bedrooms have been designed for wheelchair use. Numerous short breaks are offered, including family breaks at times when special children's entertainment is available. • Acc£££ • Open all year • Amex, Diners, MasterCard, Visa •

Westport

Matt Molloy's Bar

Bridge Street Westport Co Mayo

PUB   **Tel: 098 26655**

If you had to pick one pub in this pretty town, this soothingly dark atmospheric one would do very nicely – not least because it is owned by Matt Molloy of The Chieftains, a man who clearly has respect for the real pub: no TV (and no children after 9 pm). Musical memorabilia add to the interest, but there's also the real thing as traditional music is a major feature in the back room or out at the back in fine weather. It's worth noting that normal pub hours don't apply – this is an afternoon into evening place, not somewhere for morning coffee. • Closed 25 Dec & Good Fri • No credit cards •

Westport

Olde Railway Hotel

The Mal Westport Co Mayo

HOTEL   **Tel: 098 25166   Fax: 098 25090**

email: railway@anu.ie   www.westport.mayo-ireland.ie/railway.htm

Once described by William Thackeray as 'one of the prettiest, comfortablist hotels in Ireland', The Olde Railway Hotel was built in 1780 as a coaching inn for guests of Lord Sligo. Attractively situated along the tree-lined Carrowbeg River, on the Mall in the centre of Westport, it is an hotel of character, well known for its antique furniture and a slightly eccentric atmosphere. It has been owned by the Rosenkranz family since 1983. Certain concessions have been made to the demands of modern travellers, including en-suite bathrooms, satellite television and private car parking. There's a conservatory dining room quietly situated at the back of the hotel and a recently restored function room with original stone walls. The large bar, which is the public face of an otherwise quite private hotel, serves very acceptable bar food. • Meals£-££ • Acc££ • Closed 25 Dec & mid-Jan-mid-Feb • Amex, Diners, MasterCard, Visa •

Westport

Quay Cottage

The Harbour Westport Co Mayo

RESTAURANT   **Tel: 098 26412   Fax: 098 28120**

Kirstin and Peter MacDonagh have been running this charming stone quayside restaurant since 1984, and it never fails to delight. It's cosy and informal, with scrubbed pine tables and an appropriate maritime decor, which is also reflected in the menu (although there is also much else of interest, including mountain lamb served with lentils and a thyme and smoked bacon sauce, steaks and imaginative vegetarian options such as a spring roll of cottage cheese and crunchy vegetables with pineapple and red onion salsa). But seafood really stars, be it in a starter of Quay Cottage chowder special or oysters (plain or grilled). Main courses might include monkfish tandoori (with basmati rice and raita dressing) or pan-fried scallops with a saffron sauce. There are nice homely desserts – or a plated farmhouse cheese selection such as Cashel Blue, smoked Gubbeen and an Irish brie – and freshly-brewed coffee by the cup. There is now a full restaurant licence (allowing draught beers, spirits, liqueurs etc to be served) and, from an interesting but not overlong wine list, a Lamberti house wine is a very order-friendly £8.90. • D££ daily • Closed 24-26 Dec & 2 wks in winter • Amex, MasterCard, Visa •

Westport

Westport Woods Hotel

Quay Road Westport Co Mayo

HOTEL   **Tel: 098 25811   Fax: 098 26212**

email: woodshotel@anu.ie

Situated in seven acres of woodland just behind Westport House the Westport Woods hotel has benefited from investment recently. Substantial improvements have been made, including upgrading of the frontage. The hotel is best known for its exceptional range of special breaks: mid-week and weekend breaks, off-peak breaks, golden holidays, family holidays, special interest breaks of every kind – murder mystery, bridge, set dancing, painting, gardening, golf, wine, even one on making a will. If there is a special break to be had, this is where it is most likely to be. • Acc£££ • Amex, Diners, MasterCard, Visa •

MEATH

Royal Meath, Meath of the Pastures. The word associations which spring readily to mind perfectly evoke a county which is comfortable with itself, and rightly so. The evidence of an affluent history is everywhere in Meath, but it's a history which sits lightly on a county which is enjoying its own contemporary prosperity at a pace which belies the bustle of Dublin just down the road. That said, anyone with an interest in the past will find paradise in Meath, for along the Boyne Valley the neolithic tumuli at Knowth, Newgrange and Dowth are awe-inspiring, Newgrange in particular having its unique central chamber which is reached by the rays of sun at the winter solstice. Just 16 kilometres to the southwest is another place of fascination, the Hill of Tara. Royal Tara was for centuries the cultural and religious capital of pre-Christian Ireland. It fortunes began to wane with the coming of Christianity, which gradually moved the religious focal point to Armagh, but nevertheless Tara was a place of national significance until it was finally abandoned in 1022 AD. Little now remains of the ancient structures, but it is a magical place, for the approach by the road on its eastern flank gives little indication of the wonderful view of the central plain which the hill suddenly provides. It is truly inspiring, and many Irish people reckon the year is incomplete without a visit to Tara, where the view is to eternity and infinity, and the imagination takes flight.

Local Attractions and Information

Navan	Tourist Information 046 73442
Hill of Tara	Interpretative Centre 041 24824
Trim	Butterstream Garden 046 36017
Newgrange	prehistoric, incl Dowth & Knowth 041 28824

Bettystown — Bacchus at the Coastguard

Bayview Bettystown Co Meath

RESTAURANT   Tel: 041 28251   Fax: 041 28236

Kieran Greenway and Anne Hardy's fine seafood restaurant is right beside the beach, with views over Bettystown Bay where, even at night, it is interesting to see the lights of the ships waiting in the bay for the tide to allow them up the river to the port at Drogheda. The entrance is from the road side (actually the back of the building, as the sea is at the front) and the door opens into a cosy bar where aperitifs are served. The menu majors in seafood, supplied by local fishermen and from the west coast – in starters like croûtes of smoked Donegal salmon with blue cheese set on ginger butter sauce, perhaps, and main courses such as roast monkfish dressed with vegetable julienne on chive beurre blanc. But the choice is far from being restricted to seafood; vegetarian options are included and there's a good selection of poultry and red meats. The restaurant is well-appointed and cosy, food well-cooked and attractively presented, service friendly and efficient. The wine list would benefit from tasting notes. • D££ Tue-Sat, L£ Sun only • Amex, MasterCard, Visa •

Dunshaughlin — Gaulstown House

Dunshaughlin Co Meath

FARM STAY   Tel/Fax: 01 825 9147

Built in 1829, this fine farmhouse is surrounded by mature trees and set on a working farm. It also overlooks a golf course and is within a short walk of Dunshaughlin village. Spacious en-suite accommodation has all the necessary amenities and good home cooking is Kathryn Delaney's particular interest – be it a really good breakfast to set guests up for the day, afternoon tea on the lawn or – the speciality of the house – dinner for residents, which is served at 6.30 pm if booked in advance. Home -reared lamb, local sausages, home-grown vegetables, free range eggs and local honey are all used in everyday cooking. All baking is done in the farm kitchen and an Irish farmhouse cheeseboard is offered at dinner. Traditional dishes like Irish stew and bacon and cabbage are served with pride and there are country puddings such as apple pie. • D£ • Acc£ • Closed Oct-Mar • MasterCard, Visa •

Establishment reports for Dublin City and Greater Dublin can be found on the Dublin Live section of The Irish Times On Line site (www.irish-times.com).

Dunshaughlin

ACCOMMODATION

The Old Workhouse
Ballinlough Dunshaughlin Co Meath
Tel/Fax: 01 825 9251
email: comfort@a-vip.com

It's hard to imagine that this striking cut-stone listed building was once a workhouse – it has now been restored by Niamh and Dermod Colgan to make a beautiful old house of great character and charm, with five highly individual bedrooms. Each bedroom has been furnished and decorated with great attention to detail, using carefully sourced antiques and an ever-growing collection of old plates. Of the five rooms three are officially shower-only but the Colgans have got around the problem of space with ingenuity by installing half-baths instead of shower trays. More power to them for their thoughtfulness (others please take note). Niamh is an enthusiastic cook and dinners worthy of any restaurant are served to residents at 7.30pm if bookings are received by noon. She also lavishes attention on breakfast, sourcing ingredients with great care. • Residents D££ • Acc££ • Closed Nov-mid Mar • MasterCard, Visa •

Kells

FARM STAY

Boltown House
Kells Co Meath
Tel: 046 43605   Fax: 046 43036

Jean and Susan Wilson's family home is a lovely eighteenth century house 4 miles from Kells. Apart from the appeal of endless countryside, hunting, fishing, golfing and touring the historic sites of the area, the real attraction here is the Wilson's exceptional food. Scones appear straight from the Aga when guests arrive and are served with homemade jam and tea from wonderful china cups. Everything served here – especially the baking – is absolutely delicious. Breakfast is a feast of plums stewed with orange zest, homemade brown bread, free range eggs – the works. Dinner (£24) is available to residents by arrangement. Accommodation is old-fashioned country – well-worn but immaculately clean throughout; bedrooms have electric blankets, crisp white sheets and lots of towels, but a shared (slightly chilly) bathroom. Absolutely authentic. • D££ • Acc££ • Closed Xmas • Amex •

Kells

RESTAURANT/CAFE

Penny's Place
Market Street Kells Co Meath
Tel: 046 41630

Penny McGowan's cheerful coffee shop has gorgeous hanging baskets outside in summer, a warm-toned interior featuring local art, fresh flowers on the tables and very friendly staff. Penny keeps a close eye on everything herself and produces a large variety of homemade food. The selection, which is displayed on a blackboard, changes each day and typically includes main dishes such as chicken curry and rice, Normandy pork, homemade quiche and salads as well as the home baked cakes and desserts which are a speciality. Good quality food (from breakfast at 9 am) and speedy service make this a very popular place among locals. • Open daily meals£ • Closed Xmas & New Year •

Kilmessan

RESTAURANT

Station House Hotel
Kilmessan Co Meath
Tel: 046 25239   Fax: 046 25588

Chris and Thelma Slattery's unique establishment is an old railway junction and all the various buildings have been converted to a new use: the old shelters are now a reception area, the waiting room has become a cosy lounge (complete with coal fire) and the ticket office serves as the restaurant. Outside, the signal box is used as an office and the platforms have been transformed into patios and lawns; even the old turntable is still intact. A major development on the hotel side, including 85 new bedrooms, awaits planning permission at the time of going to press. Our present recommendation is for the restaurant. After aperitifs in the bar, diners move through to a long traditionally furnished restaurant overlooking gardens at the back of the station. Wholesome fare is provided by Thelma Slattery, who has overseen the kitchen since 1984 and presents both daily set dinner menus and an à la carte. Both traditional tastes and current food trends are taken into account and there is always an imaginative vegetarian choice. From a selection of about ten dishes on first and main courses, an indication of the style is seen in starters of warm pigeon breast with green salad and juniper berry sauce, or stuffed courgettes with a tomato and herb sauce, then main courses like panfried monkfish with basil pesto dressing, Kilmessan rack of lamb roasted and served with a rosemary jus or mushrooms tortellini with olives, mushrooms and chilli oil. Finish with farmhouse cheeses or desserts such as chocolate and orange parfait or warm lemon tart. Sunday lunch is extremely popular and justifies two sittings but staff remain calm and cheerful throughout. • L£ Mon-Fri & Sun, D££ daily • Closed Good Fri • Amex, Diners, MasterCard, Visa •

Navan   Ardboyne Hotel

Navan Co Meath

HOTEL/RESTAURANT   Tel: 046 23119   Fax: 046 22355

Standing in its own grounds on the outskirts of town, the Ardboyne is a modern hotel with a thriving conference and function trade. The entrance and all public areas have all been recently refurbished, giving a good initial impression of the hotel. Judging by our recent visit, bedrooms urgently need the same attention and the standard of housekeeping needs to be addressed. However, as has been the case for a number of years, food at the hotel is particularly good.

Terrace Restaurant

Although the decor is conventional 'hotel dining room', and there appears to be no restaurant manager meeting guests on arrival, the restaurant is very comfortable. The menu looks unremarkable but turns out to have hidden depths. There are, for example, plenty of options for dieters – melon starter, fresh fruit desserts and dishes served without butter or sauces. Ingredients are good quality (and include some unexpected ingredients, such as ostrich), the standard of cooking is high, presentation is stylish and service both efficient and friendly – all adding up to a good dining experience, even in a room with very little atmosphere. Particularly good desserts from the buffet continue to be one of the specialities. • Acc££ • Meals£-££ • Open all year • Amex, Diners, MasterCard, Visa •

·Navan   China Garden Restaurant

58 Brews Hill Navan Co Meath

RESTAURANT   Tel: 046 23938   Fax: 046 29107

The Yips take pride in their restaurant's reputation and it shows in good food and quietly attentive service. A fish pond in the seating area at the entrance creates a very soothing atmosphere, a feeling of calm heightened by the dim light of the restaurant interior. A wide choice is offered and the food is good – crispy lemon chicken received particular praise on the guide's visit – and well-presented. Chinese tea is served with delightful ceremony at the end of the meal. • D££ daily, L£ Mon-Sat • Amex, Diners, MasterCard, Visa •

Navan   Hudson's Bistro

30 Railway Street Navan Co Meath

RESTAURANT   Tel: 046 29231   Fax: 046 73382

Since Richard and Tricia Hudson's stylish, informal bistro opened in 1991 it has built up a strong following and is now established as a leading restaurant in the area. Richard's menus include an "Early Bird" which is excellent value at £10, followed by an exciting à la carte based on wide-ranging influences – Cal-Ital , Mexican, Thai, French and modern Italian. Appealing vegetarian and healthy options are a feature – and, traditionalists will be pleased to hear, the ever-popular sirloin steak has not been overlooked. There are Irish cheeses and/or some very tempting puds to finish. The wine list echoes the global cooking and is keenly priced, with house wine a commendable £9. • D£-££ Tues-Sun • Closed Xmas & New Year • Amex, MasterCard, Visa •

Navan   Killyon House

Dublin Road Navan Co Meath

ACCOMMODATION   Tel: 046 71224   Fax: 046 72766

Just across the road from the Ardboyne Hotel, Michael and Sheila Fogarty's modern guesthouse immediately attracts attention, with its striking array of colourful flowers and hanging baskets. The house is furnished stylishly with interesting antiques, and made comfortable by modern double glazing which reduces traffic noise. The back of the house, which leads down to the banks of the Boyne, is unexpectedly tranquil, however, and the dining room overlooks the river, giving guests the added interest of spotting wildlife, sometimes including otters and stoats, along the bank from the window. The Fogartys are extremely hospitable hosts and nothing (even doing a very early breakfast) is too much trouble. The house is very well run and rooms are all en-suite and comfortable, if on the small side and shower-only. There's also a separate guests' sitting room and, although they are too close to the restaurants of Navan to make evening meals a viable option, they do a very good breakfast. • Acc£ • Closed 24-25 Dec • MasterCard, Visa •

Navan   Newgrange Hotel
Bridge Street Navan Co Meath

HOTEL/RESTAURANT   Tel: 046 74100   Fax: 046 73977

This hotel right in the centre of Navan only opened in 1998. It replaced an existing hotel, but was virtually a reconstruction job. Given the constraints of space the results are very stylish and impressive, in both public areas and accommodation. Rooms may not be enormous but they have been furnished with care and decorated with flair; one is designed for disabled guests (there is a lift), three are designated non-smoking and even though space was at a premium, all have well-designed bathrooms with full bath and shower. Double glazing helps ease traffic noise, although this could present problems in hot weather as there is no air conditioning. Conference/banqueting facilities for up to 450.

Restaurant – The Bridge Brasserie

Like the rest of this impressive new hotel, the restaurant is smartly and quite formally decorated in luxurious fabrics, and the modish neo-gothic theme of the decor seems quite at home in this historic area. Head chef Michael O'Neill presents exciting, contemporary menus at lunch (2/3 course £12.50/13.50) and dinner (3-course £18.50) and there's also an evening à la carte menu. Set menus change daily and always include vegetarian options. Main courses could be goujons of sole with sesame and ginger dressing and oriental vegetable salad. Even the trusty steak gets an update – fillet comes with a herb topping, thyme and shallot compote, while sirloin has tarragon, mustard and shallot butter and straw potato sticks. The cooking is good and service both efficient and friendly; although quite expensive for an hotel dining room. There is a real sense of occasion in this restaurant; the adjoining brasserie is less formal (and less inexpensive). • L£ & D££ daily • Acc££ • Amex, Diners, MasterCard, Visa •

Skryne   O'Connell's
Skryne nr Tara Co Meath

PUB   Tel: 046 25122

Three generations of O'Connell's have been caretakers of this wonderfully unspoilt country pub. The present owner, Mary O'Connell, has been delighting customers old and new for over ten years now. It's all beautifully simple – two little bars with no fancy bits, lots of items of local interest, and a welcoming fire in the grate. What more could anyone want? As for directions – just head for the tower beside the pub, which is visible for miles around. • Closed 25 Dec & Good Fri •

Slane   Boyle's Licensed Tea Rooms
Main Street Slane Co Meath

CAFÉ/BAR   Tel: 041 24195

Boyles has been run for the past ten years by Josephine Boyle, the third generation of the family to do so. The tea rooms lie behind a superb traditional black shopfront with gold lettering, with an interior that has barely changed since the 1940s. Visitors from all over the world come here, often after visiting nearby Newgrange – hence the unlikely facility of menus in 12 languages! The food – which is plainly cooked and, true to the era evoked, includes bought-in cakes and shop jam – is not really the point here as people come for the character. • Meals£ • Closed Tues, 25 Dec & Good Fri • MasterCard, Visa •

Slane   Conyngham Arms Hotel
Slane Co Meath

HOTEL   Tel: 041 84444   Fax: 041 24205
email: conynghamarms@tinet.ie

Built in the middle of the last century, and located in the middle of the manor town of Slane, this attractive stone hotel has been owned and run by the Macken family since 1929. It creates a very good impression with its lovely signage and twin bay trees at the main entrance. Chintzy fabrics and wood panelling creating a cosy country feeling in the restaurant and bar areas. It's a good place to call into when travelling as the self-service counter in the bar serves lovely traditional home-made food all day (12 noon -8 pm) – roast chicken with stuffing, bacon and cabbage, delicious apple tart – and is good value. All the bedrooms have recently been refurbished; the hotel is popular for weddings and there is one suite. • Meals£-££ • Acc££ • Closed 25 Dec & Good Fri • Amex, Diners, MasterCard, Visa •

MONAGHAN

Of all Ireland's counties, it is Monaghan which is most centrally placed in the drumlin country, that strip of rounded glacial hills which runs right across the country from Strangford Lough to Clew Bay. Monaghan, in fact, is all hills. But as very few of them are over 300 m, the county takes its name from Muineachain – "Little Hills". Inevitably, the actively farmed undulating country encloses many lakes, and Monaghan in its quiet way is a coarse angler's paradise. Also looking to water sports is the line of the old Ulster Canal, much of which is in Monaghan. Once upon a time, it connected Lough Erne to Lough Neagh. It has been derelict for a very long time, but with the success of the restored Shannon-Erne Waterway along the line of the old Ballinamore-Ballyconnell canal, the even more ambitious notion of restoring the Ulster Canal is being given serious consideration, providing us with the vision of cruisers chugging through Monaghan on a fascinating inland voyage all the way from Waterford on the south coast to Coleraine on the north coast. Vision of a different sort is the theme at Annaghmakerrig House near the Quaker-named village of Newbliss in west Monaghan. The former home of theatrical producer Tyrone Guthrie, it is now a busy centre for writers and artists who can stay there to complete 'work in progress'. In the east of the county at Castleblayney, there's a particularly attractive lake district with forest park and adventure centre around the unfortunately-named Muckno Lough – surely the people at Annaghmakerrig could come up with something more inspiring? Meanwhile, north at Clontibret, there's gold in them thar little hills, and the word is that another gold mining operation may be getting under way.

Local Attractions and Information

Annaghmakerrig House	Sir Tyrone Guthrie's writers' centre
Clones	Hilton Park (restored pleasure grounds) 047 56003
Rossmore Forest Park	R189 Newbliss Road

Carrickmacross — Nuremore Hotel & Country Club

Carrickmacross Co Monaghan

HOTEL/RESTAURANT　　Tel: 042 61438　　Fax: 04261853

email: nuremore@tinet.ie

This fine, well-managed country hotel has prospered and developed over the years and is now an impressive establishment by any standards. Set in a parkland estate with its own 18-hole golf course (drivers entering the driveway should presumably keep an eye on the state of play and also watch out for the ducks which often waddle across the road), the hotel serves the sporting, leisure and business requirements of a wide area very well. The superb country club has a full leisure centre with swimming pool and a good range of related facilities, while a new conference centre (opened in 1997) boasts state-of-the-art audio-visual equipment. The hotel gives a very good impression on arrival and this sense of care and maintenance is continued throughout all the spacious areas and the bedrooms (which are of a high standard and regularly refurbished).

Restaurant

The restaurant is elegantly appointed, with a couple of steps dividing the window area and inner tables. Now well established as the leading restaurant in the area, both food and service match the high standards of the rest of the hotel. • Acc£££-££££ • Meals£-£££ • Open all year •Amex, Diners, MasterCard, Visa

Clones — Hilton Park

Clones Co Monaghan

COUNTRY HOUSE　　　Tel: 047 56007　　Fax: 047 56033

email: hilton@tempoweb.com

International Hospitality Award Winner　　www.tempoweb.com/hilton

Hilton Park, Johnny and Lucy Madden's wonderful 18th century mansion, has been described as a "capsule of social history" because of their collection of family portraits and memorabilia going back 250 years or more. In beautiful countryside, amidst 200 acres of woodland and farmland (home to Johnny's champion rare breed sheep) with lakes, Pleasure Grounds and a Lovers' Walk to set the right tone, the house is magnificent in every sense, and the experience of visiting it a rare treat. Johnny and Lucy are natural hosts and, as the house and its contents go back for so many generations, there is a strong feeling of being a privileged family guest as you wander through grandly-proportioned, beautifully furnished rooms. Another special pleasure is sitting in the dining room watching the light fading over the garden after enjoying produce from the lakes or the organic garden. Four-posters and all the unselfconscious comforts that make for a very special country house stay are part of the charm, but as visitors from all over the world have found, it's the warmth of Johnny and Lucy's welcome that lends that extra magic. International hospitality – with an Irish flavour – at its best. A worthy award winner. • Residents D££ • Acc£££ • Closed Oct-Mar • Amex, MasterCard, Visa •

Glaslough   Castle Leslie

Glaslough Co Monaghan

COUNTRY HOUSE/RESTAURANT   **Tel: 047 88109**   **Fax: 047 88256**

email: ultan@castle-leslie.ie   www.castle-leslie.ie

Castle Leslie is an extraordinary place, with a long and fascinating history to intrigue guests. Suffice it to say that it is set in a 1,000 acre estate, has been in the Leslie family for over 300 years and has changed very little in that time. There is no reception desk, just a welcoming oak-panelled hall, and there are no phones, television sets or clocks in the rooms, although concessions to the 20th century have been made in the form of generous heating and plentiful hot water. In a charming reverse of circumstances, the family lives in the servants' wing, so guests can enjoy the magnificence of the castle to the full – it has all the original furniture and family portraits. The fourteen bedrooms are all different, furnished and decorated around a particular era, with en-suite bathrooms a feature in their own right. Numerous changes and improvements are in progress at the moment: the basement is being restored as a cookery school and two of the six gate lodges are being renovated to provide students' accommodation. The greenhouses and walled gardens are also undergoing renovation, and there is a plan to make the gallery library and billiard rooms suitable for conferences and meetings. The estate has wonderful walks. Pike fishing, boating and picnic lunches on the estate are available by arrangement. Due to the nature of the castle (and the fact that the Leslies see it as a wonderful refuge from the outside world for adults) this is not a suitable place to bring children.

Restaurant

Good food is an important element of any visit to Castle Leslie and Ultan, Sammantha Leslie's partner, is the chef. Non-residents are welcome to come for dinner, by arrangement, and it is all done in fine old style with pre-dinner drinks in the drawing room (or the Fountain Garden in summer) and dinner served in the original dining room (which has remained unchanged for over a century). Waitresses wear Victorian uniforms, but guests enjoy rather more up-to-date food from an à la carte menu based on local ingredients. • Acc£££ • D££-£££ • MasterCard, Visa •

Monaghan   Andy's Bar & Restaurant

12 Market Street Monaghan Co Monaghan

PUB/RESTAURANT   **Tel: 047 82277**   **Fax: 047 89415**

The Redmond family's well-run bar and restaurant in the centre of Monaghan has a strong local following, and it is easy to see why. The high-ceilinged bar is furnished and decorated in traditional Victorian style, with a lot of fine mahogany, stained glass and mirrors. Everything is gleaming clean and arranged well for comfort, with high-backed bar seats and plenty of alcoves set up with tables for the comfortable consumption of their good bar food. Substantial bar meals include a range of mid-day specials on a blackboard as well as a concise written menu. A different, slightly more sophisticated range is offered in the evening, as well as a short children's menu. The upstairs restaurant offers a much more extensive range of popular dishes. Traditional desserts like pavlova, lemon cheesecake, fresh fruit salad and home-made ices are served from a trolley, and there might be something comforting like a hot treacle sponge pudding in cold weather. No food served on Sunday or on Monday evening. But it's not all down to the food at Andy's – they also serve a great pint of the black stuff. • L£ Mon-Sat, D££ Tues-Sun • Closed 25 Dec, Good Fri & 1-14 July • MasterCard, Visa •

Monaghan   Hillgrove Hotel

Armagh Road Monaghan Co Monaghan

HOTEL   **Tel: 047 81288**

The Hillgrove is the leading hotel in the area, overlooking the town from a fine hillside location. It is impressive, well-run, has good conference and banqueting facilities and is open all year. • Acc££ • Open all year • Amex, Diners, MasterCard, Visa •

OFFALY

Offaly is Ireland's most sky-minded county. Not only is there in Birr the Parsons family's famous 1845-vintage 1.83 m astronomical telescope through which the 3rd Earl of Rosse observed his discovery of the spiral nebulae, but as well in Tullamore there's a thriving amateur Astronomical Society whose members point out that the wide clear skies of Offaly have encouraged the regular observation of heavenly bodies since at least 1057 AD. Back in Birr meanwhile, the annual Irish Hot Air Balloon meeting has been run with increasing success since 1970. It attracts serious international balloonists who welcome the opportunity for participation in a relaxed fun event where everyone wins a prize, and is equally suitable for beginners as Offaly's bogs provide a soft landing – "there's a bit of give in a bog". Offaly is also historic hunting country. It is home to the Ormonde, which may not be Ireland's largest or richest hunt, "but it's the oldest and undoubtedly the best." Once upon a time, they invited the neighbouring County Galway Hunt for a shared meet, and afterwards the carousing in Dooley's Hotel in Birr reached such a hectic pitch that the hotel was joyously torched by the visitors. Dooley's was rebuilt to fulfill its central role in Birr, and the hunt from across the Shannon has been known as the Galway Blazers ever since. The Grand Canal finally reaches the great river at Shannon Harbour in Offaly, after crossing Ireland from Dublin, and on the river itself, waterborne travellers find that Offaly affords the opportunity of visiting Clonmacnoise, where the remains of an ancient monastic university city give pause for thought. In the south of the county, the Slieve Bloom Mountains rise attractively above Offaly's farmland and bogs. These are modest heights, as they attain just 526 m on the peak of Arderin. However, it is their understated charms which particularly appeal, and in the Slieve Blooms we find Ireland's first organised system of gites, the French concept whereby unused farmhouses have been restored to a comfortable standard for self-catering visitor accommodation.

Local Attractions and Information

Birr	Castle Demesne 0509 20336
Clonmacnoise	monastic settlements/visitor centre 0905 74195
Edenderry	3-day Canal Festival (coarse angling) (June) 0405 32071
Tullamore	Offaly Tourist Council 0506 52566

Banagher   J. J. Hough's

Main Street Banagher Co Offaly

PUB   Tel: **0509 51893**

Hidden behind a thriving vine, which threatens to take over in summer, this charming 250-year old pub is soothingly dark inside – making a fine contrast to the cheerful eccentricity of the current owner, Michael Hough. Very much a local, it's also popular with people from the river cruisers, who come up from the harbour for the pints and the craic. • Closed 25 Dec & Good Fri •

Banagher   The Vine House

Banagher Co Offaly

PUB/RESTAURANT   Tel/Fax: **0509 51463**

At the bottom of the village, very close to the harbour, this bar and restaurant is well worth knowing about (especially if you are staying overnight in a cruiser). It's an attractive place (with an interesting history too) and both food and hospitality are good. • Meals £-££ • Closed 25 Dec & Good Fri • MasterCard, Visa •

Birr   Dooly's Hotel

Emmet Square Birr Co Offaly

HOTEL   Tel: **0509 20032**   Fax: **0509 21332**

One of Ireland's oldest coaching inns, dating back to 1747, this attractive, old-fashioned hotel is right on Emmet Square, the centre of Georgian Birr. Public rooms, including two characterful bars, are traditional in furnishing style but have all been refurbished recently. Bedrooms have recently been upgraded and now include a junior suite and an executive room; all are en-suite with full bathrooms (bath and shower). Some may be noisy when there's a function on, but the hotel tries to allocate appropriate rooms if possible. A good holiday centre with plenty to do locally – Birr Castle gardens are very near, also golfing, fishing, riding and river excursions. • Meals £-££ • Acc££ • Closed 25 Dec • Amex, Diners, MasterCard, Visa •

Birr

Spinners Town House & Bistro

Castle Street Birr Co Offaly

HOTEL/BISTRO   Tel/Fax: 0509 21673

Joe and Fiona Breen's unusual establishment in the centre of Birr runs through five Georgian townhouses, which have been restored and refurbished throughout in a simple modern style. In addition to their own sitting room and breakfast room, guests have the use of an enclosed courtyard garden. The bistro, which offers eclectic menus based on fresh ingredients, local wherever possible, is also open to non-residents, from lunchtime daily. The ten bedrooms include family rooms, doubles and twins, all with en-suite or private bathrooms. • L£ & D£ daily • Acc£ • Closed Xmas, New Year, mid Jan-mid Feb • Amex, MasterCard, Visa •

Birr

The Stables Restaurant & Townhouse

Oxmantown Mall Birr Co Offaly

RESTAURANT/ACCOMMODATION   Tel: 0509 20263   Fax: 0509 21677

The Boyd family have owned and run this characterful establishment in a lovely old Georgian house overlooking the tree-lined mall since the mid '70s. It has a strong local following. The restaurant is in the converted stables and coach house and has lots of atmosphere, with attractive exposed bricks and stonework, arches and an open fire in the period drawing room (which is used as a bar and reception area). Head chef Paul Boyd offers both à la carte and weekly changing set menus at both lunch and dinner; the cooking style is quite traditional – a blend of Cordon Bleu and traditional Irish – and hearty country portions are to be expected.

Rooms

En-suite accommodation is provided in the main house, where bedrooms overlook the mall or the courtyard. • L£ & D££ Tues-Sun • Acc£ • Closed 23-28 Dec & Good Fri • Amex, Diners, MasterCard, Visa •

Birr

Tullanisk

Birr Co Offaly

COUNTRY HOUSE   Tel: 0509 20572   Fax: 0509 21783

email: tnisk@indigo.ie   www.indigo.ie/~tnisk

An 18th-century Dower House in the demesne of the Earls of Rosse (still resident at Birr Castle), Tullanisk has been carefully restored by George and Susie Gossip, who have run it as a private country house since 1989. The house is beautiful, interesting and comfortable, and the surrounding gardens and parkland lovely (and full of wildlife, which can add to the interest of dinner, served at the big mahogany dining table commanding a fine view at the back of the house). George is an excellent chef and enjoys producing memorable 'no-choice' dinners, including game in season – asparagus and spinach from Birr Castle may be whipped up into an interesting starter. followed by a main course such as roast sirloin of midland beef with a Cashel Blue sauce (served with lots of home-grown vegetables). There are home-made biscuits and farmhouse cheeses (which will probably include the local Abbey Blue as well as Gubbeen, Carrigbyrne and Cashel Blue), with a dessert like hot chocolate souffle for the grand finale. The en-suite bedrooms (one with shower only) are large, characterful and comfortable. Breakfasts provide another culinary experience to treasure. Dinner is mainly for residents, but extra guests can sometimes be included by arrangement. • D££ • Acc££ • Closed Xmas • Amex, Diners, MasterCard, Visa •

Crinkle

The Thatch Bar & Restaurant

Crinkle Birr Co Offaly

PUB/RESTAURANT ⭐   Tel: 0509 20682   Fax: 0509 21847

This characterful little thatched pub and restaurant just outside Birr shows just how good a genuine, well-run country pub with imaginative, freshly cooked food can be. Since 1991 the energetic owner Des Connole has worked tirelessly to improve standards with the help, since June 1995, of head chef James McDonnell. Five-course dinner menus change weekly and include a mixture of traditional dishes such as sirloin steaks with mushrooms in garlic and surprisingly adventurous choices like local ostrich, wild boar and even kangaroo; between the extremes there are lots of interesting things – local pigeon and rabbit terrines, roast duck with vegetable stir-fry, loin of pork with a rhubarb compote. It is to James McDonnell's credit that he's been able to steer people towards more adventurous food in an area known for its conservative tastes. Having tried it and liked it, there will be no turning back. There's also an à la carte menu and a tempting bar food menu. Sunday lunch is a speciality, attracting two sittings. • D££ Tues-Sat, L£ Sun, bar meals£ • Closed 25 Dec & Good Fri • MasterCard, Visa •

Dunkerrin   Dunkerrin Arms

Dunkerrin Birr Co Offaly
PUB   **Tel: 0505 45377/45399**
Set well back from the road, but clearly visible, this large well-managed pub makes a useful break on the Limerick-Dublin road and serves freshly-cooked food all day. Toilets equipped for disabled. • Meals£ all day • Closed 25 Dec & Good Fri • Access, Visa.

Kinnity   Kinnity Castle

Kinnity Birr Co Offaly
HOTEL 🏛   **Tel: 0509 37318   Fax: 0509 37284**
email: kinnitty@tinet.ie   www.commerce.ie
Recently refurbished in keeping with its dramatic history and theatrical character, this Gothic Revival castle has been transformed into a luxurious hotel. Set in the foothills of the Slieve Bloom Mountains, right in the middle of Ireland, the castle is at the centre of a very large estate (accessible for horseriding and walking) with 650 acres of parkland and formal gardens. There is plenty to do, with good indoor health and leisure facilities, as well as country pursuits. Public areas – a library bar, Georgian style dining room, Louis XV drawing room and an atmospheric Dungeon Bar – are mainly furnished in the style expected of a castle hotel. The accommodation, however, is slightly different: big, romantic bedrooms have stunning views over the estate (and sumptuous, dramatically styled bathrooms). Medieval-style banqueting/conference facilities for up to 220 in a courtyard at the back of the castle; new but atmospheric. • Acc££££ • Open all year • MasterCard, Visa •

Tullamore   Tullamore Court Hotel

O'Moore Street Tullamore Co Offaly
HOTEL   **Tel: 0506 46666   Fax: 0506 46677**
This big new hotel opened as recently as 1997 but it has quickly become established as the leading establishment in the area. An attractive building, set back from the road a little and softened by trees, it has a large foyer and public areas are bright and cheerful. It serves the local community well, with good conference and banqueting facilities (750/575 respectively) and has an excellent leisure centre with a wide range of facilities, including a crèche. Well-appointed bedrooms all have full bathrooms (bath and shower), are decorated in a lively contemporary style and include four rooms suitable for disabled guests. There are three junior suites and nine executive rooms – an ideal base for business or leisure. Staff are friendly and helpful. • Acc££ • Amex, Diners, MasterCard, Visa •

ROSCOMMON

Roscommon is a county much put upon by the counties about it. Or, put another way, to the casual visitor it seems that just as Roscommon is on the verge of becoming interesting, it becomes somewhere else. In one notable example – the hotel complex at Hodson's Bay on the western shores of Lough Ree – the location is actually in Roscommon, yet the exigencies of the postal service have given it to Athlone and thereby Westmeath. But Roscommon is a giving sort of county, for it gave Ireland her first President, Gaelic scholar Douglas Hyde (1860-1949), it was also the birthplace of Oscar Wilde's father, and as well the inimitable songwriter Percy French was a Roscommon man. Like everywhere else in the western half of Ireland, Roscommon suffered grievously from the Great Famine of the late 1840s, and at Strokestown, the handsome market town serving the eastern part of the county, Strokestown Park House has been sympathetically restored to include a Famine Museum. A visit to it will certainly add a thoughtful element to your meal in the house's restaurant. Roscommon town itself has a population of barely 1,500, but the presence of extensive castle ruins and a former gaol tell of a more important past. The gaol was once noted for having a female hangman. In the north of the county the town of Boyle near lovely Lough Key with its forest park is a more substantial centre with a population nearing the 2,000 mark. Boyle is coming to life, and symbolic of this was the recent re-opening of Katie Lavin's pub, a gem of an old bar which had been shut for many years. They simply opened the door, dusted it out, and hey presto! – they'd an indisputably authentic traditional pub. Lough Key is of course on one of the upper reaches of the inland waterways system, and a beautiful part it is too. In fact, all of Roscommon's eastern boundary is defined by the Shannon and its lakes, but as the towns along it tend to identify themselves with the counties across the river, Roscommon is left looking very thin on facilities. But it has much to intrigue the enquiring visitor. For instance, along the Roscommon shore of Lough Ree near the tiny village of Lecarrow, the remains of a miniature city going back to medieval times and beyond can be dimly discerned among the trees down towards Rindown Point. Such hints of a more active past serve to emphasise the fact that today, Roscommon moves at a gentler pace than the rest of Ireland, something which is reflected in its pubs to people ratio. It is second only to Leitrim in this scale, as Leitrim has just 148 people for every pub licence, while Roscommon has 170.

Local Attractions and Information

Boyle	Josie McDermott Memorial Festival (April/May) 078 47024
Boyle	King House (500 years of Irish life) 079 63242
Boyle	Lough Key Forest Park 079 62363
Castlerea	Clonalis House (ancestral home of kings of Connaught) 0907 20014
Frenchpark	Dr Douglas Hyde Interpretative Centre 0907 70016
Roscommon	Tourist Information 0903 26342
Strokestown	Park House, Garden & Famine Museum 078 33013

Boyle

Kate Lavin's

St Patrick Street Boyle Co Roscommon

PUB **Tel: 079 62855**

Although established in 1889, the survival of Marie Harvey's characterful pub is nothing less than a miracle, as it has been left virtually untouched ever since and closed for around twenty years – the two old ladies who lived here got tired of running it and simply shut the door until a younger relative took up the challenge in the late 'eighties – and had the wisdom to leave well alone. It's one of those magic places with an open fire in the sitting room and the old range in the kitchen – it's lit on St Patrick's Day every year, when a couple of big pots of stew are cooked on it. Traditional music on Wednesday nights. • Closed 25 Dec & Good Fri •

SLIGO

There's a stylish confidence to Sligo. Perhaps it's because they know that their place and their way of life have been immortalised through association with two of the outstanding creative talents of modern Ireland, W.B.Yeats and his painter brother Jack. The former's greatness is beyond question, while the latter's star was never higher than it is today. But whatever the reason for Sligo's special quality, there's certainly something about it that encourages repeat visits. The town of Sligo itself is a fine place, big enough to be reassuring, yet small enough to be comfortable. And the county in which it is set is an area in which nature has been profligate in her gifts. The mountains, with unique Ben Bulben setting the standard, are simply astonishing. The sea is vividly omnipresent, and the beaches are magnificent. Mankind has been living here with enthusiasm for a very long time indeed, for in recent years it has been demonstrated that some of County Sligo's ancient monuments are amongst the oldest in northwest Europe. Lakes abound, and there are tumbling rivers a-plenty. Yet if you wish to get away from the bustle of the regular tourist haunts, Sligo can look after your needs in this as well, for the western part of the county down through the Ox Mountains towards Mayo is an uncrowded region of wide vistas and clear roads.

Local Attractions and Information

Drumcliffe	Lissadell House 071 63150
Inniscrone	Sea Weed Bath House 096 36238
Sligo	Yeats Memorial Building, Hyde Bridge 071 42693
Sligo	County Library & Museum, Stephen Street 071 2212
Sligo	Tourist Information (June-August) 071 61201

Ballymote

Temple House
Ballymote Co Sligo

COUNTRY HOUSE   **Tel: 071 83329**   **Fax: 071 83808**
email: templehouse@tinet.ie   www.tempoweb/temple

One of Ireland's most unspoilt old houses, this is a unique place – a Georgian Mansion situated in 1,000 acres of farm and woodland, overlooking the original lakeside castle which was built by the Knights Templar in 1200 A.D. The Percevals have lived here since 1665 and the house was redesigned and refurbished in 1864 – some of the furnishings date back to that major revamp. The whole of the house has retained its old atmosphere, and in addition to central heating has log fires to cheer the enormous rooms. The five bedrooms, which are all furnished with old family furniture, include four large doubles with private bathrooms and a single room with shower. Guests have the use of two elegant sitting rooms with open fires. Deb Perceval's evening meals are served in the very elegant dining room and are a treat to look forward to – she is a Euro-Toques chef and takes pride in preparing fine meals based on produce from the estate and other local suppliers. • D££ • Acc££ • Closed Dec-Mar • Amex, MasterCard, Visa •
NB: Sandy Perceval is seriously allergic to scented products, so guests are asked to avoid all perfumes, aftershave and aerosols.

Castlebaldwin

Cromleach Lodge
Castlebaldwin via Boyle Co Sligo

HOTEL/RESTAURANT   **Tel:071 65155**   **Fax: 071 65455**
email: cromleach@iol.ie

Set in the hills just above Lough Arrow, Cromleach Lodge enjoys one of the finest views of any restaurant in Ireland. The building, which is uncompromisingly modern in style and occupies a prominent position, has been the source of some controversy – but proprietors Moira and Christy Tighe wanted to maximise the view from both restaurant and rooms and find that their design has served them very well. But it is not architecture that brings people to Cromleach, rather the drive and dedication of Christy and Moira, which translates into high standards of both food and accommodation. Most importantly, they have the magic ingredient of genuine hospitality, doing everything possible to ensure comfort and relaxation for their guests. Spacious bedrooms are thoughtfully furnished with king-size and single beds, excellent bathrooms and every comfort to please the most fastidious of guests. Housekeeping is outstanding (it is one of the few places to provide not only a mini-bar but, more importantly, a jug of fresh milk in the fridge for your tea and coffee). Other extras include a complimentary basket of fruit and miniatures of Baileys.

Restaurant

The restaurant is such a strong magnet in drawing people to Cromleach that it really feels more like a restaurant with accommodation than an hotel. The restaurant (which is totally non-smoking) is arranged as a series of rooms, creating a number of individual dining areas for varying numbers of people – a system which works well for groups but can be short on atmosphere for couples dining alone. All overlook Lough Arrow. Immaculate maintenance and lovely simple table settings – crisp linen, modern silver and crystal, fine, understated china and fresh seasonal flowers – provide a fit setting for dinner, the high point of every guest's visit to Cromleach. Moira Tighe and her personally trained all-female kitchen team work superbly well together, producing some stupendously good cooking. They have a growing number of established specialities that are in constant demand, so new menus have to include these as a base, with new dishes added in the most appropriate way. Menus offered include an 8-course Gourmet Tasting Menu (for residents only) and a 5-course table d'hôte which has a minimum charge of £25 (but also flexibility, in that courses are charged individually so you can pick and choose between them if you like). Pastry chef Sheila Sharpe has developed many of the house specialities – tartlets are much in demand, as perhaps in a starter of roquefort cheese with walnut and redcurrant dressing. Dessert could be ginger and coffee torte with whiskey caramel, possibly partnered with a home-made ice cream, or presented as part of a tasting plate with other award-winning desserts. The wine list includes two pages of accessible house recommendations from around the world, from £12.95 to £22.95, and the dessert menu comes with helpful suggestions of dessert wines and ports. • D££ daily • Acc£££ • Closed Nov-Jan • Amex, Diners, MasterCard, Visa •

Collooney   Glebe House
Collooney Co Sligo
COUNTRY HOUSE/RESTAURANT   **Tel: 071 67787   Fax: 071 30438**
email: glebehse@iol.ie

Brid and Marc Torrades have been running their renowned restaurant with rooms just outside Collooney village since 1990. It is now firmly established as a leading establishment in the area. They have done wonders with the house – which had lain empty for several years before they bought it and started renovations – and it now provides comfortable accommodation in four en-suite rooms (two shower only), comfortably done up with old furniture and lots of interesting things to read. Extensive renovations are planned for the winter of 1998/9 – these will add two new bedrooms, self-catering accommodation and a conservatory dining area suitable for small weddings. But it's mainly the restaurant which has earned Glebe House its reputation for excellence – Brid is an enthusiastic Euro-Toques chef and takes great pride in sourcing the best of local ingredients for her cooking, which is imaginative without being fussy . She offers an à la carte, and dinner menus that are changed daily always include strong vegetarian choices. Main courses could be a mixed bean goulash or a pancake of mixed vegetables in a light mustard sauce. Those who like seafood will enjoy starters such as baked Kellystown mussels with garlic and breadcrumbs or warm squid salad with lemon and fennel dressing, followed perhaps buy local meats such as sautéed fillet of beef with wild mushrooms or loin of lamb with sundried tomato stuffing and a garlic jus. Finish with a surprise sweet plate, or an Irish farmhouse cheeseboard. • Acc££ • Closed 25 Dec • Amex, Diners, MasterCard, Visa •

Collooney   Markree Castle
Collooney Co Sligo
HOTEL/RESTAURANT   **Tel: 071 67800   Fax: 071 67840**
email: markree@iol.ie   www.surfers-paradise.com/gateway/accom/markree.htm

Sligo's oldest inhabited house has been home to the Cooper family for 350 years. Set in magnificent park and farmland, this is a proper castle, with a huge portico leading to a covered stone stairway that sweeps up to an impressive hall, where an enormous log fire always burns. Everything is a on very large scale, and it is greatly to the credit of the present owners, Charles and Mary Cooper, that they have achieved the present level of renovation and comfort since they took it on in a sad state of disrepair in 1989. They have always been generous with the heating, which made a stay here surprisingly comfortable even in the early days of the restoration programme. Now it is very civilised, and although Charles is always planning another stage of the endless task, the casual observer will probably assume that everything has been done. Ground floor reception areas include a very comfortably furnished double drawing room with two fireplaces at one end of the building (where light food – such as their famous afternoon tea – is served). There is a beautiful restaurant where head chef Tom Joyce has been serving very good food since 1993. Non-residents are very welcome.(Dinner daily and Sunday lunch, reservations advised). • D£-££ daily, L£ – Sun only • Acc£££ • Closed 24-26 Dec • Amex, Diners, MasterCard, Visa •

Riverstown   Coopershill
Riverstown Co Sligo

COUNTRY HOUSE   Tel: 071 65108   Fax: 071 65466
email: ohara@coopershill.com

Undoubtedly one of the most delightful and superbly comfortable Georgian houses in Ireland, this sturdy granite mansion was built to withstand the rigours of a Sligo winter – but numerous chimneys suggest there is warmth to be found within its stern grey walls. Peacocks wander elegantly on the croquet lawns (and roost in the splendid trees around the house at night) making this lovely place, home of the O'Hara family since it was built in 1774, a particularly perfect country house. Nothing escapes Brian O'Hara's disciplined eye: in immaculate order from top to bottom, the house not only has the original eighteenth century furniture but also some fascinating features – notably an unusual Victorian free-standing rolltop bath complete with fully integrated cast-iron shower 'cubicle' and original brass rail and fittings, all in full working order. Lindy runs the house and kitchen with the seamless hospitality born of long experience, and creates deliciously wholesome, unpretentious food which is served in their lovely dining room (where the family silver is used with magnificent insouciance – even at breakfast). • D£££ • Acc£££ • Closed Nov-Mar • Amex, Diners, MasterCard, Visa •

Rosses Point   Austie's
Rosses Point Co Sligo

PUB   Tel: 071 77111

This 200 year-old pub overlooking Sligo Bay has always been associated with a seafaring family and is full of fascinating nautical memorabilia. It has a very nice ship-shape feeling about it and friendly people behind the bar. The sea stars on the simple bar menu too, with local seafood in dishes like garlic mussels, seafood chowder and in open sandwiches or salads made with crab, prawns and salmon. If you're going out to Rosses Point specially it's wise to ring ahead and check opening times off-season. • Open evenings • Meals£ daily • Closed 25 Dec & Good Fri • Amex, MasterCard, Visa •

Sligo   Bistro Bianconi
44 O'Connell Street Sligo Co Sligo

RESTAURANT   Tel: 071 41744   Fax: 071 62881

This attractive informal restaurant is very gentle on the eye, with its terracottas and soft sandy tones, gentle wall lights and large leafy plants. It has never been a restaurant with pretensions but they have always made a point of sourcing fresh ingredients, cooking to order and providing casual but efficient table service. The idea was based on Italian restaurants in Liège, Belgium, and when they first opened in 1993 menus were strictly Italian – a wide range of pizzas and good pastas and salads – but the idea has been developed and broadened recently, with new menus designed to suit the modern Irish palate. The menu is now more global – still mainly Italian but sitting easily beside spicier cuisines. Vegetarians are well catered for and 'healthy options' (low in calories, fat and cholesterol) are highlighted on the menu. The wine list has developed as well, to include a large selection of quality New World wines. • D£-££ daily • Closed 25-26 Dec & Good Fri • Amex, Diners, MasterCard, Visa •

Sligo   Hargadon's
O'Connell Street Sligo Co Sligo

PUB   Tel: 071 70933

Unquestionably one of Ireland's greatest old pubs, the best time to see Hargadon's properly is early in the day when it's quiet – they'll give you good coffee (and a newspaper to go with it) and you can relax and take in the detail of this remarkable old place. It still has the shelves which used to hold the groceries when it was a traditional grocer-bar, the snugs and the old pot belly stove – and it's still owner-run by the Hargadon family, who have maintained it, unspoilt, since 1908. Later in the day it gets very busy, especially at weekends – but by then it's time for a bit of craic anyway. • Meals£ • Closed 25 Dec & Good Fri •

Sligo

HOTEL

Sligo Park Hotel

Pearse Road Sligo Co Sligo
Tel: 071 60291   Fax: 071 69556
email: sligopk@leehotels.ie   www.iol.ie/lee

Set amongst seven acres of landscaped gardens and parkland on the edge of Sligo town, this modern hotel is the centre of local activity, serving the community well with good conference, leisure and banqueting facilities. Recent investment has seen standards improved overall, but it is especially noticeable in the refurbished rooms, which are now furnished and decorated to the standards expected of a hotel of this calibre. • Acc££ • Open all year •

Strandhill

PUB

The Strand

Sea Front Strandhill Co Sligo
Tel: 071 68140   Fax: 071 68593

Just five minutes drive from Sligo, close to the airport and one of Europe's most magnificent surfing beaches, this well-known bar has a big welcoming turf fire, cosy snugs, friendly staff – and the smell of good bar food. Extensions and alterations were in progress at the time of going to press, but if past experience is a useful guide, these will be improvements which will not spoil the character of the place. • Meals£ • Closed 25 Dec & Good Fri • MasterCard, Visa •

Tubbercurry

PUB

Killoran's Traditional Lounge

Main Street Tubbercurry Co Sligo
Tel: 071 85111   Fax: 071 86300

Killoran's is renowned (and recommended by this guide) for its traditional music – traditional Irish nights are held every Thursday from June to September. There's set dancing, ceili music, a traditional fashion show and boxty, colcannon and potato cakes are served to everyone (with samples of their country butter churned by the visitors). • Closed 25 Dec & Good Fri • Amex, Diners, MasterCard, Visa •

TIPPERARY

The cup of life overflows in Tipperary. In this wondrously fertile region there's an air of fulfilment, a happy awareness of the world in harmony – and the placenames reinforce this sense of natural bounty. Across the middle of the county there's the Golden Vale, with prosperous lands along the wide valley of the River Suir and its many tributaries, and westwards towards County Limerick across a watershed around Donohill. The county's largest town, down in the far south under the Comeragh Mountains, is the handsome borough of Clonmel – its name translates as "Honey Meadow". Yet although there are many meadows of all kinds in Tipperary, there's much more to this largest inland county in Ireland than farmland, for it is graced with some of the most elegant mountains in the country. The Comeraghs may be in Waterford, but Tipperary gets the benefit of their view. Totally in southeast Tipperary is Slievenamon (719 m) the "Mountain of the Women". Along the south of the county, the Knockmealdowns soar. Across the valley, the lovely Galtees reach 919 m on Galtymore, and on their northern flank, the Glen of Aherlow is a place of enchantment. North of the Golden Vale, the Silvermine Mountains rise to 694 m on Keeper Hill, and beyond them the farming countryside rolls on in glorious profusion to Tipperary's own "sea coast", the beautiful eastern shore of Lough Derg. Inevitably, history and historic monuments abound in such country, with the fabulous Rock of Cashel and its dramatic remains of ancient ecclesiastical buildings setting a very high standard for evoking the past. But Tipperary lends itself every bit as well to enjoyment of the here and now. Tipperary is all about living life to the full, and they do it with style in a place of abundance.

Local Attractions and Information

Cahir Castle	052 41011
Clonmel	Moortown (apple & arable farm with walks & maps) 052 41459
Glen of Aherlow	Glenbrook Trout Farm 062 56214
Thurles	Racecourse 0504 22253
Tipperary town	Tourist Information 062 5145

Ballinderry   Kylenoe

Nenagh, Co Tipperary

COUNTRY HOUSE   Tel: 067 22015   Fax: 067 22275

Pet Friendly Establishment of the Year

Located close to Lough Derg in the rolling Tipperary countryside, Virginia Moeran's lovely old stone house on 150 acres of farm and woodland offers home comforts and real country pleasures. The farm includes an international stud and the woodlands provide a haven for an abundance of wildlife, including deer, red squirrel, badgers, rabbits and foxes. With beautiful walks, riding (with or without tuition), golf and water sports available on the premises or close by, "Kylenoe" provides a most relaxing base for a break. Spacious, airy bedrooms (two of them en-suite) are furnished in gentle country house style, with antiques and family belongings, and overlook beautiful rolling countryside. Downstairs there's a delightful guests' sitting room and plenty of interesting reading. Virginia enjoys cooking – her breakfasts are a speciality – and dinner is available to residents by arrangement. Importantly for people who like to travel with their dogs, this is a place where man's best friend is also made welcome – and Kylenoe is the recipient of our Pet Friendly Establishment Award for 1999. Dogs may come into the house with their owners and there is a loose box for larger dogs at night, if required. • Acc£ • Closed 18-29 Dec & 1 Jan • MasterCard, Visa •

Birdhill   Matt The Thresher

Birdhill Co Tipperary

PUB   Tel: 061 379227   Fax: 061 379219

Ted and Kay Moynihan's large roadside pub never ceases to amaze – every year it seems to get bigger and develop more additions to the core business. One of the latest, for example, is self-catering apartments ("Matt's Resting Loft"). But it's all done with such style and confidence, it's kept so scrupulously clean and the new parts are integrated into the older ones so successfully that you can't help but admire it – even if you really prefer smaller, less energetic pubs. The bar food is very acceptable too – interesting but not too adventurous, based on freshly cooked quality ingredients and varied without offering a ridiculously long menu. Soups, home-made breads, seafood – fresh and smoked salmon, crab claws, mussels – and a good range of sandwiches. There are more substantial main meals – steaks and lamb cutlets, for example – in the evenings. • Meals£-££ • Closed 25 Dec & Good Fri • Amex, Diners, MasterCard, Visa •

Borrisokane   Ballycormac House

Aglish Borrisokane Nr Nenagh Co Tipperary

FARM STAY   Tel: 067 21129   Fax: 067 21200

John and Cheryleen Lang took over this well-known farmhouse as a going concern in the summer of 1998 and to any casual visitor previously familiar with it there are no obvious changes. This is a charming, cottagey place, delightfully furnished and very comfortable in a laid-back way – all the five bedrooms have their own bathrooms (4 en-suite, one private, and all with full bath) and one of them is a romantic suite with its own fireplace. The main change is that the Langs have their own horses on the premises and equestrian activities are now the biggest attraction. Other changes include a moderation of prices under the new management (B&B £25, no single supplement, +£5 for the suite) and children and well-behaved pets are now welcome. Cheryleen cooks dinner for guests – a simple no-choice 4-course menu (£20) in country house style, based on fresh local ingredients (including produce from their own garden). Non-residents are welcome for dinner by reservation, if there is room. If you have any special dietary requests (including vegetarian meals) please mention them when booking. No smoking in the dining room or bedrooms. •D££ • Acc£-££ • Amex, Diners, MasterCard, Visa •

Cahir   Kilcoran Lodge Hotel

Cahir Co Tipperary

HOTEL   Tel: 052 41288   Fax: 052 41994

This former hunting lodge is set in spacious grounds just off the main Dublin-Cork road – it makes a good place for a break when travelling. While it has all the comforts now expected of an hotel, Kilcoran has retained its old-world character to a remarkable degree and is very welcoming, with open fires and friendly, helpful staff. There's a leisure club on the premises, with indoor pool, gym and solarium. Outdoor activities including fishing, golf, pony trekking and hill walking in the locality. • Acc££-£££ • Open all year • Amex, Diners, MasterCard, Visa •

Cashel   Cashel Palace Hotel

Main Street Chasel Co Tipperary

HOTEL   Tel: 062 62707   Fax: 062 61521

email: reception@cashel-palace.ie   www.cashel-palace.ie

One of Ireland's most famous hotels, and originally a bishop's residence, Cashel Palace is a lovely Queen Anne style house (dating from 1730) set well back from the road in the centre of Cashel town. It is large and graciously proportioned. The beautiful reception rooms and some of the spacious, elegantly furnished bedrooms overlook the gardens and the Rock of Cashel at the rear. The informal Bishop's Buttery restaurant in the basement is a good place for a light bite to eat when travelling. The hotel has changed hands several times recently, with successive owners having contrasting views on how this wonderful building should best be restored and managed; while undoubtedly impressive, it is in need of a sure guiding hand. • Acc££££ • Closed 24-26 Dec • Amex, Diners, MasterCard, Visa •

Cashel   Chez Hans

Rockside Cashel Co Tipperary

RESTAURANT   Tel: 062 61177

Hans-Peter Matthia's dramatically converted Wesleyan chapel is tucked behind the town right under the Rock of Cashel. Although others have since followed suit, the idea of opening a restaurant in a church was highly original when he established it in 1968. The atmosphere and scale – indeed the whole style of the place – is superb and provides an excellent setting for the fine food which Hans-Peter and his son Jason prepare for appreciative diners (some of whom travel great distances for the treat). Their tempting, wide-ranging à la carte menus change with the seasons and reflect a number of styles, but the overall feeling is of local ingredients in classic French cooking. The choice of fifteen soups and starters ranges from a simple cream of mushroom soup, through luxurious pâté of chicken liver and foie gras with spiced pear chutney and toasted brioche to light choices such as ogen melon with fresh fruit and a mango sorbet. There is also seafood such as oak smoked wild Irish salmon with pickled cucumber and crème fraîche. Main courses offer an equally wide choice, always including rack of Tipperary lamb, cassoulet of seafood – a selection of half a dozen varieties of fish and shellfish with a delicate chive veloute sauce – and roast duckling with honey and thyme roasted shallots and soy and ginger sauce. Finish with a dessert tasting plate, perhaps, or a selection of continental and Irish farmhouse cheeses. • D£££ Mon-Sat • Closed 25 Dec, Good Fri, 1st-3 wks Jan • MasterCard, Visa •

Cashel   Dowling's
Cashel Co Tipperary
PUB   Tel: 062 62130
On the left (and at the bottom) of the main street heading towards Cork, Pat and Helen Dowling's unspoilt traditional pub is just the spot if you like things simple. There's an open fire, light bar food – home-made soups, salads and sandwiches – and there may be impromptu music sessions at the weekend. • Closed 25 Dec & Good Fri •

Cashel   The Spearman
97 Main Street Cashel Co Tipperary
RESTAURANT   Tel: 062 61143
Just a few steps away from the Cashel Palace Hotel, and down a slip road off the main street, David and Louise Spearman run an admirably down-to-earth operation. Menus change weekly and include an evening à la carte with about half a dozen starters and a dozen main courses. Pasta features strongly ("fresh parmesan served with all pastas"), there are a few international influences coming through (Thai chicken, for example) but it is mainly sound European cooking. Lunch menus are shorter but include some of the dinner dishes as well as lighter fare and some extra daily specials. This is a great place to break a journey at lunchtime because you can be sure of wholesome food and quick service. Sunday lunch, on the other hand, is the time to see a more leisurely side of The Spearman. • L£ & D££ daily high season, closed Sun & all Mon Oct-May • Closed 25 Dec, Good Fri & all Nov • Amex, Diners, MasterCard, Visa •

Clonmel   Hotel Minella
Clonmel Co Tipperary
HOTEL   Tel: 052 22388   Fax: 052 24381
Just on the edge of Clonmel, in its own grounds overlooking the River Suir, the original part of this hotel was built in 1863 as a private residence. It was bought in the early 1960s by John and Mary Nallen and since then has been owner-run by the Nallen family. They have expanded the hotel over the years, to provide extensive banqueting and conference facilities and high quality accommodation. Public areas in the old house, including a cocktail bar, restaurant and lounge areas, have a lovely view over well-kept lawns and the river. Bedrooms, which include three suites with steam rooms, five junior suites with jacuzzis, ten executive rooms and one suitable for disabled guests, are all furnished to a very high standard with well-finished bathrooms (three are shower-only) and housekeeping is exemplary. Excellent facilities and the romantic situation make the hotel especially popular for weddings. A leisure centre with 20 metre swimming pool is due to open in May 1999. • Acc£££ • Closed 24-28 Dec • Amex, Diners, MasterCard, Visa •

Clonmel   Knocklofty House
Knocklofty Clonmel Co Tipperary
COUNTRY HOUSE   Tel: 052 38222   Fax: 052 38300
Formerly the country residence of the Earls of Donoughmore, Knocklofty House is set in 105 acres of gardens and parkland with sweeping views over the River Suir (which runs through the demesne). The original house dates back to the 17th century, with additions following in the 18th and 19th centuries. The interior is classic Irish Georgian. Fine reception rooms include a comfortable two-storey galleried library and an oak-panelled dining room (serving excellent food) with extensive views over river and parkland to the Comeragh and Knockmealdown mountains beyond. Spacious bedrooms are decorated in sympathy with the age and style of the house, but with all the modern comforts. There are conference/banqueting facilities (60/140) and it is a romantic setting for weddings. Good on-site leisure facilities include a recently completed leisure centre. It is worth noting that there is self-catering accommodation and timeshare letting available as well as the accommodation in the house. Trout and salmon fishing is available on the premises too – Knocklofty owns the fishing rights for about a mile of the banks of the

Suir. •L£ & D££ daily • Acc£££ • Closed 24-26 Dec • Amex, MasterCard, Visa •

Clonmel   Mr Bumbles

Richmond House Kickham Street Clonmel Co Tipperary
RESTAURANT   Tel: 052 29188   Fax: 052 29007

Declan Gavigan's large bistro-style restaurant in the centre of town caters for a changing clientele throughout the day and evening, seven days a week. With a stylish seating area at reception, attractively laid tables and plenty of plants, the atmosphere is relaxed and informal. The menus – a light morning and afternoon menu with sandwiches and cakes, a fairly short à la carte lunch menu and a choice of à la carte or set dinner in the evening – offer straightforward, popular dishes with an international tone. Well-balanced choices include light and vegetarian dishes (chilled melon; Mr Bumbles salad – leaves tossed with balsamic dressing, garnished with feta cheese, cherry tomatoes and tapenade croutons; penne pasta with 'marmande' tomato sauce and tossed salad) as well as the hearty steaks (char-grilled with green peppercorn sauce) and Tipperary lamb (roasted with rosemary & thyme, served with tarragon champ and its own juices) for which the area is renowned. Poultry is good too – free range duck over caramelised pineapple with lemon grass and orange sauce, for example – and seafood choices might include unusual fish such as grey mullet. Lunchtime main courses include home-made burgers, chicken breast (typically with Mediterranean vegetables, basil and sundried tomato pesto) and a roast of the day with hot vegetables. Friendly service, fair pricing and a very drinkable house wine under £10 all help make this cheerful restaurant a great asset to the area. • L£, D££ & light meals daily •

Clonmel   Sean Tierney

13 O'Connell Street Clonmel Co Tipperary
PUB   Tel: 052 24467

What an amazing place this tall, narrow pub is. Warm, welcoming and spotlessly clean in spite of the huge amount of memorabilia and bric a brac filling every conceivable space. No "characterful" dust here; every bit of brass or copper, every glass and bottle glints and gleams to an almost unbelievable degree. The front bar, especially, is seriously packed with "artefacts of bygone days – in short a mini-museum". If curiosity prompts a tour of the premises the back bar will yield a big surprise – in the shape of a giant screen, discreetly hidden around the corner. Upstairs (and there are a lot of them – this is a four storey building) there's a relaxed traditional family-style restaurant. Food starts with breakfast at 10.30 and there are all sorts of menus for different times and occasions. Expect popular, good value food like potato wedges, mushrooms with garlic, steaks and grills rather than gourmet fare, although the evening restaurant menus are more ambitious. Loos are at the very top, but grand when you get there. • L£ & D£-££ daily • Closed 25 Dec & Good Fri • MasterCard, Visa •

Garykennedy   Ciss Ryan's Pub

Garykennedy Co Tipperary
PUB   Tel: 067 23364

Garykennedy is one of the most charming little harbours on the inland waterways. It's about six miles from Nenagh (turn right at Portroe village and it's another couple of miles) but it's really in a world of its own. Ciss Ryan's is a lovely old traditional pub, and although it changed hands in 1998 a recent visit revealed no major changes. It was very well-run, spotlessly clean and serving nice, simple home-made bar food such as chowders and smoked salmon with home-made brown bread, as well as more substantial dishes such as steaks. • Closed 25-26 Dec & Good Fri • Amex, MasterCard, Visa •

Glen of Aherlow   Aherlow House Hotel

Glen of Aherlow Co Tipperary
HOTEL   Tel: 062 56153   Fax: 065 56212
email: aherlow@iol.ie

Originally a hunting lodge, this hotel is romantically located in a forest on the slopes of this famous glen. It enjoys stunning views of the surrounding mountains and countryside. The old house is one of the loveliest of its type, with well-proportioned rooms furnished in a particularly appealing country house style. The drawing room, bar and dining room are all well-placed to take advantage of the view, and there is a large terrace which is lovely in fine weather. The bedrooms in the original house also reflect the gracious style, while those recently added are comfortably furnished and have all the modern conveniences but less character. Further developments planned for 1999 include the construction of fourteen self-catering houses and also a health and fitness club which will offer therapeutic spa baths, aromatherapy treatments, jacuzzi and steam rooms as well as a gym. Special breaks including these therapies are available. Good banqueting facilities (280) and the romantic location make this a prime spot for weddings. • Acc££ • Closed Jan-Mar • Amex, Diners, MasterCard, Visa •

Killaloe   Goosers

Ballina Killaloe Co Tipperary

PUB   **Tel: 061 376792**

Just across the road from the river and close to the bridge that links Tipperary and Clare, this pub is chameleon-like in character. At quieter times it is an orderly, welcoming place where the day's blackboard specials (soups with freshly baked brown bread, oysters, mussels, Irish stew and bacon and cabbage are typical), can be enjoyed at leisure in front of an open fire. At other times, however – as on two recent visits – it can get overcrowded. Midweek or off-season visits might be most enjoyable. There is a restaurant at the back which has a separate side entrance and is bound to be more civilised at all times – and they do a good Sunday lunch (booking advised). Outdoor seating. • Meals£ daily (Sun from 12.30pm) • Closed 25 Dec & Good Fri • MasterCard, Visa •

Killaloe   Waterman's Lodge

Ballina Killaloe Co Tipperary

HOTEL   **Tel/Fax: 061 376333**

Views down to Killaloe and across the Shannon are among the pleasant features of this delightful country house hotel and restaurant. The standard of furnishing is high throughout – public areas are both attractive and comfortable, while the bedrooms are individually decorated, each with a homelike individuality, and have all the amenities, including satellite TV, tea/coffee trays and trouser press. Golf, fishing, horse riding and pony trekking are all available nearby.

Restaurant

Head chef Thomas O'Leary's dinner menus are well-balanced and wide-ranging, based on the best of local produce. Organic salads and vegetables, Burren lamb, Ballina beef, Kenmare brill and local cheeses all feature in dishes which have some international influences but are mainly country house in style. Menus change weekly, vegetarian dishes are always available and any other dietary requirements can be met if a day's notice is given. A phone call is recommended to check opening times off-season. • Acc£££ •D£££ • Closed 20 Dec-10 Feb • Diners, MasterCard, Visa •

Nenagh   Country Choice Delicatessen & Coffee-Bar

25 Kenyon Street Nenagh Co Tipperary

CAFÉ/DELI   **Tel/Fax: 067 32596**

This magic place is a mecca for food-lovers from all over the country. If planning a journey which might take them anywhere near Nenagh they make sure they build in a visit to Peter and Mary Ward's unique shop. Old hands head for the little coffee shop at the back first, fortifying themselves with the superb, simple home-cooked food that reflects a policy of seasonality – if the range is small at a particular time of year, so be it. "We feel that a shop should reflect the time of year with goods as simple as potatoes, cabbages, lettuce and tomatoes," explains Peter, describing the coffee shop as "a mirror of the seasonal foods available". Soups, main courses and puddings all contain quality local vegetables, meats, milk, cream, eggs, butter and flour: "The economy of Tipperary is agricultural and we intend to demonstrate this with a finished product of tantalising smells and tastes." Specialities developed over the years include Cashel Blue and broccoli soup – served with their magnificent home-baked breads (made with local flours) – savoury and sweet pastry dishes (quiches, fruit tarts) and tender, gently-cooked meat dishes like lamb ragout and beef and Guinness casserole. Peter is too modest by far, and seasonal shortcomings in supply in no way diminish the appeal of the shop, which actually carries a very wide range of the finest Irish artisan produce, plus a smaller selection of specialist products from further afield, such as olive oil. But there are two specialities which attract richly deserved special mention: the home-made marmalade based on oranges left to caramelise in the Aga overnight, producing a runny but richly flavoured preserve; secondly – and most importantly – there is Peter's passion for cheese.

He is widely credited as the country's best supplier of Irish farmhouse cheeses, which he minds like babies as they ripen and, unlike most shops, only puts on display when they are mature. Do not leave this place without buying cheese! • Open shop hours, Food£ • Closed Good Fri & Bank Hols •

Terryglass   Tir na Fiuise Farmhouse
Terryglass Co Tipperary
FARM STAY   **Tel/Fax: 067 22041**
email: nheenan@tinet.ie   www//homepage.tinet.ie/~niallheenan

Just a mile or so from the pretty village of Terryglass, Niall and Inez Heenan's neat family farmhouse is on a 125 acre organic farm. They offer all the interest of a farm stay with the comfort of well-designed en-suite bedrooms and tremendous hospitality. Guests are welcomed with tea or coffee and freshly-baked muffins and scones with home-made jam. After that it's country relaxation all the way. Breakfast – fresh orange juice, porridge, home-made yoghurts, smoked salmon, farmhouse cheeses or a traditional breakfast with home-cured bacon – is served until noon. Guests are welcome to take part in activities on the farm ("help with the haymaking and let the children feed our pigs!") or lend a hand with the turf-cutting in summer. On a recent visit work was progressing well on the renovation of two self-catering cottages in old buildings behind the main house; guests in the cottages have the option of having breakfast in the farmhouse. • Acc£ • Closed Nov-Easter • MasterCard, Visa •

Thurles   Inch House
Bouladuff Thurles Co Tipperary
COUNTRY HOUSE/RESTAURANT   Tel: 0504 51348/51261   Fax: 0504 51754

Built in 1720 by John Ryan, one of the few landed Catholic gentlemen in Tipperary, this magnificent Georgian house managed to survive some of the most turbulent periods in Irish history and to remain in the Ryan family for almost 300 years. John and Norah Egan, who farm the surrounding 250 acres, took it over in a state of dereliction in 1985 and began the major restoration work which has resulted in the handsome, comfortably furnished period house which guests enjoy today. Reception rooms on either side of a welcoming hallway include an unusual William Morris-style drawing room with a tall stained glass window, a magnificent plasterwork ceiling (and adjoining library bar) and a fine dining room which is used for residents' breakfasts and is transformed into a restaurant at night. Both rooms have period fireplaces with big log fires. The five bedrooms are quite individual but all have en-suite facilities (some rather cramped) and are furnished with antiques.

Restaurant
Polished wood floors, classic dark green and red decor and tables laid with crisp white linen and fresh flowers provide a fine setting for Kieran O'Dwyer's excellent dinners, especially when the atmosphere is softened by firelight and candles. Menus are changed fortnightly and offer a well-balanced choice in a fairly traditional style that combines French country cooking and Irish influences. A typical dinner might begin with a choice of soup or sorbet followed by a light course with a choice of six dishes (such as fresh mussels gratinated with garlic butter or baked Cooleeny cheese in filo pastry with grape chutney). Main courses featuring local meats could be entrecôte steak with whiskey and cream sauce or pan roasted tenderloin of lamb with vegetable purée and red wine sauce. There are poultry dishes such as roast half duck with orange sauce and fish, typically poached filet of turbot with a white wine and cream sauce. Anyone with special dietary needs, including vegetarians, should mention this on booking to allow for preparation of extra dishes. Not suitable for children under 10. • Acc££ • D££ Tues-Sat • Closed Xmas wk & Bank Hols • Amex, Diners, MasterCard, Visa •

WATERFORD

The fine city port of Waterford was founded in 853 AD when the Vikings – Danes for the most part – established the trading settlement of Vadrefjord. Its almost perfect strategic location in a sheltered spot at the head of the estuary near the confluence of the Suir and Barrow rivers guaranteed its continuing success under different administrators, so much so that it tended to completely dominate the county of Waterford, almost all of which is actually to the west of the port. But for many years now, the County town has been Dungarvan, which is two-thirds of the way westward along Waterford's extensive south coast. This spreading of the administrative centres of gravity has to some extent balanced the life of the Waterford region. But even so, the extreme west of the county is still one of Ireland's best kept secrets, a place of remarkable beauty between the Knockmealdown, Comeragh and Monavullagh mountains, where fish-filled rivers such as the Bride, the Blackwater, and the Nire make their way seawards at different speeds through valleys of remarkable variety. West Waterford is a place of surprises. For instance, around the delightful coastal village of Ardmore, ancient little monuments suggest that the local holy man, St Declan, introduced Christianity to the area quite a few years before St Patrick went to work in the rest of Ireland. Across the bay from Ardmore, the Ring neighbourhood is a Gaeltacht (Irish-speaking) area with its own bustling fishing port at Helvick. Dungarvan itself has now relinquished its role as a commercial port, but is enthusiastically taking to recreational boating and harbourside regeneration instead. Along the bluff south coast, secret coves gave smugglers and others access to charming villages like Stradbally and Bunmahon. Further east, the increased tempo of the presence of Waterford city is felt both at the traditional resort of Tramore, and around the fishing/sailing harbour of Dunmore East, which devotees would claim as the No. 1 Fun Spot in all Ireland.

Local Attractions and Information

Dungarvan	Tourist Information 0058 41741
Lismore	Lismore Castle Gardens 058 54424
Waterford city	Tourist Information 051 875823
Waterford	Crystal Glass Factory 051 73311
Waterford	International Festival of Light Opera (September) 051 375437
Waterford	South East Regional Tourist Authority 051 875823

Annestown   Annestown House

Annestown Co Waterford

COUNTRY HOUSE   **Tel: 051 396160   Fax: 051 396474**
email: annestownhouse@tinet.ie   www.homepage.tinet.ie/~annestown
Half way up the hill on the Tramore-Dungarvan road, John and Pippa Galloway's comfortable home overlooks a small bay, with a private path leading to the beach below. In front of the house are manicured lawns – one for croquet, one for grass tennis – while inside there are several lounges with log-burning fires and a billiard room with full-size table. Everywhere you look there are books – a catholic collection ranging from classics to thrillers. For the evening meal there will be, typically, dishes such as mushroom soup, roast duck and rhubarb crumble. Annestown also has a wine license. In the morning a hearty Irish breakfast (with excellent breads) will set you up for the day ahead. All the centrally-heated bedrooms are en suite with direct-dial telephone and tea-making facilities (and hot water bottles are thoughtfully provided for those who still feel cold). • D££ • Acc££ • Amex, MasterCard, Visa •

Ballymacarbry   Melody's Nire View Bar

Ballymacarbry Co Waterford

PUB   **Tel: 052 36147**
Pat and Carmel Melody's welcoming pub has been in the family for over a hundred years and is best known as a pony-trekking and horse riding centre (an experienced guide is available). But those in the know always try to plan their routes via this neat, traditional pub to take in a bite of Carmel's home-made bar food. Something simple but good suits walkers, pony-trekkers, tourists and locals alike – and that's just what Melody's offers, with Carmel's delicious home-made soup served with freshly baked brown bread, or a scrumptious sandwich and a bit of crisp apple tart. The sandwiches – typically turkey, ham, cheese or salad – are freshly made to order. There's live music on Tuesdays, Wednesdays and (usually) Sundays in summer. Off-road parking across the road (Beware: it's on a bad bend). • Light meals£ • Closed 25 Dec & Good Fri • No credit cards •

Cappoquin

COUNTRY HOUSE/RESTAURANT

Richmond House

Cappoquin Co Waterford

Tel: 058 54278   Fax: 058 54988

www.amireland.com/richmond

Set well back, in large grounds graced by mature trees, Paul and Claire Deevy's fine 18th century country house and restaurant is very much a family affair, offering a delightful combination of warm hospitality and a high standard of comfort. Approaching through well-tended grounds, a good impression is made from the outset, a feeling confirmed by the welcoming hall, which has a wood-burning stove and well-proportioned, elegantly furnished reception rooms opening off it. Upstairs there are ten individually decorated en-suite bedrooms, which vary in size and appointments but are comfortably furnished in country house style.

Restaurant

The restaurant is the most important single element at Richmond House, and non-residents regularly make up a high proportion of the guests. Warm and friendly service begins at the front door, after which menus are presented over aperitifs, in front of the drawing room fire or in a conservatory overlooking the garden. Herbs, fruit and vegetables are grown on the premises for use in the kitchen and Paul is an ardent supporter of local produce. The cooking style is traditional country house with some global influences, presented in well-balanced 4-course dinner menus offering a choice of about six on each course (always with imaginative vegetarian choices). Start, perhaps, with half a dozen Rossmore oysters, warm organic asparagus wrapped in smoked salmon with hollandaise or Helvick prawns with basmati rice and garlic butter. Main courses might include a baked Mediterranean vegetable pie as well as local meats (eg steak with red wine and thyme essence), poultry (roast duckling on a plum and Cointreau essence) and seafood (fillets of John Dory with a herb butter sauce). Classic desserts include a tasting plate and a wide range of local cheeses which usually includes Knockalara sheep's cheese and Knockanore Smoked (which won an Irish Food Writers Guild Award in 1998). Ample private parking. • D£££ • Acc£££ • Closed 23 Dec-14 Feb • Amex, Diners, MasterCard, Visa •

Cheekpoint

PUB

Jack Meade's Bar

Cheekpoint Road Halfway House Waterford Co Waterford

Tel: 051 50950/873187   Fax: 051 843034

William and Carmel Hartley's beautiful old pub is widely known as "Meade's Under The Bridge" though it was actually established in 1705, thereby predating the bridge by over 150 years. It's been in the Hartley family since 1857, so they know a fair bit about its colourful history. In response to all the questions frequently asked by curious visitors this has all been put down in a useful little brochure. Old-fashioned this pub may be, but it's immaculate inside and out, with pretty roses around the door and everything inside gleaming. Outdoors in extensive (tidal) waterside grounds there's a mixture of heritage museum – an old lime kiln, ice house, a restored cottage and even an agricultural museum to look at – and also a large beer garden, children's playground, toilets (including wheelchair facilities) and a baby changing room. Food is available all-day in peak season, at lunchtime all year and there are barbecues on summer Sundays and bank holidays. Like any place geared for a crowd, this can be a very busy pub in high season. Quieter types will love it in the winter though, when the fires are on and there's a bit of space to relax in. • Meals£ • Closed 25 Dec & Bank Hols • Amex, MasterCard, Visa •

Cheekpoint

RESTAURANT

McAlpin's Suir Inn

Cheekpoint Co Waterford

Tel: 051 382220

email: cheekpoint@tinet.ie

This attractive 300 year-old, traditional black-and-white painted inn has been run by the McAlpin family since 1972. During that time they have earned an enviable reputation for hospitality and good food served at a moderate price, notably local seafood. It's a characterful, country style place with rustic furniture, cottagey plates and old prints decorating the walls. Seasonal menus offer a choice of about six starters (nearly all seafood and all under £5) and ten main courses, including three cold dishes and two vegetarian ones, again all moderately priced. All meals come with brown soda bread, butter and a side salad – and there's a nice little wine list including a special selection of eight good New World wines, "The £11 Cellar". • D£-££ Mon-Sat • Closed 25 Dec-1 Jan, 2 wks Jan •

Dungarvan   The Park Hotel
Dungarvan Co Waterford

HOTEL   Tel: 058 42899   Fax: 058 42969

This attractive hotel on the outskirts of Dungarvan has views over the Colligan River estuary. It is owner-run by the Flynn family, who have many years of experience in the hotel business. The hotel fits comfortably into its surroundings, with mature trees softening the approach. Public areas include a cosy traditional bar with panelled walls and a spacious, elegantly appointed dining room. Bedrooms are furnished and decorated to a high standard, with well-finished bathrooms (full bath and shower) and generous desk space as well as easy chairs. In addition to the many outdoor activities in the area – including tennis, fishing, windsurfing, walking, horseriding, pony-trekking as well as shooting and hunting, in season – there's an aqua and fitness centre with 20 metre pool, separate children's pool and many other features. Well-behaved pets are permitted in certain areas of the hotel, by arrangement. • Acc££-£££ • Closed 25-27 Dec • Amex, Diners, MasterCard, Visa •

Dungarvan   Seanachai Bar & Restaurant
Dungarvan West Co Waterford

PUB   Tel: 058 46285   Fax: 058 46305

Few could fail to be charmed by this proudly maintained traditional pub just off the main Cork road – it has white-washed walls, a well-kept thatched roof, displays of local memorabilia and a big open fire in the old kitchen complete with crane and cooking pots. Expect warm hospitality and wholesome, simply prepared fresh food offered from a choice of menus, in English or Irish. Local seafood is a speciality. There are vegetarian options and a special "children's corner". Traditional music is a big draw here – with informal sessions every night in summer and a traditional night every Saturday all year – and set dancing is so popular that a new wooden floor has had to be built in the restaurant, in addition to the flower-decked courtyard area already in use. • Meals£ • Closed 25 Dec & Good Fri • MasterCard, Visa •

Dungarvan   The Tannery
10 Quay Street Dungarvan Co Waterford

RESTAURANT   Tel: 058 45420   Fax: 058 45118

Paul and Maire Flynn's dashing contemporary restaurant echoes the building's previous life with great imagination – the leather tannery theme has been used with commendable subtlety. Paul's kitchen is open to view as guests go up to the first-floor dining area and the cooking is very much in step with this essentially minimalist atmosphere: colourful dishes look completely at home on elegant white plates set against unadorned lightwood tables. Roast red pepper soup with basil aoili will perfectly complement a delicious home-baked bread selection; local seafood features in crispy cod cakes "Nicoise" and grilled sirloin steak comes with seared vegetables, basil and chilli cream. Desserts enjoyed by our assessors included a delicious steamed individual chocolate pudding with candied orange. If there are criticisms they centre on what some see as unnecessary complications in the cooking, and "less is more" might be a useful philosophy: for example, for every diner who adores the grilled fillet steak with kidney pie, there is one who claims they are better served as two separate dishes. But controversy is the spice of restaurant life – and a visit to the Tannery is sure to be a pleasure. • L£ & D££ Tues-Sat • Closed Bank Hols & end Jan-early Feb • Amex, Diners, MasterCard, Visa •

Dunmore East   The Ship
Dunmore East Co Waterford

RESTAURANT   Tel: 051 383141/144

The Prendiville's well-known bar and restaurant is high above the harbour, in a Victorian corner house with a patio on the harbour side. This is used mainly for casual lunches in fine weather (lunch available June-August only, except for Sunday lunches in the shoulder seasons – April, May, September & October). But outside eating and sea views are secondary here – it's the seafood that draws people to this atmospheric bar and informal restaurant designed around a nautical theme. Some concessions are made to non-seafood eaters but seafood is emphatically the star. Starters might include an imaginative creation such as cured fillets of monkfish with chervil and dill, served with a sorbet "bloody mary style". Soups will usually include a good bisque and main courses range from simple pan-fried fish of the day to luxurious dishes such as poached fillets of dover sole and prawns with a lobster and brandy sauce (which might be garnished rather surprisingly with a goat's cheese lasagne). Tempting desserts tend to be variations on classic themes and there's always an Irish farmhouse cheeseboard. Set Sunday lunch menus are shorter and simpler, but also major on seafood. • L£ & D£-££ daily high season, check opening in winter • Closed Xmas & New Year • Amex, MasterCard, Visa •

Lismore   Ballyrafter House Hotel
Lismore Co Waterford
HOTEL/RESTAURANT   Tel: 058 54002   Fax: 058 53050

Set in spacious, refreshingly unmanicured grounds on the edge of the magical town of Lismore, Joe and Noreen Willoughby's comfortable country house hotel has views through tall trees to the pride of Lismore – the Duke of Devonshire's fairytale riverside castle. Although especially loved by fisherfolk, the uniquely relaxing atmosphere of Ballyrafter is attracting growing numbers of guests who have never cast a fly but who return time after time for its unpretentious comforts. Accommodation is simple but comfortable, in ten en-suite rooms (some with shower only). At night, residents and locals congregate in the bar, which is set up for informal meals and lined with photographs of happy fishermen and their catches – all, along with Joe's laid-back hospitality, creating genuine atmosphere. The dining room has an open fire, family antiques and flowers from the garden – an appropriate setting for the home cooking that features local specialities such as Carr's crabmeat (recent recipient of an Irish Food Writers' Guild Award), fresh and smoked Blackwater salmon, home-produced honey and a trio of local cheeses – Knockanore, Knockalara and Ring. • D££ daily, Sun L£ • Acc££ • Closed 25 Dec • Amex, Diners, MasterCard, Visa •

Lismore   Buggy's Glencairn Inn
Glencairn near Lismore Co Waterford
PUB/RESTAURANT ⭐⭐   Tel/Fax: 058 56232

Ken and Cathleen Buggy have created a dream of a rural pub just a couple of miles from Lismore. Their collection of rural memorabilia is at home in this bar, dining room and four delightful en-suite bedrooms. The Buggy's uniquely entertaining style of hospitality accounts for much of this attraction, but Ken's simple rustic food often draws the greatest praise – everything is based on fresh ingredients and is made on the day. Dinner – from a menu offering perhaps four choices on each course – is served in the little firelit dining room and might include specialities such as pâté de campagne or a freshly made soup of the day (served with Ken's famous brown soda bread), followed by sole on the bone or steak with mushrooms and lovely crisp little chips. Simple puddings and farmhouse cheeses are followed up with cafetiere coffee, served in the bar. Prices may seem somewhat steep for a pub, but the food is like the best home cooking and the numbers are small. There's a short wine list, but the best bet is usually something from the interesting, keenly priced blackboard. Off road parking. • L£ high season (phone ahead) D£-££ Mon-Sun • Closed 25 Dec • MasterCard, Visa •

Lismore   Eamonn's Place
Main Street Lismore Co Waterford
PUB   Tel: 058 54025

"Good food in pleasant surroundings at a reasonable price" is Eamonn Walsh's aim for his bar/restaurant in the centre of Lismore. The main bar area and dining room behind it have been refurbished in a comfortable traditional style and at the back there's a well-kept beer garden. Locals working in the town pop in for a quick, affordable lunch – soup of the day, such as parsnip and carrot perhaps, with ready-buttered bread, and inexpensive hot main course dishes such as lamb's liver and bacon casserole or chicken cordon bleu. Generous portions, wholesome quality and good value keep the regulars coming back for more – and most keep a corner to spare for tasty home-made puddings like apple tart and cream, lemon meringue pie, treacle tart or strawberries and cream in season. • Meals£ • Closed 25 Dec & Good Fri • No Credit Cards •

Lismore   Madden's Bar
Main Street Lismore Co Waterford
PUB   Tel: 058 54148
email: madden@tinet .ie

Owen and John Maddens' Bar presents a neat and colourful face to the world. Recent renovation of the interior has produced an extremely pleasant pub with due respect paid to traditional values but a distinctly youthful atmosphere. Far from the dreaded Irish "theme pub", which is taking over the island (and far beyond), this one has many genuine features – including a huge fireplace in the dining area which was found by accident during the renovation – as well as a smaller one in the "drinking" bar in the back. John's light, modern menus offer food which is nearer to modern bistro fare than traditional bar food. John and joint head chef Tanya Schleich, who are both Ballymaloe trained, serve delicious light meals in the modern idiom, featuring local produce in dishes like chargrilled breast of chicken sandwich with sundried tomatoes and pesto or smoked fish cake with coriander and lime tartare sauce with potato chips. These are followed by desserts such as classic lemon tart. • Meals£ • Closed 25 Dec & Good Fri • MasterCard, Visa •

Lismore   O'Brien's

Main Street Lismore Co Waterford

PUB   Tel: 058 54816

Lismore has a great selection of pubs, each with its own special character, but this one is the jewel in the crown. Run by sisters Joan and Mary Casey for "a very long time", it is a completely unspoilt example of how many pubs used to be. The hours are slightly unusual, described by the delightful proprietresses as 10-12 in the morning and 8-10 in the evening "give or take". Go and relish it.

Nire Valley   Hanora's Cottage

Nire Valley via Clonmel Co Waterford

ACCOMMODATION/RESTAURANT   Tel: 052 36134   Fax: 052 36540
Guesthouse of the Year

Outdoor pursuits, especially walking, bring most people up the valley to Hanora's Cottage Guesthouse. Although its size may come as a surprise, foot-weary walkers are only too delighted when the large, comfortable and modern premises of Hanora's Cottage comes into view – a warm, restoring place echoing the spirit of the ancestral home around which it is built. Many changes have taken place since Seamus and Mary Wall first opened their doors to guests in 1967 – and, as growth and improvements continue, the accommodation has become distinctly luxurious – but their hospitality never falters. The breakfast buffet at Hanora's is legendary too, featuring Crinnaughton apple juice from Lismore, home-made preserves and delicious freshly-baked breads, made early each morning by Seamus. These are also used in packed lunches provided for residents. • MasterCard, Visa •

Restaurant

The latest wave of improvements includes a newly-extended kitchen, so the restaurant side of the business – which began when Seamus and Mary's son Eoin, a keen chef, returned to the family business in 1994 – is clearly growing. Now dinner guests travel considerable distances to sample Eoin's fare, served in a dining room overlooking an immaculately kept garden, floodlit at night. An enthusiastic supporter of small suppliers, Eoin uses local produce whenever possible in imaginative, well-balanced menus that feature fresh fish from Dunmore East, free range chickens from Stradbally and local cheeses (which are also popular for breakfast). • D££ Mon-Sat, Sun res only • Acc££ • Closed Xmas & New Year • MasterCard, Visa •

Waterford   Dwyer's Restaurant

8 Mary Street Waterford Co Waterford

RESTAURANT   Tel: 051 877478   Fax: 051 877480

Quietly located in an elegantly converted old barracks, chef-proprietor Martin Dwyer and his wife Sile have been running what is now widely recognised as Waterford's leading restaurant since 1989. Without show or fuss they consistently provide dishes of high excellence. Low-key presentation of some of the country's finest food is accompanied by discreet, thoughtful service. Martin carefully sources the best seasonal local produce which he prepares in a style which is basically classic French, although with some country French and New Irish influences; he sums up his philosophy with admirable simplicity: "We feel that the basis of good food is taste rather than presentation or fashion". Menus change monthly and include a keenly-priced 3-course early dinner (6-7.30pm), then an la carte in similar style. Main courses lean towards seafood – brochettes of monkfish and scallops with honey and mustard vinaigrette and roast fillet of cod spiced with cumin and chili would both be typical – but there are good choices for carnivores and vegetarians too. Classic desserts are well worth leaving room for and there's always an

Irish cheese plate. Espresso and herbal teas are offered as well as regular cafetiere coffee and tea. Like the cooking, the wine list favours France, although Spain, Italy, Germany and the New World are also represented. • D£-££ Mon-Sat • Closed Xmas wk & Bank Hols • Amex, Diners, MasterCard, Visa •

Waterford   Foxmount Farm

Passage East off Dunmore East Road Waterford Co Waterford

FARM STAY   Tel: 051 874308   Fax: 051 854906

Foxmount Farm, the Kent family's 17th century country house and working dairy farm, is just 15 minutes drive from the centre of Waterford city. It is a haven of peace and tranquillity. Margaret Kent's hospitality is the key to Foxmount Farm's special magic, but the house is lovely too – classically proportioned reception rooms provide a fine setting for home-cooked food. Dinner is available for residents by arrangement. It is prepared personally by Margaret and based on the farm's own produce. Vegetarian or other special dietary requirements can be built into menus if mentioned on booking. Margaret is a great baker, as guests quickly discover when she serves afternoon tea in the drawing room (or in the morning, when freshly-baked breads are presented with her renowned breakfasts). Thoughtfully furnished accommodation, in six very different rooms (four en-suite, two with private bathrooms and two shower-only) is extremely comfortable and includes some family rooms – but bear in mind that peace and relaxation are the aim at Foxmount, so don't expect phones or TVs in bedrooms. There is a hard tennis court on the premises (plus table tennis). • D££ • Acc£ • Closed Nov-Mar •

Waterford   Granville Hotel

Meagher Quay Waterford Co Waterford

HOTEL   Tel: 051 305555   Fax: 051 305566

email: granvillehotel@tinet.ie

One of the country's oldest hotels, this much-loved quayside establishment in the centre of Waterford has many historical connections – with Bianconi, for example, who established Ireland's earliest transport system, and also Charles Stuart Parnell, who made many a rousing speech here. Since 1979 it's been owner-run by the Cusack family, who have overseen significant restoration and general refurbishment. It's a large hotel – bigger than it looks perhaps – with fine public areas. There are two suites and two junior suites among its hundred well-appointed bedrooms (all with well-designed bathrooms with both bath and shower) and conference/banqueting facilities for up to 200 people. • Acc£££ • Closed 25-26 Dec • Amex, Diners, MasterCard, Visa •

Waterford   Henry Downes

10 Thomas Street Waterford Co Waterford

PUB   Tel: 051 874118

In the same (eccentric) family for five generations, Jonny de Bromhead's unusual pub is one of the few remaining houses to bottle its own whiskey. Although not the easiest of places to find, once visited it will certainly not be forgotten. Large, dark and cavernous – with a squash court on the premises as well as the more predictable billiards and snooker – it consists of a series of bars of differing character, each with its own particular following. It achieves with natural grace what so-called Irish theme pubs would dearly love to capture (and can't). Friendly, humorous bar staff enjoy filling customers in on the pub's proud history – and will gladly sell you a bottle of Henry Downes No.9 to take away. Closed 25 Dec & Good Fri •

Waterford   Jurys Hotel

Ferrybank Waterford Co Waterford

HOTEL   Tel: 051 832111   Fax: 051 832863

Situated high up over the River Suir, across from the town centre, this 1960s building is set in its own grounds with ample parking space and quite impressive public areas. Bedrooms, which include one suite, all have good views over Waterford city and are comfortably furnished with darkwood furniture and full bathrooms (all have bath and shower).The well-equipped leisure centre is a popular attraction. Conference facilities for up to 800 (banquets 550). • Acc£££ • Closed 24-26 Dec • Amex, Diners, MasterCard, Visa •

Waterford   The Marina Hotel

Canada Street Waterford Co Waterford

HOTEL   Tel: 051 856600   Fax: 051 856605

Just opening as we were visiting Waterford for the 1999 guide, this stylish new hotel is attractively situated and promises well for the future. • Acc£££ • Closed 25 Dec • Amex, MasterCard, Visa •

Waterford   McCluskey's Bistro

18 High Street Waterford Co Waterford

RESTAURANT   Tel/Fax: 051 857766

Proprietor-chef Paul McCluskey's colourful bistro is near Reginald's Tower and just one street back from the post office on the quays. Paul's menus are carefully thought out, based on the traditional French themes that everyone loves (moules marinières, peppered minute steak with herb tomatoes or garlic butter and Lyonnaise potatoes, daube provençale) lightened with global influences (penne with pesto, aubergine, courgette, parmesan and scallions, roast monkfish with Thai sauce, aoili, butter beans and sauté potatoes). He relies on prime local ingredients (Knockalara cheese, local butcher Tom Phelan's sausages). The quality of ingredients is impressive, the cooking admirably simple and the whole package excellent value for money (notably for the early evening sitting) – so it's hardly surprising there's lots of return business. • L£ & D£-££ Tues-Sat • Closed 25 Dec, New Year & Good Fri • MasterCard, Visa •

Waterford   O'Grady's Restaurant & Guesthouse

Cork Road Waterford Co Waterford

RESTAURANT   Tel: 051 378851   Fax: 051 374062

Situated in a restored Gothic lodge on the main Cork road, Sue and Cornelius O'Grady have established a good local following since taking over the premises in 1997. Off-road parking and a warm reception from the proprietors get guests off to a good start. The dining area – which is fresh and bright, with booths and café curtains providing privacy without shutting diners off from the buzz – is well-situated at the rear of the building, away from the road. Menus, which change weekly and always offer tempting vegetarian dishes, include 2/3 course lunch menus, an early-bird menu (before 8 pm) and an interesting, well-balanced à la carte. Ingredients and cooking are excellent, in starters such as O'Grady's seafood soup with rouille and risotto with fresh asparagus, sundried tomatoes and parmesan wafers. Main courses include some unusual dishes – calves' liver, Alsace bacon, onion gravy and colcannon for example, as well as popular choices such as rack of lamb with provençal vegetables. Classic desserts might have a new twist – chocolate crusted lemon tart for instance. Plated farmhouse cheeses, while served in good condition, are perhaps too generous – a smaller quantity (and, at £5.75, a lower price) would be more appropriate at the end of a meal.

Accommodation

En-suite rooms (shower-only) are comfortably furnished and have all the necessary amenities but close proximity to traffic lights on a very busy road (used by lorries all night) makes a good night's sleep unlikely. Ear plugs may be the only practical solution. • Acc£ • L£ & D£-££ Mon-Sat • Closed 24-26 Dec • Amex, Diners, MasterCard, Visa •

Waterford   Waterford Castle

The Island Ballinakill Waterford Co Waterford

HOTEL   Tel: 051 878203   Fax: 051 879316

email: wdcastle@iol.ie

This beautiful hotel dates back to the 15th century. It is uniquely situated on its own wooded island (complete with 18 hole golf course) and reached by a little private ferry. It had just changed hands at the time of going to press – the new owners plan to renovate all the hotel's bedrooms and public areas in the winter of 1998-9, with a view to completion early in 1999. • Acc££££ • Amex, Diners, MasterCard, Visa •

Waterford   The Wine Vault

High Street Waterford Co Waterford

RESTAURANT   Tel: 051 853444/853777

Based in the oldest part of the city, in a building that dates back to the Elizabethan era, international sommelier David Dennison's buzzy and informal little wine bar/bistro is over a vaulted wine merchant's premises which forms part of the restaurant (and can also be used for private parties/meetings and wine tastings – Saturday tastings weekly 10 am-6 pm) Informal, bistro-style menus – international in tone and strong on vegetarian choices – might begin with marinated Wine Vault salmon with tomato tarragon horseradish or satay of quail served with rice noodles and crispy leeks on a soy dressing. Main courses could be chargrilled monktail with ratatouille ragu and salsa verdi, an updated coq au vin or imaginative vegetarian dishes such as roast vegetables with cous-cous and a tomato saffron fondue. Finish with some plated farmhouse cheeses or a classic dessert. As would be expected, experimenting with wine is a major part of the fun at the Wine Vault, where David Dennison offers a special menu of half bottles and wines by the glass (and suggestions for perfect partnerships of food and wine) in addition to an extensive main list. Lunchtime specials and early evening menu (5-7.30) are especially good value. A new restaurant area is planned for 1999. Seats 60. Parties 10. • L£-££ & D££ Mon-Sat • Closed 25 Dec, 1 Jan & Good Fri • Amex, MasterCard, Visa •

WESTMEATH

As its name suggests, in ancient times Westmeath tended to be ruled by whoever held Meath itself, but today it is a county so cheerfully and successfully developing its own identity that they should find a completely new name for the place. For Westmeath is somewhere that makes the very best of what it has to hand. Its highest "peak" is only the modest Mullaghmeen of 258 m, 10 kilometres north of Castlepollard. But this is in an area where hills of ordinary height have impressive shapes which make them appear like miniature mountains around the spectacularly beautiful Lough Derravaragh, famed for its association with the legend of the Children of Lir, who were turned into swans by their wicked step-mother Aoife, and remained as swans for 900 years until saved by the coming of Christianity. Westmeath abounds in lakes to complement Derravaragh, such as the handsome expanses of Lough Owel and Lough Ennell on either side of the fine county town of Mullingar, where they've been making life even more watery in recent years with schemes to speed the restoration of the Royal Canal on its way through town from Dublin to the north Shannon. Meanwhile, Westmeath's other main urban centre of Athlone has, like Mullingar, greatly benefited from having a by-pass built to remove through traffic bound for the west coast. Thus Athlone is confidently developing as Ireland's main inland river town, its Shannonside prosperity growing on a useful mixture of electronics, pharmaceuticals and the healthcare industry. Despite such modern trends, this remains a very rural place – immediately south of the town, you can still hear the haunting call of the corncrake coming across the callows (water meadows). But Athlone itself has a real buzz, and north of it there's Lough Ree in all its glory, wonderful for boating in an area where, near the delightful village of Glasson, they also have a monument to mark what some enthusiasts reckon to be the geographical centre of all Ireland. You really can't get more utterly rural than that.

Local Attractions and Information

Athlone	Youth Festival (April) 0902 73358
Heineken	Athlone River Festival & Regatta (June) 0902 94981
Athlone	All Ireland Drama Festival (May) 0902 72333
Athlone	Tourist Information 0902 94630
Clonmellon	Ballinlough Castle Gardens & Demesne 046 33135

Athlone   Higgins'

2 Pearse Street Athlone Co Westmeath

PUB   **Tel: 0902 92519**

The Higgins' well-run, hospitable pub is near the Norman castle and provides comfortable inexpensive accommodation in a very central location. The four bedrooms range from a single room to a large family room, all with en-suite shower, hair dryer, TV and access to tea and coffee-making facilities in the breakfast room. Bedrooms have secondary glazing to reduce the possibility of disturbance at night and there's a residents' lounge, also with television. The pub only does light bar food, such as soup and sandwiches and plated salads, but there are several good restaurants nearby for inexpensive family meals. • Acc£ • Closed 25 Dec & Good Fri •

Athlone   Hodson Bay Hotel

Hodson Bay Athlone Co Westmeath

HOTEL/RESTAURANT   **Tel: 0902 92444   Fax: 0902 92688**

email: hodson@iol.ie   www.hodsonbayhotel.com

Very much the centre of local activities, this well-located modern hotel adjoins Athlone Golf Club on the shores of Lough Ree, just three miles outside Athlone town. With lovely lake and island views and a wide range of leisure activities on site – including boating and fishing and a fine leisure centre – it is very much in demand as a venue for both business and social occasions. The hotel has grown considerably since opening in 1992 and there are currently plans for further expansion, this time to expand the bar (which can seem very crowded on busy weekends), to create a second restaurant and to add a further 20 bedrooms. Bedrooms, which are accessible by lift and include one room designed for disabled guests, are bright and comfortable, with contemporary decor, well-finished en-suite bathrooms and double and single beds in most rooms. Phone, TV, hairdryer, trouser press and tea/coffee trays are standard. Excellent banqueting/conference facilities can cater for 600/700 respectively. Helipad.

L'Escale Restaurant

The restaurant is on the lake side of the hotel, well-appointed in traditional style. Head chef Tony Hanevy has been at the hotel since 1992 and recent visits have indicated a standard of cooking which is well above the usual expectation for hotels. In addition to the basic à la carte daily set menus ensure variety for residents. While not adventurous, the quality of ingredients, cooking, presentation and service all ensure an enjoyable meal. Expect popular dishes such as wild Irish smoked salmon served traditionally with lemon and capers, and deep-fried mushrooms on crispy salad with garlic mayonnaise; steaks may be predictable but this is great beef country and they are well-cooked, with a choice of sauces. The seafood selection can sometimes include lobster, along with several fish. Vegetarians get a choice of three or four dishes (on the carte) and farmhouse cheese is always available in addition to traditional desserts. Both the dinner menu (£22) and house wines (eight, £11.50-£15) are good value. • L£ & D££ daily • Acc£££ • Open all year • Amex, Diners, MasterCard, Visa •

Athlone   Left Bank Bistro

Bastion Street Athlone Co Westmeath
HOTEL/RESTAURANT   Tel: 0902 94446   Fax: 0902 94509

Annie McNamara and Mary McCullough's wacky little restaurant on the bohemian side of the river is a great place for a most entertaining evening out. If you can plan a journey across Ireland to suit, it is also a fine place to stop for lunch when travelling. Old stone walls, oil-clothed tables and paper napkins create an informal atmosphere with loads of character – just right for the enjoyment of Annie's lively food. A wide range of delicious-sounding dishes – from menus described as a multicultural mix including contemporary Australian – make choices difficult. Whether you start with Tiger prawns with Thai sweet chili dip or today's homemade soup (with crispy garlic focaccia bread) it will be a good decision as the quality of ingredients and cooking is consistently high. Main courses might include char-grilled duck breast with plum and ginger compote and a delicious vegetarian special, Left Bank vegetable and creamy garlic burrito topped with red cheddar. Fresh fish dishes are on a specials board, changed daily – which might also have char-grilled kangaroo on offer. Desserts are more traditional. Lunches offer less choice but in the same style and light snacks are available morning and afternoon. • Summer Mon-Sat all day – check times off season L£ & D££ • Closed 24 Dec-6 Jan •

Athlone   The Olive Grove

Custume Place Athlone Co Westmeath
RESTAURANT   Tel: 0902 76946

Garry Hughes and Gael Buckley opened their charming little restaurant in the autumn of 1997 and it has quickly built up a following for its pleasant, informal atmosphere (seasoned with a good dash of style), excellent home-cooked food from noon until late (light food in the afternoon) and a great willingness to do anything which will ensure a good time being had by all. The style is vaguely Mediterranean and youthful – as seen in starters such as bruschetta and vegetarian specials like Greek salad – but this is beef country and the speciality of the house is chargrilled steaks. At the time of going to press Garry and Gael were in the process of introducing live jazz into the restaurant. • L£ & D£-££ • Closed Xmas & New Year • Amex, Diners, MasterCard, Visa •

Athlone   Restaurant Le Chateau

Athlone Co Westmeath
RESTAURANT   Tel: 0902 94517   Fax: 0902 73885
Atmospheric Restaurant of the Year   www.lechateau.ie

When Steven and Martina Linehan moved Le Chateau – the restaurant they first opened in 1989 – a couple of hundred yards down the hill to its present quayside location, a Presbyterian church in Athlone was given a new lease of life (and a very different character). The church, which was closed in the early 1970s, has been magnificently transformed into a two-storey restaurant of great character. As well as the couple's established reputation for excellent food and hospitality an additional attraction is now the atmosphere created by this dramatic conversion. Designed around the joint themes of church and river, the upstairs section has raised floors at each end, like the deck of a galleon, while the church theme is reflected in the windows – notably an original "Star of David" at the back of the restaurant – and the general ambience, which is extremely atmospheric. Candles are used generously to create a relaxed, romantic atmosphere, as they were in the old Restaurant le Chateau, where the Linehans had already established the Candlelight Dinner Menu for which they are now renowned. Additional facilities also now include wheelchair access, air conditioning and a full bar. • D££ daily, L£ Sun only • Closed 25 Dec & 1 Jan • MasterCard, Visa •

Athlone   Sean's Bar

13 Main Street Athlone Co Westmeath

PUB   **Tel: 0902 92358**

West of the river, in the interesting old part of the town near the Norman castle (which has a particularly good visitors' centre for history and information on the area, including flora and fauna of the Shannon), Sean Fitzsimons' seriously historic bar claims to be the pub with the longest continuous use in Ireland – all owners since 1630 are on record. Dimly-lit, with a fine mahogany bar, mirrored shelving and an enormous settle bed, the bar has become popular with the local student population and is very handy for visitors cruising the Shannon (who have direct access to the river through the back bar and beer garden). The sloping floor is a particularly interesting feature, cleverly constructed to ensure that flood water drained back down to the river as the waters subsided (it still works). A glass case containing a section of old wattle wall original to the building highlights the age of the bar, but it's far from being a museum piece. Food is restricted to sandwiches, but the proper priorities are observed and they serve a good pint. • Closed 25 Dec & Good Fri •

Glasson   Glasson Village Restaurant

Glasson Co Westmeath

RESTAURANT   **Tel: 0902 85001**

In an attractive stone building which formerly served as an RIC barracks, chef-proprietor Michael Brooks opened the Village Restaurant in 1986, making his mark as something of a culinary pioneer in the area. On the edge of the village, there's a real country atmosphere about the place, enhanced by old pine furniture and a conservatory which is particularly pleasant for Sunday lunch. As has been the case since they opened, fresh fish features strongly on the menu – Michael takes pride in having introduced fresh seafood at a time when it wasn't popular locally, and aims to maintain the special reputation earned for fresh fish (including shellfish in season and freshwater fish like Lough Ree eel). The cooking style is imaginative and fairly traditional – country French meets modern Irish perhaps. à la carte menus change with the seasons, set menus daily and there are always a couple of vegetarian dishes. • D££ Tues-Sat, L£ Sun • Closed 3 wks Oct, 24-25 Dec & Bank Hols • Amex, Diners, MasterCard, Visa •

Glasson   Grogan's Pub

Nr Athlone Co Westmeath

PUB   **Tel: 0902 85158**

It's hard to cross the midlands without being drawn into at least a short visit to this magic pub in the "village of the roses". One of those proudly-run, traditional places with two little bars at the front (one with a welcome open fire in winter) and everything gleaming, it was established in 1750 and feels as if the fundamentals haven't changed too much since then. There's an informal bar/restaurant at the back, known as "Nannie Murph's".• Closed 25 Dec & Good Fri •

Glasson   Wineport Restaurant

Glasson Nr Athlone Co Westmeath

RESTAURANT   **Tel: 0902 85466   Fax: 0902 85471**

Hosts of the Year   email: wineport@iol.ie

Since opening Wineport, their wonderful lakeside restaurant in 1993, Ray Byrne and Jane English have worked tirelessly on improvements – the restaurant is now much bigger and includes a private dining room, The Chart Room. Wineport is almost a second home to many of their regulars. Its stunning location and exceptional hospitality draw guests back time and again – guests who return with additions to the now famous Wineport collections (nauticalia, cats) and find the combination of the view, the company and a good meal irresistible. Head chef Feargal O'Donnell is a member of Euro-Toques, the organisation committed to defending local and artisan produce and suppliers. He presents strongly seasonal menus based on local ingredients including Irish Angus beef, game in season, eels, home-grown herbs, free range eggs and wild mushrooms. There are New Irish Cuisine dishes such as confit of salmon with a black pudding champ, braised lamb shank with a spicy butterbean cassoulet and smoked ham hocks with a sweet mustard scallion béarnaise. There are always one or two vegetarian dishes for each course and an Irish cheeseboard that usually includes smoked Gubbeen, St Killian, Cooleeney and Cashel Blue. A new bar menu has recently been introduced (4-6 pm Mon-Sat in summer). • D££ daily, L£ Sun (in summer) • Closed 25-26 Dec, closed Mon & Tues Nov-Feb • Amex, MasterCard, Visa •

Kilbeggan   Locke's Distillery

Main Street Lower Kilbeggan Co Westmeath

CAFÉ/BAR   Tel: 0506 32154   Fax: 0506 32139

email: lockes@tinet.ie

Founded in 1757, and possibly the oldest licensed pot distillery in the world, Locke's has been imaginatively restored with a museum and bar open to the public all year round, seven days a week. It makes an interesting break en route between Dublin and Galway. The Distillery Kitchen – a characterful stone-walled place with big refectory tables and a welcoming fire – offers wholesome home-cooked food and good coffee. • Closed 25 Dec, Good Fri & 1 Jan • MasterCard, Visa •

Kinnegad   The Cottage

Kinnegad Co Westmeath

RESTAURANT   Tel: 044 75284

In the village of Kinnegad, just at the point where the Galway road forks to the left, this delightful homely cottage restaurant is one of Ireland's best-loved stopping places, with comfy traditional armchairs and real home-made food – anything from proper meals with a glass of wine at given times to snacks at any time and a really great afternoon tea. Baking is a speciality, with scones and home-made preserves, a wide variety of cakes and irresistible cookies always available. Home-made soups, hot dishes like poached salmon, quiches and omelettes served with a salad are all typical, along with desserts such as apple pie or gateaux. The only sad thing is that they're closed on Sundays, when so many people have to head back to the East coast after a weekend of sanity out West. • Mon-Sat daytime meals£ • Closed Xmas week • No credit cards •

Moate   Castledaly Manor

Castledaly Moate Co Westmeath

COUNTRY HOUSE   Tel: 0902 81221   Fax: 0902 81600

email: castledaly@tinet.ie

Located just off the main Dublin road between Moate and Athlone, this Georgian manor house is set in 36 acres of mature woods and parkland. The guide's visit coincided with its opening in the summer of 1998, and although not quite fully operational, it was clear that the extensive renovation and refurbishment undertaken by the new owners had resulted in an impressive country house that will complement facilities in the area very well. Furnished in period style, there's a clubby bar, traditional drawing room and a restaurant (which has opened since our visit) on the ground floor. There are twelve large bedrooms (four wheelchair friendly), all furnished to a very high standard in period style (some with four-posters) and all en-suite (although eight are shower-only). Conference/meeting facilities are also planned. • Acc£££ • Closed 25 Dec • Amex, Diners, MasterCard, Visa •

Moate   Temple Country House

Horseleap Moate Co Westmeath

COUNTRY HOUSE   Tel: 0506 35118   Fax: 0506 35008

email: templespa@spiders.ie   www.spiders.ie/templespa

Relaxation is the essence of Declan and Bernadette Fagan's philosophy at Temple, their charming and immaculately maintained 200 year-old farmhouse in the unspoilt Westmeath countryside. On its own farmland – where guests are welcome to walk – close to peat bogs, lakes and historical sites, outdoor activities such as walking, cycling and riding are all at hand. There are three lovely country style en-suite rooms in the house and, since the opening of a Spa in summer 1998, a further five in the courtyard. Relaxation programmes and healthy eating have always been available at Temple, but the new Spa has moved this side of the operation into a new phase, offering yoga, hydrotherapy, massage, reflexology and specialist treatments such as Yon-Ka spa facial and seaweed body contour wraps. Temple is a member of the Health Farms of Ireland Association, which means that Bernadette gives special attention to healthy eating guidelines (and caters for vegetarian, vegan and other special diets). She uses the best of local produce – lamb from the farm, their own garden vegetables, best midland beef, cheese and yogurts – in good home cooking. And, although the Spa is a major attraction, you do not have to be a Spa guest to enjoy a stay at Temple. • Acc££ • Closed Xmas & New Year • MasterCard, Visa •

Mullingar   The Austin Friar Hotel

Austin Friar Street Mullingar Co Westmeath

HOTEL   Tel: 044 45777   Fax: 044 45880

Built near the recently discovered ruins of an Augustinian friary, this unusual new hotel right in the middle of Mullingar opened in 1998 and has made quite an impact. The design – which is elliptical and features a central atrium – is very striking, even slightly disorientating at first, but interesting and pleasing once you have a feeling of how the building works. The very close proximity to the supermarket next door – or, for that matter the poky reception area and narrow stairs – do nothing to prepare visitors for the more stylish elements of the hotel, which blossoms into the bright first floor atrium with contemporary seating areas. Bedrooms opening off this area are furnished to a high standard in a sophisticated modern style, with quality fabrics in warm, simple designs and good amenities; most rooms have full en-suite bathrooms, although three have shower only. On the ground floor there is a rather dashing modern restaurant, Austin's. • Acc££ • Amex, MasterCard, Visa •

Mullingar   Crookedwood House

Crookedwood Mullingar Co Westmeath

COUNTRY HOUSE/RESTAURANT ☆   Tel: 044 72165   Fax: 044 72166

email: cwoodhse@iol.ie

Noel and Julie Kenny's handsome 18th century rectory is set in lush rolling farmland with views over Lough Derravaragh. It is a handsome setting for a thoroughly professional restaurant. Julie welcomes guests to the bar for aperitifs (and a chance to consider Noel's strongly seasonal menus) before proceeding to the characterful white-washed basement restaurant. Noel is a prominent Euro-Toques chef and his distinctive style of cooking favours local ingredients – including their own garden produce and food from the wild such as mushrooms, blackberries and damsons. There is also beef, for which the area is famous, Wicklow venison and fresh seafood – all of which translate into punchy, colourful dishes that are always interesting but totally innocent of gimmicks. Noel presents a well-balanced 4-course table d'hôte dinner menu (£25),with vegetarian options on all courses, a more limited early evening menu (Tue-Fri 6-7.15, £14.95) and a sensibly concise à la carte. Most dishes appeal in varying degrees to traditional tastes and are cooked and presented with attention to detail. Sunday lunch (£14.95) is a speciality and always a treat. Service, under Julie's hospitable direction, is excellent.

Accommodation

There are eight spacious, thoughtfully planned rooms (six non-smoking) with well-designed bathrooms (£55 pps). Delicious breakfasts include freshly baked bread and home-made preserves. A sister property, Clonkill House, opened in 1998 to provide additional accommodation near the restaurant; it is finished to a similar standard and has a peaceful countryside setting, with a sun room and sitting room where guests can unwind. (£35pps high season). • Acc£££ • D££ Tues-Sat • L£ Sun • Closed Xmas, New Year & 2 wks Jan • Amex, Diners, MasterCard, Visa •

Mullingar   The Greville Arms Hotel

Pearse St Mullingar Co Westmeath

HOTEL   Tel: 044 48563   Fax: 044 48052

Right at the heart of Mullingar's shopping area, this privately owned hotel is old-fashioned in the best sense of the word – well-maintained and well-run, with a strong sense of pride, friendly staff and a good deal of natural charm. Renovation and refurbishment have been undertaken on an ongoing basis over the years and housekeeping is of a high standard throughout. Public areas are in excellent order, including a lovely garden (with William Turner athenaeum) and, newly opened in 1998, a rooftop garden and conservatory. The lounge bar, which was undergoing renovation at the time of our visit, has since re-opened and the hotel has good conference and banqueting facilities. Bedrooms are comfortably furnished with good amenities and are well organised for the hotel's many business guests; all have full en-suite bathrooms. An attractive, well-run carvery and food bar is open all day, making it a good place to break a journey. • Acc££ • Closed 25 Dec • Amex, Diners, MasterCard, Visa •

Mullingar

Meares Court
Rathconrath Nr Mullingar Co Westmeath

COUNTRY HOUSE   Tel: 044 55112

Nine miles west of Mullingar, Meares Court is a magnificent Georgian mansion set tranquilly in acres of sweeping parkland. It is the kind of place people fall in love with, as Eithne and Brendan Pendred found when they "retired" here after many years in the hotel business. The house was in good order when they took it over, although they have made (and continue to make) many improvements, including the recent installation of lovely bathrooms for the comfortable bedrooms which are furnished with great style. Reception rooms include a large, elegant drawing room and a cosy study at the back of the house. There is a dining room where residents' dinners are served at 7.30 pm (book by noon). • Acc£-££ • Closed 20 Dec-2 Jan • MasterCard, Visa •

Multyfarnham

Mornington
Multyfarnham Co Westmeath

COUNTRY HOUSE   Tel: 044 72191   Fax: 044 72338
email: morning@indigo.ie   www.indigo.ie/morning

Warwick and Anne O'Hara's gracious Victorian house is surrounded by mature trees and is just a meadow's walk away from Lough Derravarragh where the mythical Children of Lir spent 300 years of their 900 year exile. The Lough is now occupied by a pleasing population of brown trout, pike, eels and other coarse fish. It has been the O'Hara family home since 1858 and is still furnished with much of the original furniture and family portraits and, although centrally heated, log fires remain an essential feature. Bedrooms are typical of this type of country house – spacious and well-appointed, with old furniture (three have brass beds) – but with comfortable modern mattresses. Bathrooms vary: each room has one of its own, although not necessarily en-suite and two are shower only. Anne cooks proper country breakfasts and country house dinners for residents (please let her know by 2 pm) and Warwick does the honours front of house. Well-behaved pets allowed by arrangement. • Acc££ • Closed Nov-Mar • Amex, Diners, MasterCard, Visa •

WEXFORD

For most people, when they think of Wexford, the thoughts are of beaches, sunshine and opera. The longest continuous beach in all Ireland runs along Wexford's east coast, an astonishing 27 kilometres from Cahore Point south to Raven Point, which marks the northern side of the entrance to Wexford's shallow harbour. As for sunshine, while areas further north along the east coast may record less rainfall, in the very maritime climate of the "Sunny Southeast" around Wexford the clouds seem to clear more quickly, so the chances of seeing the elusive orb are much improved. As for opera, well, the annual Wexford Opera Festival every October is a byword for entertaining eccentricity – as international enthusiasts put it, "we go to Wexford in the Autumn to take in operas written by people we've never heard of, and have ourselves a thoroughly good time." But there's much more to the intriguing county of Wexford than sun, sand and singing. Wexford town itself is but one of three substantial towns in the county, the other two being the market town of Enniscorthy, and the river port of New Ross. While much of the county is low-lying, to the northwest it rises towards the handsome Blackstairs Mountains, where the 793 m peak of Mount Leinster may be just over the boundary in Carlow, but one of the most attractive little hill towns in all Ireland, Bunclody, is most definitely in Wexford. In the north of the county, Gorey is a pleasant and prosperous place, and for connoisseurs of coastlines, the entire south coast of Wexford is a fascinating area of living history, shellfish-filled shallow estuaries, and an excellent little harbour at the much-thatched village of Kilmore Quay inside the Saltee Islands. Round the corner beyond the impressive Hook Head, home to Ireland's oldest lighthouse, Wexford faces west across its own shoreline along the beauties of Waterford estuary, with sheltered little ports of County Wexford such as Duncannon and Ballyhack moving at their own gentle pace.

Local Attractions and Information

Ballygarrett	Shrule Deer Farm 055 27277
Ballyhack	Castle (renovated tower house c 1459) 051 389468
Coolgreaney	Gorey, Ram House Gardens (garden "rooms") 0402 37238
Dunbrody	Abbey & Visitor Centre 051 388603
Johnstown	Castle Demesne & Agricultural Museum 053 42888
New Ross	John F Kennedy Arboretum 051 388171
Rosslare	Harbour (terminal building) 053 33622
Tintern	Abbey 051 397124
Wexford	Opera Festival (October), Theatre Royal, 053 22144
Wexford	Tourism Information, 053 23111

Arthurstown

Dunbrody Country House

Arthurstown Co Wexford

HOTEL/RESTAURANT   **Tel: 051 389600   Fax: 051 389601**
email: dunbrody@indigo.ie   www.dunbrodyhouse.com

Located on the R733 (just before you reach the Passage East car ferry at Ballyhack to cross over to Waterford), Kevin and Catherine Dundon's Georgian manor, built in 1830, is set in twenty acres of parkland and gardens. It is a short stroll from Duncannon beach. Though not yet the completely finished article – this, after all, is only their second year – the house is being elegantly restored. Public rooms, including a large entrance hall and gracious drawing room, are well-proportioned and have been tastefully furnished and decorated. The large bedrooms (with fine views) offer all the comforts expected of such a house. Wake up to an exceptional breakfast, a gargantuan affair this, seductively laid out in the dining room – and that's before you choose something cooked from the kitchen! • Acc£££ • Closed 24-30 Dec • Amex, Diners, MasterCard, Visa •

The Harvest Room

A large, uncarpeted room with draped windows looking onto the terrace beneath the croquet lawn. In winter months a huge fireplace supplements the central heating. Musical guests may care to use the grand piano. An organic vegetable and fruit garden is presently being created, with a view to almost total self-sufficiency in the future. Chef/proprietor Kevin offers a very reasonable nightly-changing £20 table d'hôte menu alongside the à la carte. From the carte you could choose a warm leek and potato cake with pieces of pan-fried crab and topped with crème fraîche, and oven-roasted rack of Wexford lamb with an orange and marmalade glaze. A lemon torte ends the meal in style. A variety of breads is baked daily on the premises and the wine list is taking shape.

Catherine leads the dining room staff with charm and panache. D££ daily, L£ Sun only • Closed 24-30 Dec • Amex, Diners, MasterCard, Visa •

Ballyhack

Neptune Restaurant & Ballyhack Cookery School

Ballyhack Co Wexford

RESTAURANT   **Tel: 051 389284   Fax: 051 389356**

Near the Passage East car ferry, just under the recently restored Ballyhack Castle, this welcoming restaurant has been run with style by Pierce and Valerie McAuliffe since 1983. Pierce, a Euro-Toques chef, takes pride in using the best of fresh local ingredients, especially the seafood (for which the restaurant is renowned) in delicious, imaginative meals that somehow reflect the sunny temperament of this south-eastern corner. Likewise Valerie, an interior designer, has created a cheerful, slightly Mediterranean atmosphere and relaxed ambience in the three rooms which make up the restaurant – a main dining room with open kitchen (used for the cookery demonstrations), a cosy snug (where smoking is allowed) and a non-smoking conservatory with views over the river. Pierce's strongly seasonal à la carte menus and daily short dinner menus reflect his interest in traditional Irish food but have a modern slant and include quite a few French classics too. Good soups include a special Neptune creamy fish soup (with delicious brown bread), there's a luscious hot crab bake with gin that has become synonymous with the restaurant, also seafood pancakes, local salmon and much else besides, including steaks, duckling and vegetarian dishes – and, of course, a Wexford cheeseboard. The cookery school – of which Martin Dwyer, of Dwyers Restaurant in Waterford city is a co-owner – offers a wide range of courses and is unusual in addressing the training needs of caterers in the pub and accommodation sectors as well as amateur enthusiasts, both Irish and foreign. (A morning demonstration of traditional Irish dishes with recipes and lunch is £20). • D£-££ Mon-Sat • Closed Nov-Apr • Amex, Diners, MasterCard, Visa •

Ballymurn

Ballinkeele House

Ballymurn Co Wexford

FARM STAY   **Tel: 053 38105   Fax: 053 38468**

email: balnkeel@indigo.ie   www.indigo.ie~balnkeel

Set in 350 acres of game-filled woods and farmland, this fine big house – which was designed by Daniel Robertson and has been the Maher family home since it was built in 1840 – is very much the centre of a working farm. It is a grand house, with some wonderful features, including a lofty columned hall with a big open fire in the colder months, the original billiards room, beautifully proportioned reception rooms with fine ceilings and furnishings which have changed very little since the house was built. Nevertheless, it is essentially a family house and has a refreshingly hospitable and down to earth atmosphere. Large bedrooms (all no smoking) have wonderful countryside views; all have en-suite bathrooms and are furnished with antiques. Margaret is a keen amateur painter and plans to run small art workshops at Ballinkeele. (Residents dinner 7.30, please book by noon). • Acc££-£££ • Amex, MasterCard, Visa •

Campile

Kilmokea Country House

Campile Co Wexford

COUNTRY HOUSE   **Tel: 051 388109   Fax: 051 388776**

email: kilmokea@indigo.ie

Follow the signs to Kilmokea Gardens on the R733 between New Ross and Ballyhack (car ferry) to find this most peaceful and relaxing late Georgian country house set in formal walled gardens. The gardens (open to the public between 9-5) hold an Irish Heritage Garden certificate; it's hard to believe they were created only fifty years ago. The house itself is most tastefully and comfortably furnished, with a drawing room overlooking the Italian Loggia, an honesty library bar, and an elegant dining room. Cream teas, shared with garden visitors, are served in a delightful conservatory. The four individually-designed and immaculately maintained bedrooms, all with their own bathroom (two shower only), command lovely views over the gardens and towards the estuary beyond. They have no TVs to disturb the tranquillity (though there's one in the lounge). Owner Emma Hewlett (husband Mark helps out at weekends) does practically everything herself, from preparing and cooking the evening meal on the trusty Aga (a typical dinner might include asparagus hollandaise, honeyed trout, rhubarb compote with home-made orange biscuits and Irish farmhouse cheeses) to offering aromatherapy treatments (for which she holds several qualifications) during the day. • Acc££-£££ • Open all year • MasterCard, Visa •

Carne   The Lobster Pot

Carne Co Wexford

PUB/RESTAURANT ⭐   Tel: 053 31110   Fax: 053 31401

Near Carnsore Point, Ciaran and Anne Hearne's fine, good-looking country pub – in elegant dark green with lots of well maintained plants – is a welcome sight indeed. Inside the long, low building several interconnecting bar areas are furnished in simple, practical style, with sturdy furniture designed for comfortable eating. For fine summer days there are picnic tables outside at the front. One room is a slightly more formal restaurant, but the atmosphere throughout is very relaxed and the emphasis is on putting local seafood to the best possible use, providing good value and efficient service. There's fresh lobster and some more unusual choices, such as Lobster Pot Pot-Pourri (an assortment of seafood served in a white wine sauce) plus half a dozen options "for landlubbers". • Meals£-££ • Closed 25 Dec & Good Fri • Amex, MasterCard, Visa •

Courtown Harbour   Harbour House

Courtown Harbour Co Wexford

ACCOMMODATION   Tel/Fax: 055 25117

Four miles from Gorey, off the N11 Dublin/Wexford/Rosslare road, Donal and Margaret O'Gorman's spick-and-span guesthouse is situated a stone's throw from the harbourside marina and a few minutes from the resort's sandy beaches. Comfortable bedrooms (all en-suite, some shower only) offer TV, tea- making facilities and hairdryer, and there's a well-appointed residents' lounge. Start the day with a substantial breakfast, sensibly served until 10am – a traditional Celtic affair this, with all the trimmings from Irish soda bread to black pudding.. As an alternative, ask about their self-catering mobile homes. Own car park. • Acc£ • Closed Nov-Feb • MasterCard, Visa •

Ferrycarrig Bridge   Ferrycarrig Hotel

Ferrycarrig Bridge Co Wexford

HOTEL/RESTAURANT   Tel: 053 20999   Fax: 053 20982

email: ferrycarrig@griffingroup.ie   www.griffingroup.ie

The recent addition of 51 bedrooms (including several suites) and an award-winning leisure centre have enhanced the appeal of this modern hotel overlooking the Slaney estuary. Outside, a new terrace patio has been constructed, and the steeply sloping gardens re-landscaped, with (many!) steps up to the car park. The old conservatory restaurant has been transformed into a lounge, and in its place are two new restaurants: the 160-seater informal Bistro, serving new Irish cuisine, and the more formal Tides (45 seats) where guests can enjoy modern French dishes. One of the great advantages of this hotel is that all bedrooms (some with balconies) have splendid views across the water. It's a few minutes' drive from Wexford, and about twenty minutes from Rosslare Harbour, where guests can enjoy a round of golf at the cliff-top St Helen's Bay course. Extensive conference facilities for up to 400. The leisure centre boasts a heated floor, alongside a 20-metre swimming pool, children's splash pool, fully equipped gym and saunas. • Acc£££ • Meals£-£££ • Amex, Diners, MasterCard, Visa •

Gorey   Marlfield House

Courtown Rd Gory Co Wexford

COUNTRY HOUSE/RESTAURANT 🏛️🏛️   Tel: 055 21124   Fax: 055 21572

email: marlf@iol.ie

Twenty years on and the Bowe family is still running the country house hotel par excellence. Marlfield House remains at the forefront of Irish hospitality. This is no ordinary hotel, but an example of how to transform a fine 19th-century house into an elegant oasis of unashamed luxury, where guests are cosseted and pampered in surroundings that can only be described as sumptuous. Signposted off the N11 (from Dublin turn left just before Gorey towards Courtown Harbour), you enter the wooded drive through imposing gates, observing the enclosed wildfowl reserve with its own island and lake. To the rear of the house are further well-maintained gardens and manicured lawns, including a fine kitchen garden that provides much of the produce used in the restaurant. The house itself features marble fireplaces, antiques, notable paintings, glittering chandeliers and fine fabrics. The hand of Mary Bowe is very much in evidence, perhaps even more noticeable in the bedrooms (including four-posters and half-testers), six of which are on the ground floor. These are 'State Rooms', larger and even more grand than those upstairs. All offer fine bedding and exquisite furnishings, plus every conceivable amenity, from fresh flowers and fruit to books and magazines. Bathrooms, many in marble, some with separate walk-in shower and spa tub, are equally luxurious and well-appointed, naturally providing bathrobes and top-quality toiletries. Housekeeping is immaculate throughout, service from committed staff thoughtful and unobtrusive. The house is now under the direction of daughter Margaret Bowe, continuing the family tradition. Dogs and children are welcome by prior arrangement.

Restaurant

The graceful dining-room and resplendent conservatory merge into one, allowing views out across the gardens. The conservatory, with its hanging baskets, plants and fresh flowers (not to mention the odd stone statue), is one of the most romantic spots in the whole of Ireland, further enhanced at night by candlelight – a wonderful setting in which to enjoy chef Jo Ryan's accomplished cooking. The fixed-price dinner (£35) offers firstly an amuse-gueule, then four courses with choices, perhaps starters such as a creamed risotto of leeks with vegetable ravioli and poached bantam eggs or a cassoulet of seafood with basil and spring onion sauce. This will be followed by a soup, sorbet or salad. Main courses might include baked monkfish with ratatouille and potato cake or perfect roast loin of spring lamb with a ragout of vegetables, herby croquette potatoes and a port jus. Desserts are particularly impressive: warm apple tartlet with vanilla ice cream and caramel sauce, and chilled ice nougatine with a citrus salad. Alternatively, you can select Irish cheeses from the board. The extensive wine list, long on burgundies and clarets, is informative. • Acc£££-££££ • D£££ daily, L££ Sun only • Closed mid Dec-1 Feb • Amex, Diners, MasterCard, Visa •

Kilmore Quay   Kehoe's Pub & Parlour

Kilmore Quay Co Wexford

PUB   **Tel: 053 29830**

Recent harbour developments, and especially the new marina, have brought an extra surge of activity to this thriving fishing village – and well-informed visitors all head straight for Kehoe's – family-owned for generations (James and Eleanor Kehoe have been running it since 1987). Changes have been made over the years, the most obvious being in 1994 when they decided to do a really good refurbishment job, to enhance the pub's traditional ambience – everything was done correctly, from the roof slates to the old pitchpine flooring (and ceiling in the Parlour). At the same time the interior was used to display a huge range of maritime artefacts, some of them recovered from local wrecks by James and his diving colleagues. They have created what amounts to a maritime museum; even the beer garden at the back of the pub is constructed from a mast and boom discarded by local trawlers. The other major change has been to the food side of the business, which has crept up on Kehoe's gradually: a few years ago they did little more than soup and sandwiches but now the pub has a growing reputation for the quality and range of its bar meals – seafood, as well as vegetarian dishes and other main courses such as lasagne and stuffed chicken breasts wrapped in bacon. There's a short but very adequate wine list in addition to normal bar drinks. • Meals£-££ • Closed 25 Dec & Good Fri •

Kilmore Quay   Quay House

Kilmore Quay Co Wexford

ACCOMMODATION/CAFÉ   **Tel: 053 29988   Fax: 053 29808**

Siobhan and Pat McDonnell's pristine guesthouse is centrally located in the village (not on the quay as might be expected) and especially famous for its support of sea angling and diving – they have an annexe especially geared for anglers with drying/storage room, fridges and freezers, live bait and tackle sales. They can also provide packed lunches as well as evening meals. The whole place is ship shape, with attractive, slightly nautical bedrooms ("a place for everything and everything in its place"), practical pine floors (a bit cold underfoot) and neat en-suite facilities (most shower only). The breakfast room/coffee shop has a floor, a maritime theme and a patio with a view of the village's pretty thatched cottages, the sea and beach; food, ranging from breakfast to bar-style meals – home-made soups with brown breads, lasagne etc – is available all day (7.30 am-6 pm). • Acc£ • Meals£ • Closed 2 wks Nov •

The best – independently assessed

Kilmore Quay

The Silver Fox
Kilmore Quay Co Wexford
Tel: 053 29888

RESTAURANT

Absolute freshness is what has made chef Nicky Cullen's reputation at this middle-market seafood restaurant close to the harbour, where popular dishes and more ambitious seafood creations appear unselfconsciously side by side. Harbour developments, which included the opening of the Kilmore Quay marina a couple of years ago, were done with an admirable regard for the size and character of the village. Menus at The Silver Fox are wide-ranging and include a sprinkling of poultry and meat dishes (also vegetarian dishes, by arrangement) as well as the wide choice of seafood for which they have become famous. Booking is almost essential now that the restaurant is becoming more widely known.• Daytime meals£, L£ & D££ daily • Closed 25 Dec & Good Fri •

Rosslare

Churchtown House
Tagoat Rosslare Co Wexford
Tel/Fax: 053 32555

COUNTRY HOUSE

Patricia and Austin Cody's converted Georgian house, set in some 8 acres of wooded gardens, is a well-run and comfortable country guesthouse, (extremely handy for the Rosslare ferryport about five minutes away). The house is just off the N25 (turn right onto the R736 between a pub and the church if coming from the harbour). If you're lucky enough to arrive at around teatime, you'll be served delicious home-made cake and tea in the drawing room. A fine Irish breakfast and dinner (notice required) is served in the bright dining room. En-suite bedrooms, with pretty co-ordinating fabrics and TV, are protected against often heavy winds by sealed windows.• Acc££-£££ • Closed Nov-mid Mar • MasterCard, Visa •

Rosslare

Great Southern Hotel
Rosslare Co Wexford
Tel: 053 33233   Fax: 053 33543
email: res@rosslare.gsh.ie   www.gsh.ie

HOTEL

A popular family venue, this 1960s hotel is perched on a clifftop overlooking the harbour – very handy for the port and an excellent place to get a fortifying breakfast if you're coming off an overnight ferry. It has good facilities and recent refurbishment has included the exterior, all public areas, the restaurant, maritime bar (with extensive collection of memorabilia covering the history of shipping in the area), function rooms and 62 of the 99 bedrooms. • Acc£££ • Closed Jan-early Mar • Amex, MasterCard, Visa •

Rosslare

Kelly's Resort Hotel
Rosslare Co Wexford
Tel: 053 32114   Fax: 053 32222
email: kellyhot@iol.ie   www.kellys.ie

HOTEL/RESTAURANT

Every year this hotel improves, if improve it can after a hundred years plus in the same family! During the off-season (and it's only closed for ten weeks) they work feverishly; renovating, refurbishing and, this past winter, building. New bedrooms have been added, public rooms have been altered and new areas created. The snooker room has grown up and an Italian lunchtime buffet bar has been installed next to the Ivy Room. This complements the existing dining room, La Marine bistro, with its stunning zinc bar imported from France – typically, managing director William Kelly is one step ahead of the rest and has reversed the trend for 'all things Irish'. Note, too, the adjacent wine cellar, visible through a large glass window; several wines are own-label (William's wife is French and her family own vineyards in the Cotes-du-Rhone). Others are imported directly. Quite simply, the hotel has everything, for both individuals and families, many of whom return year after year (the number of children is limited at any one time, so as not to create an imbalance). There is a wide variety of public rooms, ranging from a quiet reading room and the aforementioned snooker room to a supervised crèche and gallery lounge. All the walls feature pictures (mostly modern) from the outstanding art collection. Many of the well-maintained bedrooms, some with balconies, all with bathrooms, have sea views and housekeeping throughout is immaculate. Leisure facilities are second to none, including a therapeutic spa and beauty centre, two indoor swimming pools, indoor tennis, and, continuing the French theme, boules. Outside the summer holiday season (end June-early Sept), ask about activity and special interest midweek spring/autumn breaks, weekends and Bank Holidays when rates are reduced.

Restaurant

In 1998 chef de cuisine Jim Aherne celebrated 25 years at the helm, and he continues to satisfy literally hundreds of guests (hotel and locals) daily. A typical table d'hôte dinner menu – note the use of local ingredients – might include Bannow oysters or St Helen's white crabmeat with couscous and spring greens to start, followed by roast Rosslare spring lamb (an 'uncle' Kelly rears the lamb) or steamed turbot with dill hollandaise. Orange parfait with rhubarb compote or a selection of Irish cheeses finishes the meal in style, and after coffee you can dance the night away to live music in the Ivy Room.

La Marine

Now in its second year, the bistro has proved to be an unqualified success, offering an alternative, more casual option for dining. Chef Eugene Callaghan is one of a new breed of young Irish chefs with the confidence to adapt traditional continental/Mediterranean dishes to Irish produce; thus pasta quills with fresh crab, cream and chives; escalopes of veal Parmigiano with buttered tagliatelle, tomato and parsley, or crusted fillet of salmon served on a bed of champ with a scallion cream sauce. Pear and cinnamon crème brûlée or a chocolate cappuccino cup round off things nicely. Sunday lunch (three courses for a bargain £10.95) features roast rib of beef. Wines (a selection off the main restaurant list), reflecting the style of food, are fairly priced. Service is swift and friendly. • Acc£££ • L£, D££ daily • Closed Dec-end Feb • Amex, MasterCard, Visa •

Wexford   La Dolce Vita

Westgate Wexford Co Wexford

RESTAURANT   **Tel: 053 23935**

Roberto Pons – who will be remembered from the successful Dalkey restaurant, Il Ristorante, that he and his wife Celine ran a few years ago and, until recently, as restaurant manager at Dublin's Shelbourne Hotel – is once again a chef-proprietor at this new Wexford restaurant. It opened to immediate acclaim just before we went to press. A committed Euro-Toques chef, Roberto cooks in traditional Italian style and, except for necessary Italian imports, everything is based on the freshest and best of local Irish produce. • D£-££ Mon-Sat • Closed Xmas & New Year • MasterCard, Visa •

Wexford   McMenamin's Townhouse

3 Auburn Tee Redmond Rd Wexford Co Wexford

ACCOMMODATION   **Tel/Fax: 0503 46442**

Seamus and Kay McMenamin's redbrick end-of-terrace Victorian house is one of the most highly-regarded places to stay in this area. It makes an excellent first or last night overnight stop for travellers on the Rosslare ferry, a fine base for the Wexford Opera or simply an excellent base for a short break in this undervalued corner of Ireland. It's a lovely house throughout, notable for the fine beds the McMenamins provide for their five en-suite bedrooms (all except one shower only, alas). There's a special quality of hospitality provided by these outstanding hosts – the local knowledge passed on to guests to help them make the most of every day out and the terrific breakfasts, which include old-fashioned treats like kippers and lambs' kidneys in sherry sauce, as well as all the other usual breakfast dishes, served with freshly baked breads and home-made preserves. • Acc£ • Closed 25-30 Dec • MasterCard, Visa •

Wexford   La Riva

Crescent Quay Wexford Co Wexford

RESTAURANT   **Tel: 053 24330**

Just off the quays, Frank and Anne Chamberlaine's first floor restaurant has been doing a good job since 1991. It's up a steep flight of stairs – which do not give a very good first impression – however, once inside, a warm welcome offsets any negative impressions. The restaurant itself is delightful in a bright, informal way, with views through to the kitchen. A blackboard menu offers tempting specials. Eclectic menus are the speciality here, but head chef Richard Trappe tempers this with a welcome restraint (ie he doesn't give in to the current wave of increasingly absurd food combinations) and his food is well cooked with real flavour. There is good, freshly-baked soda bread (white, which makes a change) to mop up the juices. Pasta dishes can be starters or main courses, and there are more serious main courses also, like rack of lamb (with roast shallots and garlic) and monkfish (with melted parmesan and garlic cream sauce). • D££ daily • Closed 25 Dec & 3 wks Jan • MasterCard, Visa •

Wexford

White's Hotel

George Street Wexford Co Wexford

HOTEL   **Tel: 053 22311   Fax: 053 45000**

New owners are carrying out an extensive refurbishment programme at this hotel in the centre of town. From the outside it looks relatively modern, certainly when approached from the car park, but the reality is that there was a hostelry on this site in the late 18th century, which is more apparent when viewed from George Street. Bedrooms have been modernised, there's a health and fitness club (but no swimming pool) in the basement and a substantial conference centre. • Acc£££ • Amex, Diners, MasterCard, Visa •

WICKLOW

Wicklow is a miracle. Although the booming presence of Dublin is right next door, this sublimely and spectacularly lovely county is very much its own place, a totally away-from-it-all world of moorland and mountain, farmland and garden, forest and lake, seashore and river. It's all right there, just over the nearest hill, yet it all seems so gloriously different. In times past, Wicklow may have been a mountain stronghold where rebels and hermits alike could keep their distance from the capital. But modern Wicklow has no need to be in a state of rebellion, for it is an invigorating and inspiring place which captivates everyone who lives there, so much so that while many of its citizens inevitably work in Dublin, they're Wicklow people a very long way first and associate Dubs – if at all – an extremely long way down the line. Their attitude is easily understood, for even with today's traffic, it is still only a very short drive to transform your world from the crowded city streets right into the heart of some of the most heart-stoppingly beautiful scenery in all Ireland. Such scenery generates its own strong loyalties and sense of identity, and Wicklow folk are rightly and proudly a race apart. Drawing strength from their wonderful environment, they have a vigorous local life which keeps metropolitan blandness well at bay. And though being in a place so beautiful is almost sufficient reason for existence in itself, they're busy people too, with sheep farming and forestry and all sorts of light industries, while down in the workaday harbour of Arklow in the south of the county – a port with a long and splendid maritime history – they've been so successful in organising their own seagoing fleet of freighters that there are now more ships registered in Arklow than any other Irish port.

Local Attractions and Information

Ashford	Mount Usher Gardens 0404 40116
Blessington	Russborough (Beit Collection) 045 865239
Bray	Kilruddery House & Gardens 01 2863405
Enniskerry	Powerscourt Gardens & House Exhibition 01 204 6000
Wicklow	Gardens Festival (May-July) Wicklow Co Tourism 0404 66058
Wicklow Mountains	May & Autumn Walking Festivals 0404 66058

Arklow

Plattenstown House
Coolgreaney Rd Arklow Co Wicklow
FARM STAY — Tel/Fax: 0402 37822

Margaret McDowell describes her period farmhouse accurately when she says it has "the soft charm typical of the mid 19th century houses built in scenic Wicklow". About halfway between Dublin and Rosslare (each about an hour's drive away) and overlooking parkland, this quiet, peaceful place is set in 50 acres of land amidst its own lovely gardens close to the sea. There are riding stables, forest walks and golf. The house has a traditional drawing room overlooking the back garden and a dining room where breakfast is served (and evening meals provided by arrangement). There are four bedrooms, all of which are very different but comfortably furnished with en-suite or private bathrooms (one with a bath, the others shower only). Children over 5 are welcome. • Acc£ • Closed Nov-Feb • MasterCard, Visa •

Ashford

Il Cacciatore
Ashford Co Wicklow
RESTAURANT — Tel: 0404 40054

The locals are pleased enough to keep this unpretentious little restaurant a closely guarded secret – but we can reveal it is on the main road as you drive through Ashford. It's furnished and decorated in trattoria style, with simple wooden furniture and a decorative roman-tiled "roof" and scenic Italian pictures. Expect simple Italian classics – starters include insalata di mare (a salad of crab claws, prawns and squid rings) and spaghetti alla carbonara, followed perhaps by a mixture of grilled fish or veal Milanese. Desserts, in true Italian fashion, are not quite so interesting (even tiramisu is not on the menu) but you can finish with an excellent espresso anyway. Since our visit the restaurant closed for renovations, but at the time of going to press we've been assured that the only major change is that the kitchen – which was open to view – is now away from the distraction of curious diners. Service is swift and cheerful, carafe wine admirably cheap and very drinkable (there is a wine list as well) and the whole experience makes everybody rush back – which is why the locals like to keep it to themselves and booking is essential, especially at weekends. • D£ Tues-Sun • MasterCard, Visa •

Aughrim

Lawless Hotel

Aughrim Co Wicklow

HOTEL   Tel: 0402 36146   Fax: 0402 36384

email: lawhotel@iol.ie

Picturesquely situated beside the river in the lovely village of Aughrim, this delightful hotel dates back to 1787. Under the energetic management of the O'Toole family since 1990, the hotel has undergone major refurbishment, and some degree of extension recently. It is to the credit of the proprietors that everything has been done with great respect for the character of the original building. On a recent visit we were able to see completed work; the bedrooms, for example – which are limited in size (unfortunately resulting in 10 of the 14 rooms having shower only) – very cosily done up, in character with a country inn. The "Thirsty Trout" bar and the "Snug" lounge are also very appealing and a lovely dining room overlooking the river had also been completed. A new entrance/reception was under construction – no ordinary new entrance, as every care was being taken to match both design and materials with the original building – and it was clearly going to be an improvement rather than an extension. There's an attractive paved area at the back beside the river, and as the hotel is understandably popular for weddings (300), this makes a romantic spot for photographs as well as informal summer food. No children under 12 after 8 pm. Self-catering accommodation is also available in a holiday village owned by the hotel. • Acc££ • L£ & D££ daily • Closed 24-26 Dec • Amex, MasterCard, Visa •

Blessington

Downshire House

Blessington Co Wicklow

HOTEL   Tel: 045 865199   Fax: 045 865335

Situated just 18 miles from Dublin on the N81, in the tree-lined main street of Blessington, this friendly village hotel offers unpretentious comfort which is very winning. Blessington is an attractive village in an area of great natural beauty and archaeological interest – and it's also very close to Ireland's great Palladian mansion, Russborough House, home of the world-famous Beit art collection. The present owner, Rhoda Byrne, has run the hotel since 1959 and instigated many improvements, including conference facilities for up to 200 and refurbishment of public areas. Simply furnished bedrooms, which include two single rooms, all have en-suite bathrooms with full bath and shower. • Acc££ • Closed 22 Dec-6 Jan • MasterCard, Visa •

Bray

The Tree of Idleness

The Seafront Bray Co Wicklow

RESTAURANT   Tel: 01 286 3498/282 8183   Fax: 01 282 8183

This much-loved seafront restaurant opened in 1979 when the owners, Akis and Susan Courtells, arrived from Cyprus bringing with them the name of their previous restaurant (now in Turkish-held north Cyprus). A collection of photographs of old Cyprus in the reception area establishes the traditional Mediterranean atmosphere of the restaurant – and the menu cover bears a drawing of the original Tree of Idleness. Since Akis' death six years ago, Susan has run the restaurant herself with the help of her trusty head chef Ismail Basaran (who trained under Akis) and long-serving manager Tom Monaghan. Their work is a great tribute to the memory of Akis, who would be delighted with the consistently high standards and loyal following the team has maintained (both locally and from much further afield). Ismail sources the best of Irish ingredients for his modern Greek Cypriot/Mediterranean menus. Many of the classics are there – tzatziki, humus, taramosalata, Greek salad, dolmades, moussaka (including a vegetarian variation), souvlaki – and they are unfailingly excellent. But there are a couple of specialities which have the world beating a path to their door. First, there is the suckling pig. Boned and stuffed with apple and apricot stuffing, it is served crisp-skinned and tender, with a wonderful wine and wild mushroom sauce. Then there is the dessert trolley, which is nothing less than temptation on wheels: it always carries a range of fresh and exotic fruits, baklava, home-made ice creams, several chocolate desserts, Greek yogurt mousse and much else besides. Service is excellent and the wine list includes many rare vintages. No children under 12 after 8 pm. • D££ daily • Closed Bank Hols & 2 wks Aug • Amex, MasterCard, Visa •

Dunlavin

COUNTRY HOUSE

Grangebeg House

Grangebeg Dunlavin Co Wicklow
Tel/Fax: 045 401367

Set amidst 86 acres of parkland (with its own 4 acre lake available for coarse fishing), Aine McGrane's elegant Georgian house offers spacious, comfortable accommodation in an informal atmosphere. It is very well located for touring this beautiful area, or for enjoying a wide range of country pursuits. There is an equestrian centre on the premises, several golf courses nearby (Rathsallagh is only 5 minutes' drive, for example; Mount Juliet an hour), watersports on the Blessington lakes, famous gardens at Mount Usher, Kilruddery and Powerscourt, and there's the Beit Collection at Russborough house for art lovers. Hunting with local packs can also be arranged in the season. Very much a family home, Grangebeg is an unselfconscious place and the six bedrooms (five en-suite, one private bathroom – three have shower only) offer real country house style without too many frills. No evening meals, but good restaurants (including Rathsallagh House) nearby. Not suitable for very young children (under 3). No dogs in the house (kennels available). • D££ daily • Closed Xmas • MasterCard, Visa •

Dunlavin

COUNTRY HOUSE/RESTAURANT 🏛

Rathsallagh House

Dunlavin Co Wicklow
Tel: 045 403112   Fax: 045 403343

This large, rambling country house is just an hour from Dublin, but it could be in a different world. Although it's very professionally operated, the O'Flynn family insists it is not an hotel and – despite the relatively recent addition of an 18-hole golf course with clubhouse in the grounds – the gentle rhythms of life around the country house and gardens ensure that the atmosphere is kept decidedly low-key. Day rooms are elegantly furnished in country house style, with lots of comfortable seating areas and open fires. Accommodation includes one suite and is generally comfortable to the point of being luxurious, although, as in all old houses, rooms do vary; some are very spacious with lovely country views while other smaller, simpler rooms in the stable yard have a special cottagey charm. The Edwardian breakfast buffet, with its whole ham and silver chafing dishes full of good things like liver, kidneys and juicy field mushrooms, is a sight to gladden the heart of any guest, especially if they are about to embark on a day of some of the energetic country pursuits for which Rathsallagh is famous: horseriding, hunting, deer-stalking in the nearby Wicklow Mountains or a round of golf. There is a completely separate private conference facility for up to 30 in a courtyard conversion at the back. Not suitable for children under 12.

Restaurant

Head chef Niall Hill creates interesting menus based on local produce, much of it from Rathsallagh's own walled garden. A drink in the old kitchen bar is recommended while reading the 4-course menu – country house with world influences – then guests can settle down in the graciously furnished dining room overlooking the gardens and the golf course. Roast local beef is a speciality, as is Wicklow lamb. Leave some room for a treat from the magnificent traditional dessert trolley, or some Irish farmhouse cheese. • Acc£££-££££ • D££-£££ daily • Closed 23-27 Dec • Amex, Diners, MasterCard, Visa •

Enniskerry

HOTEL/RESTAURANT

Enniscree Lodge Hotel & Restaurant

Enniskerry Co Wicklow
Tel: 01 286 3542   Fax: 01 286 6037
email: enniscre@iol.ie

Raymond and Josephine Power took over this comfortable inn in 1996. It is beautifully located, high up on the sunny side of Glencree. Since the Powers took it over they have been steadily renovating and refurbishing, but to the relief of its many fans they have not made any radical changes. Attractive features of this former hunting lodge include a cosy bar with open log fire for winter and a south-facing terrace for warm days. More important, perhaps, is the relaxed rural atmosphere. Most of the comfortably furnished, individually decorated bedrooms have lovely views and all of the en-suite bathrooms were refurbished in 1998 (two are shower only). A residents' sitting room can be used for small conferences or meetings (14). • Acc££ • Open all year • Amex, Diners, MasterCard, Visa •

Restaurant

Sweeping views across Glencree to the Tanduff, Kippure and Sugarloaf peaks provide a dramatic outlook for this well-appointed dining room. In daily lunch and dinner menus head chef Jason Wall bases his cooking on local produce – Wicklow lamb, fresh fish and game in season – and offers a well-balanced choice on tempting menus that are not overlong. Dishes such as pan fried kidneys with buttered onions, roast pigeon breast with rosti potatoes, roast Wicklow lamb with rosemary and shallot jus and baked escalope of salmon with herb butter sauce all have a comfortable country ring about them. If a recent visit was typical, however, what arrives on the plate is dressier cosmopolitan cooking – a pity perhaps, as a more relaxed style that allows the goodness of local ingredients to speak for themselves might be more appropriate in this lovely mountain retreat. No children under 10 after 8.30 pm. • L£ & D££ daily • Amex, Diners, MasterCard, Visa •

Enniskerry

Powerscourt Terrace Café

Powerscourt House Enniskerry Co Wicklow

RESTAURANT/CAFE   **Tel: 01 2046070   Fax: 01 2046072**

Situated in a stunning location overlooking the famous gardens and fountains of Powerscourt House, the Pratt family of Avoca Handweavers opened this self-service restaurant in the summer of 1997, under the management of head chef Leylie Hayes. It is a delightfully relaxed space, with a large outdoor eating area as well as the 160-seater café, and the style and standard of food is similar to the original Avoca restaurant at Kilmacanogue. So expect everything to be freshly made, using as many local ingredients as possible – including organic herbs and vegetables – with lots of healthy food, especially interesting salads and good pastries, and including vegetarian dishes such as oven-roasted vegetable and goat's cheese tart. • Daytime meals£ • Closed 25 Dec • Amex, MasterCard, Visa •

Glen O'The Downs

Glenview Hotel

Glen O'The Downs Delgany Co Wicklow

HOTEL   **Tel: 01 287 3399   Fax: 01 287 7511**

email: glenview@iol.ie

Famous for its views over the Glen O'The Downs, this well-located hotel has all the advantages of a beautiful rural location, yet is just a half hour's drive from Dublin. Major renovations and additions to the hotel have just been completed, resulting in a dramatic upgrade of all facilities. Over the last few years a new conference area, with state-of-the-art facilities, has been added as well as a superb Health and Leisure Club (complimentary to hotel residents and conveniently accessible for membership in most of south county Dublin and north Wicklow). Most recently a new reception area and 35 new bedrooms (including a penthouse suite) were completed and this, together with landscaping and upgrading of the hotel exterior, combine to give a vastly improved impression of the hotel on arrival. Bedrooms and public areas are now all of a high standard, making this an especially attractive venue for the special breaks offered (golf, health and fitness, riding), as well as a good choice for conferences and (especially due to the romantic location) weddings. • Acc£££ • Diners, MasterCard, Visa •

Glendalough

Derrybawn House

Laragh nr Glendalough Co Wicklow

COUNTRY HOUSE   **Tel: 0404 45134   Fax: 0404 45109**

This appealing house was built in the style of a north Italian villa in the early 19th century, to replace an earlier one burnt down at the time of the 1798 rising. Just south of Laragh village, set well back from the road in its own parkland, the house is approached by a sweeping drive; it has an elegant overhanging roof, shuttered windows and elegant wisteria-covered verandah. Very much a family home, reception rooms and the main bedrooms are large, gracious and furnished with antiques, but not too grand. Back bedrooms are smaller but have an appealing country character. All bedrooms have country views or a pleasant outlook over a courtyard garden. All have their own bathroom (private or en-suite – four shower only). Evening meals are available by arrangement – please book a day ahead. Children over 12 are welcome. Dogs permitted in some areas by arrangement. • Acc£-££ • Closed Xmas wk •

The guide aims to provide comprehensive recommendations of the best places to eat, drink and stay throughout Ireland. We welcome suggestions from readers. If you think an establishment merits assessment , please write or email us.

Glendalough

Mitchell's of Laragh

The Old Schoolhouse Laragh nr Glendalough Co Wicklow

RESTAURANT   Tel/Fax: 0404 45302

Providing a quiet adult retreat from the world of family outings, this old cut-stone schoolhouse was painstakingly restored by Jerry and Margaret Mitchell over several years before they opened it as a restaurant in 1992. Since then they've built up a reputation for Margaret's good home cooking and the attractive country feeling of the place, with its leaded windows, pine furniture and the old dresser beside the door laden with home-made preserves and baking (including their famous brown bread with sunflower seeds), all for sale. Although more formal meals at dinner time are an important part of their business, it's for the all-day food that they are best known – people out walking know they'll find a tempting little à la carte menu here, offering really good soups, light hot dishes like sautéed lamb's kidneys with whiskey and orange, warm chicken liver salads, florentine tartlets. tagliatelle carbonara and gratin of seafood mornay – and the wines to make the most of them. No children under 12. • L£ & D££ daily • Closed 25-26 Dec, New Year, 3 wks Jan & Good Fri • Amex, MasterCard, Visa •

Greystones

The Hungry Monk

Greystones Co Wicklow

RESTAURANT   Tel: 01 287 5759   Fax: 01 287 7183

Well-known wine buff Pat Keown has run this hospitable first floor restaurant on the main street since 1988. Pat is a great and enthusiastic host; his love of wine is infectious and the place is spick and span – and the monk-related decor is a bit of fun. It all adds up to a great winding-down exercise. A combination of hospitality and interesting good quality food at affordable prices are at the heart of this restaurant's success – sheer generosity of spirit ensures value for money as well as a good meal. Seasonal menus offered include a well-priced Sunday lunch (£12.95) – a particularly popular event running from 12.30 to 8pm – and an evening à la carte menu. Main courses include traditional dishes – rack of Aughrim lamb, roast Cavan duck – as well as more adventurous ones such as chorizo risotto diablo (arborio rice, prawns, red beans and chilli), chicken pak choi (wrapped in cabbage and served with a five-spice and star anise sauce) and a couple of vegetarian dishes. There is also the golfers' special: an incredible 18 oz T-bone steak served with peppercorn sauce and vegetables at a very reasonable £17.95. Blackboard specials include the day's seafood dishes and also any special wine offers. Desserts tend to be classical, there's always a farmhouse cheese plate and the outstanding wine list includes a choice of 50 half bottles. • D£-££ Wed-Sun, L£ Sun only • Closed Xmas, New Year & Bank Hols • Amex, MasterCard, Visa •

Kilmacanogue

Avoca Handweavers

Kilmacanogue Co Wicklow

RESTAURANT/CAFE   Tel: 01 286 7466   Fax: 01 286 2367

Avoca Handweavers is one of the country's most famous craft shops but it is also well worth allowing time for a meal when you visit. Head chef Johanna Hill has been supervising the production of their famously wholesome home-cooked food since 1995 and people come here from miles around to tuck into delicious fare. Hot food includes traditional dishes such as beef and Guinness casserole. Vegetarians are especially well catered for, both in special dishes – nut loaf, vegetable-based soups – and the many that just happen to be meatless, including a wide range of salads, tarts and quiches – typically piperade (chevre, pepper and tomato) or 3-cheese and red onion – and stuffed baked potatoes. Farmhouses cheeses are another strong point, as is the baking – typical breads made daily include traditional brown soda, cheese bread and a popular multigrain loaf. There is also a wide range of excellent delicatessen fare for sale in the shop. • Daytime meals£ • Closed 25-26 Dec • Amex, Diners, MasterCard, Visa •

Establishments recommended have all met our stringent entry requirements at the time of assessment. However, standards are sometimes not always as consistent as they should be. If you are disappointed by any aspect of a visit to a listed establishment, we suggest that you try to sort it out at the time if possible, as speedy, amicable solutions are by far the best. If you are still dissatisfied, put your complaints in writing to the proprietor or manager as soon as possible after the event - and send a copy to the guide if you wish.

Kiltegan

COUNTRY HOUSE

Romantic Hideaway of the Year

Humewood Castle

Kiltegan Co Wicklow
Tel: 0508 73215   Fax: 0508 73382
email: humewood@iol.ie
www.herbestgroup.com/humewood

You arrive on a perfectly ordinary Irish country road, stop at a large (but not especially impressive) gate and press the intercom button, as instructed. Slowly the gate creaks open – and you are transported into a world of make-believe. It's impossible to imagine anywhere more romantic to stay than Humewood Castle (and hence its Romantic Hideaway Award). A fairytale 19th-century Gothic Revival castle in private ownership set in beautiful parkland in the Wicklow Hills, it has been extensively renovated and stunningly decorated. While the castle is very large by any standards, many of the rooms are of surprisingly human proportions. Thus, for example, while the main dining room provides a fine setting for some two dozen or more guests, there are more intimate rooms suitable for smaller numbers. Similarly, the luxuriously appointed bedrooms and bathrooms, while indisputably grand, are also very comfortable. Under the professional management of Chris Vos, formerly of The Stafford at St James's Place London, Hume Castle can also offer fine food prepared by Peter Barfoot, a talented chef who has already made a mark elsewhere in Ireland. Country pursuits are an important part of life at Humewood too, but even if you do nothing more energetic than just relaxing beside the fire, this is a really special place for a weekend. Not suitable for children under 12. • Acc££££ • D£££ • Amex, MasterCard, Visa •

Rathdrum

ACCOMMODATION

Avonbrae Guesthouse

Laragh Road Rathdrum Co Wicklow
Tel/Fax: 0404 46198

Paddy Geoghegan's hospitable guesthouse makes a comfortable and relaxed base for a visit to this beautiful area. Walkers and cyclists are among the most frequent guests, although riding, pony-trekking, golf and fishing are also popular – not to mention people who have no sporting interest but who just want a quiet break. Simply furnished bedrooms vary in size and outlook but all have tea and coffee trays and en-suite facilities (only the smallest room has a bath). There are open fires as well as central heating and a comfortable guest sitting room. For fine weather there's a tennis court in the well-kept garden, and although this sounds grander than it is (the pool is small and the building it is in requires renovation) there is even a nice little indoor swimming pool. Evening meals £14 at 6.30pm) and packed lunches (from £3.50) are available by arrangement. • Acc£ • MasterCard, Visa •

Rathnew

HOTEL/RESTAURANT

Hunter's Hotel

Newrath Bridge Rathnew Co Wicklow
Tel: 0404 40106   Fax: 0404 40338

A rambling old coaching inn set in lovely gardens alongside the River Vartry, this much-loved hotel has a long and fascinating history – it's one of Ireland's oldest coaching inns, with records indicating that it was built around 1720. In the same family now for five generations, the colourful Mrs Maureen Gelletlie is currently at the helm and takes pride in running the place on traditional lines. This means old-fashioned comfort and food based on local and home-grown produce – with the emphasis very much on 'old fashioned' – which is where its character lies. There's a proper little bar, with chintzy loose-covered furniture and an open fire, a traditional dining room with fresh flowers – from the riverside garden where their famous afternoon tea is served in summer – and comfortable country bedrooms (all en-suite with full bath and shower). There is now a small conference centre (max 40), which has been thoughtfully designed and built with great care to blend in with the existing building.

Restaurant

Seasonal lunch and dinner menus change daily. In tune with the spirit of the hotel, the style is traditional country house cooking: simple food with a real home-made feeling about it. Expect classics such as chicken liver pâté with melba toast, soups based on fish or garden produce, traditional roasts – rib beef, with Yorkshire pudding or old-fashioned roast stuffed chicken with bacon – and probably several fish dishes, possibly including poached salmon with hollandaise and chive sauce. Desserts are often based on what the garden has to offer, and baking is good, so fresh raspberries and cream or baked apple and rhubarb tart could be wise choices. A very fair wine list includes a modestly-priced French house wine at £8.95. • Acc£££ • L£ & D£-££ daily • Closed 25 Dec • Amex, Diners, MasterCard, Visa •

Rathnew

COUNTRY HOUSE/RESTAURANT

Tinakilly House

Rathnew Co Wicklow
Tel: 0404 69274   Fax: 0404 67806
email: wpower@tinakilly.ie

A house with a history, Tinakilly was built in the 1870s for Captain Robert Halpin, a local man who made fame and fortune as Commander of The Great Eastern, which laid the first telegraph cable linking Europe and America. Now sensitively restored and extended by William and Bee Power, who have run it as an hotel since 1983, there's always a welcoming fire burning in the lofty entrance hall, where a fascinating collection of Halpin memorabilia adds greatly to the interest. Fine antiques include an original chandelier. Extremely professional management with a strongly personal touch, an appealing balance between Victorian charm and modern comfort – and, of course, an excellent location easily accessible to Dublin, yet definitely "in the country" – have combined to make Tinakilly one of Ireland's most successful country house hotels, temporary home to a long line of the rich and famous. Accommodation includes two suites and 28 junior suites, all with views across a bird sanctuary to the sea, and period rooms, some with four-posters. Proximity to Dublin and excellent facilities for small conferences (80) and meetings have made Tinakilly one of the country's top business and corporate venues. In addition to restaurant meals, light lunches are available in the bar. • Acc£££-££££ • Open all year • Amex, Diners, MasterCard, Visa •

Restaurant

Dining arrangements at Tinakilly have improved since the completion of a panelled split level restaurant in the west wing, which seats 80 but has a more relaxed, intimate atmosphere than the design of the old restaurant allowed. John Moloney, head chef since 1989, presents a range of menus including a seasonal à la carte and a daily table d'hôte. The kitchen garden produces an abundance of fruit, vegetables and herbs for most of the year and this, plus local meats – notably Wicklow lamb and venison – and seafood, provides the basis for his cooking. An old-fashioned chef in the best sense of the term, John oversees everything from the stockpots through to the preparation of preserves and chocolates. On a recent visit "global" influences were perhaps more prominent than usual but, at its best, Tinakilly's very successful house style is sophisticated country house cooking with the main influence – classic French – showing in well-made sauces and elegant presentation. • L££ & D£££ daily • Open all year • Amex, Diners, MasterCard, Visa •

Roundwood

PUB/RESTAURANT

Roundwood Inn

Roundwood Co Wicklow
Tel: 01 281 8107

Jurgen and Aine Schwalm have owned this 17th century inn in the highest village in the Wicklow Hills since 1985. There's a public bar at one end, with a snug and an open fire, and in the middle of the building the main bar food area, furnished in traditional style with wooden floors and big sturdy tables. The style that the Schwalms and head chef Paul Taube have developed over the years is their own unique blend of Irish and German influences. Excellent bar food includes substantial soups, specialities such as Galway oysters, smoked Wicklow trout, smoked salmon and hearty hot meals such as the house variation on Irish stew. Blackboard specials often include home-made gravad lachs, lobster salad and a speciality dessert, Triple Liqueur Parfait. The food at Roundwood has always had a special character which, together with the place itself and a consistently high standard of hospitality, has earned it an enviable reputation with hillwalkers, Dubliners out for the day and visitors alike. • Closed 25 Dec & Good Fri • Amex, MasterCard, Visa •

Restaurant

The restaurant is in the same style and only slightly more formal than the main bar, with fires at each end of the room (now converted to gas, alas) and is available by reservation right through the week except Sunday night and Monday. Restaurant menus overlap somewhat with the bar food, but offer a much wider choice, leaning towards bigger dishes such as rack of Wicklow lamb, roast wild Wicklow venison, venison ragout and other game in season. German influences are again evident in long-established specialities such as smoked Westphalian ham and wiener schnitzel and a feather-light Baileys Cream gateau which is not to be missed. A mainly European wine list favours France and Germany; house wine £12.95. • Meals£-££ • Closed 25 Dec & Good Fri • Amex, MasterCard, Visa •

Wicklow   The Bakery Restaurant & Café

Church Street Wicklow Co Wicklow

RESTAURANT/CAFE   Tel: 0404 66770

Table Presentation of the Year

Sally Stevens' lovely restaurant has great character – the fine stone building has retained some of its old bakery artefacts, including the original ovens in the café downstairs. Lots of candles in the reception area and restaurant set a warm tone which is then complemented by an admirably restrained theme – stone walls and beams provide a dark background for quite austere table settings which work wonderfully well in this room. There is also a separate vegetarian menu, but the regular one offers eight starters – typically including an interesting Blue Rathgore cheesecake with pears and balsamic vinaigrette and (a house speciality) Sushi Nori, a selection of three traditional Japanese seaweed-wrapped rice cakes stuffed with smoked salmon, crab and prawn respectively, served with a soy vinaigrette. Main courses could include a generous rack of Wicklow spring lamb with a light garlic and rosemary jus and good fish dishes such as baked silver hake with a herby pesto crust – strong flavours that balance well with a parmesan cream sauce. Mixed seasonal vegetables are served in a big dish to help yourselves. To finish, a Bakery Tasting Plate, perhaps, or plated farmhouse cheeses. Good coffee and friendly service.

* Downstairs, the Café serves an eclectic, moderately priced menu eg light dishes such as crostini (£3.50) or soup of the day (£2.50) and main courses all under £10, eg warm confit of duck leg salad, £8. • Meals£ ££ • Closed 25 Dec & Good Fri • MasterCard, Visa •

Wicklow   The Grand Hotel

Abbey Street Wicklow Co Wicklow

HOTEL   Tel: 0404 67337   Fax: 0404 69607

email: grandhotel@tinet.ie   www.grandhotel.ie

Very much the centre of local activities, this friendly hotel has large public areas including the Glebe Bar, which is very popular for bar meals (especially the lunchtime carvery). The conference/banqueting facilities for up to 300/350 are in constant use, especially for weddings. Pleasant, comfortably furnished bedrooms are all en-suite (two with shower only) and warm, with all the necessary amenities. • Acc££ • Meals£ • Amex, Diners, MasterCard, Visa •

Wicklow   The Old Rectory

Wicklow Co Wicklow

COUNTRY HOUSE/RESTAURANT   Tel: 0404 67048   Fax: 0404 69181

email: mail@oldrectory.ie   http://indigo.ie/~oldrec

Flowers, flowers, flowers – whether in the area as a whole (Wicklow is after all the "garden of Ireland") or at The Old Rectory itself, it is undoubtedly through flowers that you will best remember a visit to the Saunders' home. (Unless, of course, it is ex-fireman Paul's collection of fireman's hats and related paraphernalia that captures your attention instead.) This pretty early Victorian house is quite small but makes up for its size through great attention to detail. Colourfully decorated bedrooms are all en-suite and have many homely extras – including fresh flowers, of course. Breakfast – served with your choice of newspapers – offers many unusual options, and vegetarian and other special dietary requirements will be met by Linda with exceptional creativity and enthusiasm. A new Garden Wing has provided a boardroom for small meetings (16) and a fitness suite with sauna.

Restaurant

Linda's imaginative food provides a gastronomic treat. It is prepared with an artist's eye, most especially in her amazing floral dinners, held in conjunction with the County Wicklow Gardens Festival each summer. Dinner is served by Paul in an attractive new Victorian style conservatory called the Orangery, which provides a fitting setting for this ornamental fare. (No smoking.) Interest in The Old Rectory's food is so great that Linda runs a series of full and half-day cookery courses on topics such as wild food, vegetarian food, and Christmas cookery. • Acc££ • D£££ daily • Closed 25 Dec, Jan & Feb • Amex, Diners, MasterCard, Visa •

Northern Ireland

Entries
1999

BELFAST

The cities of Ireland tend to be relatively recent developments which started as Viking trading settlements that later "had manners put on them" by the Normans. But Belfast is even newer than that. When the Vikings in the 9th century raided what is now known as Belfast Lough, their target was the wealthy monastery at Bangor, and thus their bases were at Ballyholme and Groomsport further east. Then when the Normans held sway in the 13th Century, their main stronghold was at Carrickfergus on the northern shore of the commodious inlet known for several centuries as Carrickfergus Bay.

At the head of that inlet beside the shallow River Lagan, the tiny settlement of beal feirste – the 'mouth of the Farset or the sandspit' – wasn't named on maps at all until the 15th Century. But Belfast proved to be the perfect greenfield site for rapid development as the industrial revolution got under way. Its rocketing growth began with linen manufacture in the 17th Century, and this was accelerated by the arrival of skilled Huguenot refugees in 1685. There was also scope for ship-building on the shorelines in the valleymouth between the high peaks crowding in on the Antrim side on the northwest, and the Holywood Hills to the southeast, though the first shipyard of any significant size wasn't in being until 1791, when William and Hugh Ritchie opened for business. The Lagan Valley gave convenient access to the rest of Ireland for the increase of trade and commerce to encourage development of the port, while the prosperous farms of Down and Antrim fed a rapidly expanding population.

So, at the head of what was becoming known as Belfast Lough, Belfast took off in a big way, a focus for industrial ingenuity and manufacturing inventiveness, and a magnet for entrepreneurs and innovators from the entire north of Ireland, and the world beyond. Its population in 1600 had been less than 500, yet by 1700 it was 2,000, and by 1800 it was 25,000. The city's growth was prodigious, such that by the end of the 19th Century it could claim with justifiable pride to have the largest shipyard in the world, the largest ropeworks, the largest linen mills, the largest tobacco factory, and the largest heavy engineering works, all served by a greater mileage of quays than anywhere comparable, and all contributing to a situation whereby, in 1900, the population had soared through the 300,000 mark.

Expansion had become so rapid in the latter half of the 19th Century that it tended to obliterate the influence of the gentler intellectual and philosophical legacies inspired by the Huguenots and other earlier developers, a case in point being the gloriously flamboyant and baroque new Rennaissance-style City Hall, which was completed in 1906. It was the perfect expression of that late-Victorian energy and confidence in which Belfast shared with total enthusiasm. But its site had only become available because the City Fathers authorised the demolition of the quietly elegant White Linen Hall which had been a symbol of Belfast's more thoughtful period of development in the 18th Century.

However, Belfast Corporation was only fulfilling the spirit of the times. And in such a busy city, there was always a strongly human dimension to everyday life. Thus the City Hall may have been on the grand scale, but it was nevertheless right at the heart of the city itself. Equally, while the gantries of the shipyard may have loomed overhead as they still do today, they do so near the houses of the workers in a manner which softens their sheer size. Admittedly this theme of giving great projects a human dimension seems to have been forgotten in the later design and location of the Government Building at Stormont east of the city. But back in the vibrant heart of Belfast there is continuing entertainment and accessible interest in buildings as various as the Grand Opera House, St Anne's Cathedral, the Crown Liquor Saloon, Sinclair Seamen's Church, the Linenhall Library, and Smithfield Market, not to mention some of the impressive Victorian banking halls.

In more modern times, aerospace manufacture has displaced many of the old smokestack industries in the forefront of the city's work patterns, and some of the energy of former times has been channelled into impressive urban regeneration along the River Lagan. Here, the flagship building is the new Waterfront Hall, a large state-of-the-art concert venue which has won international praise. In the southern part of the city, Queen's University (founded 1849) is at the heart of a pleasant university district which includes two of the city's four theatres – the Lyric and the Arts – as well as the respected Ulster Museum & Art Gallery, while the university itself is particularly noted for its pioneering work in medicine and engineering.

Thus there's a buzz to Belfast which is reflected in its own cultural and warmly sociable life, which includes the innovative energy of its young chefs. Yet in some ways it is still has marked elements of a country town and port strongly rooted in land and sea. The hills of Antrim can be glimpsed from most streets, and the farmland of Down makes its presence felt. They are quickly reached by a somewhat ruthlessly implemented motorway system. So although Belfast may have a clearly defined character, it is also very much part of the country around it, and is all the better for that.

Local Attractions and Information

Arts Theatre	Botanic Avenue 01232 316900
Belfast Garden Festival	Balmoral (June)
Belfast Zoo & Castle	Antrim Road 01232 776277
Grand Opera House	Great Victoria St Tel 01232 241919
King's Hall (exhibitions, concerts)	Lisburn Road 01232 665225
Lyric Theatre	Ridgeway Street 01232 381081
Palm House Botanic Gardens	01232 324902
Pat's Bar	Prince's Dock(traditional music) 01232 744525
Tourist Information	01232 246609
Ulster Hall	Bedford Street 01232 323900
Ulster Museum	Stranmillis Road 01232 383000
Waterfront Hall	Laganside 01232 334455

Belfast   Ashoka

363 Lisburn Road Belfast BT9 7EP
RESTAURANT   Tel: 01232 660362   Fax: 01232 660228
This long-established Indian restaurant came into new ownership in late 1996 and since then it has undergone extensive refurbishment. Loyal customers will be pleased to know that head chef Ishtiaque Mohammed, who has been here since 1983, still rules the kitchen. Often described as a "popular" restaurant, Ashoka can put a different spin on the term, by listing an impressive array of celebrities it has entertained, so you never know who you might meet here. Billy Connolly, perhaps, or Lenny Henry, or Chris Patten....
• Restaurant D only £ • Closed 12-13 Jul • Amex, MasterCard, Visa •

Belfast   La Belle Epoque

61 Dublin Road Belfast BT2 7HE
RESTAURANT   Tel: 01232 323244   Fax: 01232 203111
Since 1984 Alain Rousse's authentic French cooking has been giving Belfast diners a flavour of old Paris. Set menus include "Le Petit Lunch" (Mon-Sat, which is terrific value at £5.95) and a keenly priced set dinner at £15, which offers a choice of three options within each course and is augmented by an equally fairly priced à la carte. • Open all day
• Sat D only • L£ & D££ • Amex, Diners, MasterCard, Visa •

Belfast   Café Altos

Unit 6 Fountain Street Belfast 1
RESTAURANT   Tel: 01232 323087   Fax: 0044 (0) 468 269043
email: cafealtos@hotmail.com
Café Altos is a buzzy, high-ceilinged daytime place in the city centre, near the City Hall. Sister restaurant to Dieter Bergmann's Dublin establishment, Il Primo, it shares some of the same unusual qualities – Dieter, an importer of French and Italian wines, has always offered some special vinous treats in any restaurant he has been involved in, and here, in addition to an exceptional main list, there are 25 wines available by the glass. Dubliners will also remember the head chef, Eamonn O Cathain, who cooked exciting food at another of Dieter's enterprises, Shay Beano in St Stephen Street, long before the arrival of the recent café-brasseries. So, although the menu at Altos may seem to offer the same international food as many other restaurants, remember that it comes with a special pedigree.• Meals£-££ • Restaurant open all day • MasterCard, Visa •

Belfast   Café Society

3 Donegall Square East Belfast 1
RESTAURANT   Tel: 01232 439525   Fax: 01232 233749
www.cafesociety.co.uk
Handy to the main shopping area, the ground floor bistro is ideal for a quick bite during the day (from 8.30 am) and there's outside summer eating on the pavement if the weather's fine. The stylish first floor restaurant overlooks the City Hall and is popular for

dinner and more leisurely lunches. Business lunch is treated seriously (special 2/3 course menu at £14.50/£16.50) and there's a separate room suitable for private dining or small conferences (up to 40), with projection and secretarial services available Monday-Thursday. Alexander Plums, who has been head chef since the restaurant opened in 1995, presents lively, international menus and includes some excellent dishes Examples might include smoked haddock & potato chowder with spiced harrisa, char-grilled sirloin beef with tapenad mash, mustard butter & wild mushrooms and lovely desserts such as burnt orange crème brûlée. Good details include home-baked bread, freshly brewed coffee and home-made truffles to finish. Tapas bar and live jazz, Thursdays and Fridays 5.30-8. House wines from £9.95. • Open all day • L£, D££ • Closed 25-26 Dec • MasterCard, Visa •

Belfast   Cargoes

613 Lisburn Road Belfast BT9 7GT

CAFÉ   Tel: 01232 665451

This is a special little place run by partners Radha Patterson and Mary Maw, who take a lot of trouble sourcing fine produce for the delicatessen side of the business and apply the same philosophy to the food served in the café. Simple preparation and good seasonal ingredients dictate menus, which might include dishes like smoky bacon & potato soup, Moroccan chicken with couscous, vegetarian dishes such as goats cheese & tarragon tart or wild mushroom risotto. There are classic desserts like lemon tart or apple flan, and a range of stylish sandwiches. • Open all day Mon-Sat • Meals£ • Closed Sun & Bank Hols • Amex, Diners, MasterCard, Visa •

Belfast   The Crescent Townhouse & Metro Brasserie

13 Lower Crescent Belfast BT7 1NR

HOTEL/RESTAURANT   Tel: 01232 323349   Fax: 01232 320646

This is an elegant building on the corner of Botanic Avenue, just a short stroll from the city centre,. The ground floor is taken up by the Metro Brasserie and Bar/Twelve, a stylish club-like bar with oak panelling and snugs, particularly lively and popular at night (necessitating 'greeters' for the entrance). The reception lounge is on the first floor. Bedrooms are furnished in country house style, with practical furniture, colourful fabrics and good tiled bathrooms. In addition, there are two luxury suites, decorated in a more period style with canopied beds. Breakfast is taken in the contemporary split-level Metro Brasserie, which also serves competently-cooked dishes, typically pan-seared breast of pigeon with caramelised apples and a port jus, stir-fry chicken with Asian vegetables and noodles, rice pudding and stewed rhubarb. Several wines by the glass. Street parking free from 6pm-8am, otherwise ticketed. • Acc££ • L£ & D££ • Amex, MasterCard, Visa •

Belfast   Crown Liquor Saloon

46 Great Victoria Street Belfast BT2 7BA

PUB   Tel: 01232 279901   Fax: 01232 279902

www.belfasttelegraph.co.uk/crown

Belfast's most famous pub, The Crown Liquor Salon, was perhaps the greatest of all the Victorian gin palaces which once flourished in Britain's industrial cities. Remarkably, considering its central location close to the Europa Hotel, it has survived The Troubles virtually unscathed. Although now owned by the National Trust (and run by Bass Taverns) the Crown is far from being a museum piece and attracts a wide clientele of locals and visitors. A visit to one of its famous snugs for a pint and half a dozen oysters served on crushed ice, or a bowl of Irish Stew, is a must. Upstairs, The Brittanic Lounge is built with original timbers from the SS Britannic, sister ship to the Titanic. • Meals£ daily • MasterCard, Visa •

Belfast   Deanes

38-40 Howard Street Belfast

RESTAURANT/BRASSERIE   ★   Tel: 01232 560000   Fax: 01232 560001

Restaurant of the Year

Chef-proprietor Michael Deane made his mark at St Helen's Bay in Co Down, but now that he has moved into the city centre, his cooking seems also to have moved up several notches. This is seriously good cooking in exceedingly grand and elegant surroundings. The main restaurant is on the first floor (downstairs there is a more informal brasserie), and is almost club-like, with various hues of brown and subdued lighting. The dining area is small, the table settings smart, and there is an open kitchen in which the chefs

can be observed at work. Supremely professional staff are well attired and polite, enhancing the atmosphere of fine and elegant dining. The style and presentation of cooking is modern, with prime ingredients given influences from around the world; Michael Deane's special talent for" fusion food" is given full rein in exciting, wide-ranging menus that represent good value for a restaurant of this class. For example, the fixed-price lunch (four choices in each course and quite a bargain at £19) offers starters that include lobster sausage and scallion cream, a terrine of squab and foie gras with a herb jelly or open pasta of goat's cheese served with basil and tomatoes. For a main course, a more traditional chicken, mushroom and potato pie; confit of duck with a curry and soya dressing or roast salmon, served with chorizo risotto and oil. For dessert, there's an unusual gin and tonic citrus brûlée accompanied by peppered fruit, an almost classic rhubarb crumble with cinnamon ice cream or a selection of international cheeses. A three-course dinner with coffee and delectable petits fours works out at £35.50, which makes the £45 tasting menu an absolute snip. Dishes are similar to those at lunchtime: a starter of Japanese-style salmon, served with chili, cucumber, ratatouille and ginger or a mulligatawny of quail broth with all things quail (a drumstick and egg), followed by a lamb casserole with baby vegetable won tons; local venison that comes with curry mash and garnished with horseradish, pancetta and sage. Alongside this, a pigeon and cabbage tart with foie gras and Madeira sauce seems almost commonplace! Desserts are similar to those at lunch: perhaps a chocolate and raspberry casket with raspberry sorbet or a plate of exotic Asian fruits. The extensive wine list is quite grand and particularly impressive are the temperature-controlled wine cabinets. • D£££ • L£ Thurs & Fri only • Amex, MasterCard, Visa •
* The Brasserie, on the ground floor, is open Monday-Saturday, L 12.00-2.45 (no reservations) and D 5-10.45. Head chef Raymond McArdle's "Thai-influenced modern British" menu includes vegetarian dishes. Cooking is stylish and prices reasonable. •

Belfast   Dukes Hotel

65/67 University Street Belfast BT7 1HL
HOTEL   **Tel: 01232 236666   Fax: 01232 237177**
First opened in 1990, within an imposing Victorian building, the hotel is modern inside with an interesting waterfall descending down one wall, floor by floor, into a rock pool in the foyer. This is flanked on either side by a restaurant/mezzanine bar and the intriguingly-shaped Dukes Bar, a popular rendezvous for locals. The recently refurbished double-glazed bedrooms are spacious with practical furniture and good fabrics, and in addition to the usual facilities there's an ironing board and iron hidden in the wardrobe. At the time of our visit the mini-gym was closed (but due to re-open in autumn 1998), though the saunas were operational. Street parking (ticketed 8am-6pm). • Acc£££ • Amex, Diners, MasterCard, Visa •

Belfast   Europa Hotel

Great Victoria Street Belfast BT2 7AP
HOTEL   **Tel: 01232 327000   Fax: 01232 327800**
email: res.euro@hastingshotels.com   www.hastingshotels.com

Belfast's tall, central landmark hotel has undergone many changes since it first opened in the '70s. Now owned by Hastings Hotels, it has been renovated and refurbished to a high standard, with a facade that is particularly striking when illuminated at night. Off the entrance foyer, with its tall columns, is the all-day brasserie (6am-midnight) and the lobby bar, featuring Saturday afternoon jazz and other live musical entertainment. Upstairs on the first floor you'll find the Gallery lounge (afternoon teas served here to the accompaniment of a pianist) and a cocktail bar with circular marble-topped counter. Attractive and practical bedrooms offer the usual up-to-date facilities, but perhaps the hotel's greatest assets are the function suites, ranging from the Grand Ballroom (1,000 theatre-style, 600 banqueting) to the twelfth floor Edinburgh Suite (120 banqueting) with its panoramic views of the city. Additionally, there's the self-contained Eurobusiness Centre, providing several meeting rooms and full secretarial services. Nearby parking (special rates apply) can be added to your account. Staff are excellent (porters offer valet parking), and standards of housekeeping and maintenance very good. • Acc££££ • Amex, Diners, MasterCard, Visa •

Belfast   Holiday Inn Express

106 University Street Belfast BT7 1HP

HOTEL   Tel: 01232 311909   Fax: 01232 311910

Close to the city centre, off Botanic Avenue and up from Shaftesbury Square, this is an environmentally-friendly hotel (where long-term guests are asked if they want their bed linen – duvets here – and towels changed daily, in order to save energy and water resources and reduce detergent pollution). Good-size bedrooms offer plenty of workspace, multi-channel satellite TV (including payable in-house movies and radio) and compact bathrooms (most with shower). Guests can use the small business centre and there are conference facilities for up to 250. A modest continental breakfast is included in the rate. Secure parking to the rear. Although the hotel had been open some time, landscaping was still taking place at the time of our visit in summer 1998.• Acc££ • Open all year • Amex, Diners, MasterCard, Visa •

Belfast   Jurys Belfast Inn

Fisherwick Place Great Victoria Street Belfast BT2 7AP

HOTEL   Tel: 01232 533500   Fax: 01232 533511

email: bookings@jurys.com   email: info@jurys.com

Located in the heart of the city, close to the Grand Opera House and City Hall and just a couple of minutes walk from the major shopping areas of Donegall Place and the Castlecourt Centre, Jurys Belfast Inn opened in 1997, setting new standards for the city's budget accommodation. The high standards and excellent value of all Jurys Inns applies here too: all rooms are en-suite (with bath and shower) and spacious enough to accommodate two adults and two children (or three adults) at a fixed price. Rooms are well-designed and furnished to a high standard, with outstanding amenities for a hotel in the budget class. • Acc£ • Closed 24-25 Dec • Amex, Diners, MasterCard, Visa •

Belfast   Manor House Cantonese Restaurant

43/47 Donegal Pass Belfast BT7 1DQ

RESTAURANT   Tel/Fax:01232 238755

Easily found just off Shaftesbury Square, this well-established restaurant has been in the Wong family since 1982, with expansion and renovation in 1989. In common with many other Chinese restaurants the menu is long, but in addition to the many well-known popular dishes, Joyce Wong's menu also offers more unusual choices. There is, for example, a wide range of soups and specialities include Cantonese-style crispy chicken and seafood dishes like steamed whole seafish with ginger and scallions. • L & D daily ££ • MasterCard, Visa •

Belfast   The McCausland Hotel

34–38 Victoria Street Belfast BT1 3GH

HOTEL   Tel: 01232 220200   Fax: 01232 220220

email: info@mccauslandhotel

Just about to open as we went to press, the McCausland Hotel is a sister establishment to The Hibernian Hotel in Dublin. Close to the Waterfront Hall, it is in a magnificent landmark building designed by William Hastings in the 1850s in Italianate style, with an ornate four storey facade (with carvings depicting the five continents). Classic contemporary design and high quality materials combine to create an exclusive venue for business and leisure guests. Individually appointed bedrooms include wheelchair-friendly and lady executive rooms. They also have fax/modem points and entertainment systems which include TV/CD/ radio and VCR. State-of-the-art conference facilities, business centre and highly trained secretarial support will all be available. • Acc££££ • Amex, Diners, MasterCard, Visa •

Belfast   Mizuna

99 Botanic Avenue Belfast BT7 1JN

RESTAURANT   Tel: 01232 230063

Interesting contemporary decor gives this traditional red-brick house a thoroughly modern feel, an impression backed up by eclectic menus and confident cooking. Well-sourced ingredients – organic salads, wild salmon – feature in lively menus that change once or twice a week. A slightly wider choice is offered in the evening than at lunchtime. Strikingly simple presentation and careful flavour combinations characterise a style that has impact without artifice. Good soups and salads – always a sign of a sure hand in the kitchen – imaginative fish dishes and old favourites are presented in an interesting combination of traditional and modish ingredients that works well. Good service from friendly staff. • L & D Tues-Sat ££ • Closed Sun, Mon & 12-13 Jul, 25-26 Dec • MasterCard, Visa •

Belfast   The Morning Star

17-19 Pottinger's Entry Belfast BT1 4DT

PUB   Tel: 01232 235986   Fax: 01232 438696

Situated in a laneway in the middle of the city, The Morning Star is a listed building and has been trading as a public house since about 1840 (although it was mentioned even earlier in the Belfast Newsletter of 1810 as a terminal for the Belfast to Dublin mail coach). Special features of the pub include an original Victorian hanging sign and bracket and, in the downstairs bar, the original mahogany bar and terrazzo floor. Corinne and Seamus McAlister took over the business in 1989 and, with due respect for the special character of the pub, immediately started on improvements. The Morning Star always had a good name for food, albeit with a limited choice, and the McAlisters wanted to build on that. They now run an impressive range of menus through the day, beginning with breakfast at 9.30, then Morning Star 'Morning Tea' with a full range of teas and coffees, on to lunch and so on. Between them, an astonishing range of food is served, including traditional specialities like Irish stew, champ and sausage, local Strangford mussels, roast Antrim pork and aged Northern Ireland beef (which is a particular source of pride), as well as many universal pub dishes. Daily chef's specials, blackboard specials, there seems no end to the choices offered each day. • Bar food daily £ • Amex, MasterCard, Visa •

Belfast   Nick's Warehouse

35/39 Hill Street Belfast 1

RESTAURANT   Tel: 01232 439690   Fax: 01232 230514

Nick's Warehouse is a clever conversion on two floors, with particularly interesting lighting and efficient aluminium duct air-conditioning. It's a lively spot, notable for attentive, friendly service and excellent food, in both the wine bar and the restaurant. A typical three-course meal (dishes are perhaps simpler and less expensive than in the restaurant) from the wine bar menu might consist of courgette and leek soup, venison, lamb and mushroom casserole with mash, and orange cheesecake for dessert. A meal in the restaurant might include local rainbow trout with spiced polenta and a ginger and lentil dressing, breast of duck with mash and a red wine and green peppercorn sauce, ending with a fine panacotta with stewed rhubarb, or a good selection of half a dozen Irish and continental cheeses. There's a sensible wine list, featuring several by the glass and some 'finer' wines at very fair prices. Open all day Mon-Fri ££ • Sat D only ££ • Closed Sun • Amex, Diners, MasterCard, Visa •

Belfast   Roscoff

7 Lesley House Shaftesbury Square Belfast BT2 7DB

RESTAURANT   ★   Tel: 01232 331532   Fax: 01232 312093

Approaching its tenth anniversary, Paul and Jeanne Rankin's chic and modern restaurant continues to make culinary waves. The dining area is long and on the narrow side, while the track spot lighting highlights some interesting artwork, complemented by the colourful waistcoats worn by the excellent staff. One of Britain's busiest chefs, with his own TV series and cookery books, plus other regular TV appearances, Paul has nevertheless cut down on these activities to spend more time in the kitchen again – and to establish a small chain of cafés around the city. The couple spearheaded Californian cuisine when they first opened, to which they have added modern European and Asian touches alongside the very freshest Irish ingredients. Though still relatively young, Paul has trained a number of fine chefs, who have gone on to make their mark in their own right, and the Roscoff kitchen is still one that young chefs aspire to join. Menus are fixed-price, the business lunch (three choices for each course) almost a steal at £17.50. Start, perhaps, with fish cakes served with a spiced rocket salad or poached eggs with black pudding, Parma ham and a bearnaise sauce, followed by pan-fried fillet of cod with saute potatoes and langoustine cream or confit leg of rabbit with saffron barley risotto and basil. Lemon tart with fresh strawberries or date and apple pudding with coffee sauce and crème fraiche make for an excellent finish. There's more choice at dinner – starters such as risotto primavera with asparagus, peas and broad beans, goat's cheese ravioli with sweet peppers and basil or a classic fish soup with rouille and garlic croutons. Main courses include glazed duck breast with aubergines and Chinese spices, roast monkfish with Mediterranean vegetables or escalopes of veal served with artichokes, tomatoes and basil. Desserts follow a similar and interesting pattern: rhubarb pizza with fresh ginger ice cream, brûléed rice pudding with roast plums or a gooey chocolate cake with Grand Marnier ice cream. Alternatively, Irish and British cheeses are served in tip-top condition. The wine list is so-so, with several available by the glass. • Mon-Fri L££ & D£££ • Sat D only • Closed Sun & Xmas • Amex, Diners, MasterCard, Visa •

Belfast   Stormont Hotel

Upper Newtownards Road Belfast BT4 3LP

HOTEL   Tel: 01232 658621   Fax: 01232 480240

email: conf.stor@hastingshotels.com   www.hastingshotels.com

Four miles east of the city centre, the hotel is directly opposite the imposing gates leading to Stormont Castle and Parliament Buildings. There's a huge entrance lounge, with stairs up to a more intimate mezzanine area overlooking the castle grounds. The main restaurant and informal modern bistro are pleasantly located. Bedrooms, most with co-ordinating fabrics, are spacious and practical with good worktops and offer the usual facilities. Several rooms are designated for female executives. The hotel also has eight self-catering apartments with their own car parking area, featuring a twin bedroom, lounge and kitchen/dinette, available for short stays or long periods. The self-contained Confex Centre, comprising ten trade rooms, complements the function suites in the main building. • Acc££ • Amex, Diners, MasterCard, Visa •

Belfast   Wellington Park Hotel

21 Malone Road Belfast BT9 6RU

HOTEL   Tel: 01232 381111   Fax: 01232 665410

Situated in the University area of South Belfast, but only five minutes away from the city centre, the redevelopment of this hotel at the time of writing is just about complete, with the addition of twenty-five bedrooms and a dedicated business centre with its own secure parking (the main conference facilities remain on the first floor of the redesigned building). Individual guests need not worry about being overrun by conference delegates, since one of the bars is exclusively for their use. The spacious foyer and public areas are comfortably furnished, as are the refurbished bedrooms, featuring the usual facilities, some with modem points and voice-mail. Guests have free use of Queen's University sports centre, a few minutes from the hotel. The Dunadry Hotel & Country Club, a fifteen minute drive from the city, is in the same ownership. • Acc££ • Closed Xmas • Amex, Diners, MasterCard, Visa •

ANTRIM

With its boundaries naturally defined by the sea, the River Bann, Lough Neagh and the River Lagan, County Antrim has always had a strong sense of its own clearcut geographical identity. This is further emphasised by the extensive uplands of the Antrim Plateau, wonderful for the sense of space with the moorland sweeping upwards to heights such as Trostan (551m) and the distinctive Slemish (438m), famed for its association with St Patrick. The plateau eases down to fertile valleys and bustling inland towns such as Ballymena, Antrim and Ballymoney, while the coastal towns ring the changes between the traditional resort of Portrush in the far north, the ferryport of Larne in the east, and historic Carrickfergus with its well-preserved Norman castle overlooking a harbour complex which today places its emphasis on recreation. In the spectacularly beautiful northeast of the county, the most rugged heights of the Plateau are softened by the nine Glens of Antrim, havens of beauty descending gently from the moorland down through small farms to hospitable villages clustered at the shoreline and connected by the renowned Antrim Coast Road. Between these sheltered bays at the foot of the Glens, the sea cliffs of the headlands soar with remarkable rock formations which, on the North Coast, provide the setting for the Carrick-a-Rede rope bridge and the Giant's Causeway. From the charming town of Ballycastle, Northern Ireland's only inhabited offshore island of Rathlin is within easy reach by ferry, a mecca for ornithologists and perfect for days away from the pressures of mainstream life.

Local Attractions and Information

Annaghmore	Ardress (Stapleton decor) 01762 851236
Antrim	Castle Gardens 01849 428000
Bushmills	World's Oldest Distillery
Carrickfergus Castle	01960 351273
Giant's Causeway Centre	012657 31855
Moy, Dungannon	The Argory ("time capsule") 018687 84753
Lisburn	Irish Linen Centre/Lisburn Museum 01846 663377
Portrush	Dunluce Castle 012657 31206

Ballycastle   House of McDonnell

71 Castle Street Ballycastle Co Antrim BT64 6AS

PUB   **Tel: 012657 62586/0411 668797**

The House of McDonnell has been in the caring hands of Tom and Eileen O'Neill since 1979 and in Tom's mother's family for generations before that – they can even tell you not just the year, but the month the pub first opened (April 1766). Tom and Eileen (who is a character known as "the Tipperary tinker") delight in sharing the history of their long, narrow bar with its tiled floor and mahogany bar (which was once a traditional grocery-bar and is now a listed building). The only change in the last hundred years or so, says Tom, has been a toilet block "but outside the premises you understand". Music is important too – they have a good traditional music session every Friday and love to see musicians coming along and joining in. • Open Mon-Thurs eves, Fri/Sat & Sun 12pm & 1pm respectively •

Ballymena   Adair Arms Hotel

Ballymoney Road Ballymena Co Antrim BT43 4BS

HOTEL   01266 653674   01266 40436

Located in the centre of Ballymena town, this attractive creeper-covered hotel has been owned and managed by the McLarnon family since 1995. Very much the centre of local activities – the bar and lounge make handy meeting places, and there are good conference and banqueting facilities – it's also a popular base for visitors touring the Glens of Antrim and the coastal beauty spots. Bedrooms are not especially big, but they are comfortably furnished and well-maintained, with all the usual amenities. • Acc££ • Amex, Diners, MasterCard, Visa •

Ballymena   Galgorm Manor Hotel

136 Fenaghy Road Ballymena Co Antrim BT42 1EA

HOTEL   **Tel: 01266 881001**   **Fax: 01266 880080**

email: mail@galgorm.com   www.galgorm.com

Set amidst beautiful scenery, with the River Maine running through the grounds, this converted gentleman's residence was completely refurbished before opening under the present management in 1993. It is now one of Ireland's leading country house hotels. Approaching through well-tended parkland, one passes the separate banqueting and conference facilities to arrive at the front door of the original house, (which is a mere 100 yards from the river). An impressive reception area with antiques and a welcoming log fire sets the tone of the hotel, which is quite grand but also friendly and relaxed. Day rooms include an elegant drawing room and a traditional bar, as well as the more informal Ghillies Bar in characterful converted buildings at the back of the hotel (where light meals are also served). Accommodation includes three suites; two rooms have four-posters. All rooms are very comfortably furnished with good bathrooms, and most have views over the river.

Restaurant

Galgorm Manor has had a good reputation for its food since opening. The Dining Room seats 75 and head chef Alistair Fullerton (who joined the hotel in July 1998) offers table d'hôte menus for lunch and dinner, with an emphasis on local produce. Menus are changed weekly and there are always vegetarian dishes offered. Private dining is available in the Board Room, which is panelled and has an antique dining table seating 12. • Acc£££ • Amex, Diners, MasterCard, Visa •

Bushmills   Bushmills Inn

25 Main Street Bushmills Co Antrim BT57 8QA

HOTEL   **Tel: O12657 32339**   **Fax: 012657 32048**

www.bushmills-inn.com

Only a couple of miles from the Giant's Causeway, Bushmills is home to the world's oldest distillery – a tour of the immaculately maintained distillery is highly recommended. The Bushmills Inn is one of Ireland's best-loved hotels. It has grown since its establishment as a 19th-century coaching inn, but its development under the current ownership – including complete restoration before re-opening in 1987 – has been thoughtful. The latest addition, a completely new wing (with 22 bedrooms, a conference centre, new kitchen and staff facilities, car park and an additional entrance) has been so skilfully done that it is hard to work out where the old ends and the new begins. Inside, it's the same story: all the features which made the old Inn special have been carried through and blended with new amenities. The tone is set by the turf fire and country seating in the hall and public rooms – bars, the famous circular library, the restaurant, even the Pine Room conference room – carry on the same theme. Bedrooms are individually furnished in a comfortable cottage style and even have "antiqued" bathrooms – but it's all very well done and avoids a theme park feel. Conferences are held in an oak-beamed loft. • Acc££-£££ • Meals£-££ • Open all year • Amex, Diners, MasterCard, Visa •

Carnlough   Londonderry Arms Hotel

Harbour Road Carnlough Co Antrim BT44 0EU

HOTEL   **Tel: 01574 885255   Fax: 01574 885263**

email: ida@glensofantrim.com   www.glensofantrim.com

Carnlough, with its charming little harbour and genuinely old-fashioned atmosphere (they still sell things like candyfloss in the little shops) is one of the most delightful places in Northern Ireland – and, to many people, the Londonderry Arms Hotel is Carnlough. Built by the Marchioness of Londonderry in 1848 as a coaching inn, it was inherited by her great grandson, Sir Winston Churchill, in 1921. Since 1948 it has been in the caring hands of the O'Neill family. The original building and interior remain intact, giving the hotel great character. Guests can enjoy good home-made bar meals or afternoon tea. There is also a restaurant, providing lunch, high tea and dinner, where unpretentious well-cooked food, much of it based on local ingredients – wild salmon , crab, lobster and mountain lamb – is served. Bedrooms, which are all en-suite and include 14 recently added at the back of the hotel, are comfortable and well-furnished in keeping with the character of the building. Many of the older rooms have sea views. • Acc££ • Meals£-££ • Closed 25 Dec • Amex, Diners, MasterCard, Visa •

Carnlough   The Waterfall

1 High Street Carnlough Co Antrim BT44 0EU

PUB   **No phone**

One row back from the harbour, this friendly pub has a welcoming atmosphere. Although much of the work has been done more recently than it might appear, its red tiled floor and low beamed ceiling are authentic enough, and both the fireplace and the bar itself are made of reclaimed bricks from an old mill across the road. Behind, there's a cosy lounge bar with a stained glass window, decorative plates and another brick fireplace. All very cosy and relaxed. • No credit cards •

Carrickfergus   Quality Hotel

75 Belfast Road Carrickfergus Co Antrim BT38 8PH
HOTEL   Tel: 01960 364556   Fax: 01960 351620

The opening of the Quality Hotel in 1997 added a much needed boost to accommodation in this area – and at prices which are far from outrageous. Conveniently located to Belfast airport (10 miles) and the scenic attractions of the Antrim coast, the hotel makes a good base for business and leisure visitors. It has good conference facilities (600), meeting rooms (max 60) and in-room amenities (desk, fax/modem line) for business guests. Bedrooms include three suitable for disabled guests, two suites, two junior suites and 20 non-smoking rooms; all are furnished to a high standard with good en-suite bathrooms (all with bath and shower). The Glennan Suite ("simply the best suite on the island") has jacuzzi bath and separate shower, his & hers washbasins, private dining room, leather furniture and a raised American king size bed overlooking Belfast Lough through balcony doors. • Acc££ • Open all year • Amex, Diners, MasterCard, Visa •

Coleraine   Greenhill House

24 Greenhill Road Aghadowey Co Antrim BT51 4EU
FARMHOUSE   Tel: 01265 868241   Fax: 01265 868365

Framed by trees with lovely country views, the Hegarty family's Georgian farmhouse is at the centre of a large working farm. In true Northern tradition, Elizabeth Hegarty is a great baker and greets guests in the drawing room with an afternoon tea which includes a vast array of home-made teabreads, cakes and biscuits. There are two large family rooms (6 in total) and, although not luxurious, the thoughtfulness that has gone into their furnishing makes them exceptionally comfortable – everything is in just the right place to be convenient. Little touches like fresh flowers, a fruit basket, After Eights, tea & coffee making facilities, hair dryer, bathrobe, good quality clothes hangers and even a torch are way above the standard expected of farmhouse accommodation. Elizabeth provides dinner for residents by arrangement – please book by noon. (No wine.) • D££ • Acc£ • Closed Oct-Mar • MasterCard, Visa •

Crumlin   Aldergrove Airport Hotel

Belfast International Airport Crumlin Co Antrim BT49 4ZY
HOTEL   Tel: 01849 422033   Fax: 01849 423500

This pleasant modern hotel opened in 1993 and is just 50 metres from the main terminal entrance at Belfast International Airport (and 17 miles from Belfast city centre). Spacious, attractively furnished bedrooms include three designed for disabled guests and a non-smoking floor; all are double-glazed, sound-proofed and have good bathrooms with bath and shower. Fully air-conditioned throughout, the hotel has spacious public areas and good facilities, including a fitness suite with sauna, conference and banqueting facilities, ample parking, a sun terrace and garden. At the time of going to press plans were in hand for an extra 60 bedrooms. To address the needs of longstay business guests, a full leisure centre and games room will also be added, plus a public bar to meet local demand. High security around the airport is seen as a bonus by the hotel, as it helps guests to feel relaxed. • Acc££ • Open all year • Amex, Diners, MasterCard, Visa •

Dunadry   Dunadry Hotel & Country Club

2 Islandreagh Drive Dunadry Co Antrim BT412HA
HOTEL   Tel: 01849 432474   Fax: 01849 433389

The riverside Dunadry Hotel & Country Club was formerly a mill and it succeeds very well in combining the character of its old buildings with the comfort and efficiency of an international hotel. Set in ten acres of grounds, the hotel has excellent business and leisure facilities, plus banqueting for 180. Stylish, spacious bedrooms include three suites and eleven executive rooms – all have good amenities, including satellite TV, and executive rooms have computer points and fax machines. The most desirable rooms have French windows opening onto the gardens or the inner courtyard. Leisure facilities within the grounds include a professional croquet lawn, fun bowling, trout fishing and cycling, as well as a leisure centre which rates as one of the best in Britain and Ireland. Sister establishment to the Wellington Park Hotel in Belfast city (see entry). • Acc£££ • Closed 25-26 Dec • Amex, Diners, MasterCard, Visa •

Portballintrae   Sweeney's Public House & Wine Bar

6b Seaport Avenue Portballintrae Co Antrim BT57 8SB

RESTAURANT   Tel: 012657 32405   Fax: 012657 31279

This attractive stone building is on the sea side of the road as you drive into Portballintrae and is very handy to both the Royal Portrush Golf Club and the Giant's Causeway. It's a pleasant place, with a welcoming open fire in the bar and a choice of places to drink or have a bite to eat. During the day the conservatory is an attractive option. On chillier days, however, the fireside in the main bar wins over the conservatory and its view. The food, prepared by Pauline Gallagher, is in the modern international café/bar style with no gourmet pretensions. Although likely to suit all age groups during the day, it can get very busy during the evening, especially on live music nights (there is a late licence to 1 am on Friday and Saturday). Toilet facilities for disabled. No reservations and, unusually for a food establishment, no credit cards. • Restaurant open all day Mon-Sun •

Portglenone   Crosskeys Inn

Portglenone Ballymena Co Antrim BT42

PUB   Tel: 01648 50694

This pretty thatched country pub dates back to 1740. It is one of Ireland's most famous pubs for traditional music, with sessions every Saturday night (and other impromptu sessions, with singing and storytelling, that happen at the drop of a hat). There are occasional blues sessions as well as traditional Irish. It's a charackterel cottagey place, with a fire in the old kitchen and several small, low-ceilinged rooms that fill up easily on a busy night. • Open all day, all wk • No credit cards •

Portrush   Maddybenny Farmhouse

18 Maddybenny Park off Loguestown Road Portrush Co Antrim BT52 2PT

FARM STAY   Tel/Fax: 01265 823394

Just two miles from Portrush, Rosemary White's Plantation Period farmhouse was built before 1650. Since extended and now modernised, it makes a very comfortable and hospitable place to stay, with a family-run equestrian centre nearby (including stabling for guests' own horses). There is also snooker, a games room and quiet sitting places, as well as an area for outdoor children's games. The accommodation is just as thoughtful. The bedrooms are all en-suite and there are all sorts of useful extras – electric blankets, a comfortable armchair, hospitality tray complete with teacosy, a torch and alarm clock beside the bed, trouser press, hair dryer – and, on the landing, an ironing board, fridge and pay phone for guest use. Across the yard there are also six self-catering cottages, open all year (one wheelchair friendly). Golf, fishing, tennis and pitch & putt nearby. No evening meals, but Rosemary guides guests to the local eating places that will suit them best. • Acc££ • Closed 15 Dec-6 Jan • MasterCard, Visa •

Portrush   Ramore

The Harbour Portrush Co Antrim BT56 8VM

RESTAURANT 🕯️   Tel: 01265 824313   Fax: 01265 823194

This remarkable restaurant is in a first-floor room with views over Portrush harbour. Established well ahead of the other "new wave" restaurants in Northern Ireland, such as Roscoff and Shanks, the sheer cosmopolitan buzz of the place – sleek modern style, well-dressed tables and the drama of an open kitchen – is impressive. High demand means two sittings are the norm and booking well ahead is essential. Freshly-baked breads accompany aperitifs (at the table unless a delay means waiting at the bar), giving time to consider a combination of owner-chef George McAlpin's written and blackboard menus. Typical starters might be Dublin Bay prawn croissants with garlic cream sauce or a terrine of foie gras, Parma ham and duck served with a mixed leaf salad. Main courses include fish of the day and duck done two ways (roasted and 'confit' i.e. preserved in its own fat, then reheated until crisp) which could be partnered with Jerusalem artichokes, mushrooms and shallots. Dressy desserts always include a speciality hot souffle and excellent cheese – a selection of five, served with salad and fresh fruit. Service is quite efficient on the whole, but can at times be brusque and impersonal. [Major changes were due for this year but the anticipated building work was delayed; it is to be hoped that the slightly off-hand attitude of the staff we experienced – possibly due to their frustration with delayed improvements – will improve when the work is complete.] A compact, well-balanced wine list offers good value – 'house selection' wines, for instance start at stg £7.75; good choice of half bottles.

*Before entering the rarefied atmosphere of Ramore, allow time to have a drink down

below at the Harbour Bar – or escape there for 15 minutes perhaps, if there's a delay on tables and a queue at the bar in the restaurant. • D only Tues-Sat ££-£££ • Closed Sun & Mon, 2 weeks Feb, Christmas/New Year • MasterCard, Visa •

Portrush   The Royal Court Hotel

233 Ballybogey Road Whiterocks Portrush Co Antrim BT56 8NF

HOTEL   Tel: 01265 822236   Fax: 01265 823176

Set in a spectacular clifftop location just outside Portrush, and a 10 minute drive from the Giant's Causeway, the Royal Court offers the most desirable hotel accommodation in the area. Public areas are spacious and comfortable – the dining room has the sea view. Bedrooms are all well-furnished with good bathrooms, but vary considerably in size and outlook – the most desirable are on the sea side and have little private balconies. Very handy to a number of golf links including the Royal Portrush and an excellent base for touring this lovely area. • Acc££ • Amex, Diners, MasterCard, Visa •

ARMAGH

Mention Armagh, and most people will think of apples and archbishops. In the more fertile northern part of the county, orchards are traditionally important in the local economy, and the lore of apple growing and their use is part of County Armagh life. As for the pleasant town of Armagh itself – recently restored to its ancient status as a city – it is of course the ecclesiastical capital of all Ireland, and many a mitre is seen about it. But in fact Armagh city's significance long pre-dates Christian times. Emhain Macha – Navan Fort- to the west of the town, was a royal stronghold and centre of civilisation more than 4,000 years ago. As with anywhere in Ireland, we are never far from water, and even inland Armagh has its own "coastline" of 25 kilometres along the southern shores of Lough Neagh, Ireland's most extensive lake and Europe's largest eel fishery. Today, Lough Neagh provides sand for the construction industry, eels for gourmets, and recreational boating of all sorts. In times past, it was part of the route which brought coal to Dublin from the mines in Coalisland in Tyrone, the main link to the seaport of Newry being the canal from Portadown which, when opened in 1742, was in the forefront of canal technology. That County Armagh was a leader in canal technology is only one of its many surprises – the discerning traveller will find much of interest, whether it be in the undulating farmland and orchards, the pretty villages, or the handsome uplands rising to Carrigatuke above Newtownhamilton, and the fine peak of Slieve Gullion in the south of the county.

Local Attractions and Information

Armagh	County Museum 01861 523070
Armagh	Planetarium 01861 523689
Armagh	Apple Blossom Time; May trail in apple country (signed) 01861 521800
Armagh	Navan Fort (prehistoric) 01861 525550
Armagh	Palace Stables (18c stables, carriage rides) 01861 5299629
Lough Neagh	Discovery Centre, Oxford Island 01762 322205
Portadown	Moneypenny's Lock (restored lock keeper's house) 01762 322205
Tourist Information	01861 521800

Armagh   Navan Centre

Killylea Road Armagh Co Armagh

VISITOR CENTRE/CAFÉ   **Tel: 01861 525550**

In the Navan Centre the coffee shop in the interpretative centre serves wholesome hot food and light snacks. • All day Mon-Sun, light meals£ •

Mullaghbane   O'Hanlon's Bar

Mullaghbane Co Armagh

PUB   **Tel: 01693 888284**

Near the Ti Chuainn heritage centre (which has accommodation), this pub has a pedigree to beat them all, with 15 generations and 400 years in the same family. Its Stray Leaf Folk Club is the premier venue for traditional music in the area. Ringed by an attractive river walk, it has the charm of the surrounding Ring of Slaigh Cuillion, an area of outstanding beauty. • Normal pub hours •

DOWN

You can expect to find more scenic variety in County Down than most other Irish counties as it rings the changes in its own quiet way from the affluent southern shoreline of Belfast Lough – the "Gold Coast" – through the rolling drumlin country which provides Strangford Lough's many islands, and on then past the uplands around Slieve Croob with the view southward increasingly dominated by the soft purple slopes of the Mountains of Mourne. But although the Mournes may soar to Northern Ireland's highest peak of Slieve Donard (850m), and provide within them some excellent hill-walking and challenging climbing, nevertheless when seen across Down's patchwork of prosperous farmland they have a gentleness which is in keeping with the county's well-groomed style. In the same vein, Down is home to some of Ireland's finest gardens, notably Mount Stewart on the eastern shore of Strangford Lough, and Rowallane at Saintfield, while the selection of forest and country parks is also exceptional. Throughout the contemporary landscape, history is much in evidence. St Patrick's grave is in Downpatrick, while the Ulster Folk and Transport Museum near Holywood provides an unrivalled overview of the region's past. The coastline is much-indented, so much so that when measured in detail County Down provides more than half of Northern Ireland's entire shoreline. Within it, the jewel of Strangford Lough is an unmatched attraction for naturalists and boat enthusiasts. There is greater interaction with the sea than anywhere else in Northern Ireland. Bangor in the north of the county has Ireland's largest marina, an award-winning facility, while all three of Northern Ireland's main fishing ports – Portavogie, Ardglass and Kilkeel – are in County Down.

Local Attractions and Information

Ballycopeland	Windmill, Millisle 01247 861413
Castle Espie	Wildfowl and Wetlands Centre 01247 874146
Cultra	Ulster Folk & Transport Museum 01232 428428
Downpatrick Cathedral	01396 614922
Newtownards	
	Mount Stewart (house, gardens & Temple of the Winds) 012477 88387
Portaferry	Aquarium (Exploris) 012477 28062
Rathfriland	Bronte Interpretive Centre 018206 31152
Saintfield, Ballynahinch	Rowallane (National Trust garden) 01238 51031
Strangford	Castle Ward National Trust house, Opera Festival June 01396 881204

Annalong   Glassdrumman Lodge

85 Mill Road Annalong Co Down BT34 4RH

COUNTRY HOUSE   Tel: 013967 68451   Fax: 013967 67041

Nestling between the magnificent Mountains of Mourne and the surging east coast seas, in an area where you could be forgiven for thinking that they 'grow' the boulders for dry stone walls, is Glassdrumman Lodge. Proprietors Graeme and Joan Hall have transformed what was once a typical Mourne farmhouse into a particularly comfortable small hotel; luxurious bedrooms have fresh flowers, fruit, and exceptionally well-appointed bathrooms. There is 24 hour room service, laundry and secretarial support. Breakfast is a speciality, taken communally round a big country table. Non-residents are welcome to join guests for dinner at 8 pm. Special note – directions, turn up the hill at Halfway House in Annalong. (£32, reservations essential). • Acc££-£££ • D only £££ • Open all year • Amex, Diners, MasterCard, Visa •

Bangor   Clandeboye Lodge Hotel

10 Estate Road Clandeboye Bangor Co Down BT19 1UR

HOTEL   Tel: 01247 852500   Fax: 01247 852772

Set in woodland on the edge of the Clandeboye estate, this comfortable modern hotel fits in well with its rural surroundings. The stylish foyer creates a good impression, with its welcoming fire and plentiful seating areas. Off it is the Lodge Restaurant with gothic-style windows and furnishings (where breakfast is also served). Good-sized, attractively decorated bedrooms are accessible by lift and have neat, well-planned bathrooms and quality furnishings and amenities including orthopaedic mattresses and phones with voicemail and fax/modem points. Extras supplied as standard include robes, mineral water, tea/coffee trays neatly stowed behind doors, a turn-down service and complimentary morning newspaper. Two suites have whirlpool baths and there are also two wheelchair-friendly rooms. A country-style pub, The Poacher's Arms, is in an original Victorian building beside the hotel. • Acc££ • Closed 25-26 Dec • Amex, Diners, MasterCard, Visa •

Bangor   Marine Court Hotel

The Marina Bangor Co Down BT20 5ED

HOTEL   Tel: 01247 451100   Fax: 01247 451200

email: marine.court@dial.pipex.com   www.nova.co.uk/nova/marine

Excellent leisure facilities at the Marine Court's Oceanis Health & Fitness Club are this hotel's greatest strength – these include an 18 metre pool, steam room, whirlpool and sunbeds, plus a well-equipped, professionally-staffed gym. As a result the club is extremely popular with locals as well as hotel residents. The hotel overlooks the marina (beyond a public carpark) but the first-floor restaurant is the only public room with a real view and only a few bedrooms are on the front – most have views of dull but tidy service areas. Decor is rather unimaginative but rooms are quite a good size and amenities above-average, with king-size beds and orthopaedic mattresses (but very large, hard pillows). Plenty of shelf/desk space and tea/coffee tray, hair dryer and trouser press are standard in all rooms. Noise from a disco at the back of the hotel can be a problem on certain nights. There is 24hr room service but only continental breakfast is served in the rooms. Good conference/banqueting facilities (350) with secretarial and other back-up services for business requirements. Patrick McCrystal, head chef at the hotel since 1995, oversees three restaurants in the hotel, two informal ones and the first-floor Lord Nelson's Bistro, overlooking the marina. • Acc££ • Closed 1 Jan • Amex, Diners, MasterCard, Visa •

Bangor   Shanks

150 Crawfordsburn Road Bangor Co Down BT19 1GB

RESTAURANT ★   Tel: 01247 853313   Fax: 02147 852493

Follow signs to the golf centre on the Clandeboye Estate, about three miles off the A2 just outside Bangor. This is an unlikely setting in which to find one of Ireland's finest restaurants, let alone one designed by Sir Terence Conran's company. On two floors (the first floor is mostly taken up by the bar and reception area, with some tables in use for extra-busy sittings, and a balcony for al fresco eating), the main restaurant is downstairs, simple, minimalist and bright. There is lots of light wood, some banquette seating and smart table settings, in addition to the windowed kitchen where you can observe the chefs at work. Chef-patron Robbie Millar first trained as a butcher, so you can be assured of prime-quality meat, especially the venison that comes from the estate. Fish is treated with no less respect. His effervescent wife Shirley orchestrates the well-drilled front-of-house team, perfectly complementing the assured, often brilliant cooking that emanates from the kitchen. Since the cooking is in the modern style, influences are often Mediterranean and Asian, aligning the best local ingredients with produce from afar. On arrival, a basket of home-made breads is served with tapenade, followed by an amuse-gueule. Main courses include sliced loin of lamb with crunchy polenta, red onion marmalade and Roquefort butter; steamed turbot with English asparagus, new potatoes and grain mustard cream; pecan-crusted salmon with saffron orzo and peas, lobster, basil and tomato vinaigrette or fillet of fallow deer with noodle pancakes, fondant sweet potato and shitake mushrooms. A wide-ranging selection of desserts rounds off the meal nicely; rhubarb and ginger crème brûlée, a gratin of raspberries with an apricot compote and apricot sorbet or a warm fresh cherry tart with almond ice cream. Cheeses (and there are plenty to choose from) are in tip-top condition, though they do attract a supplement. Two- or three-course lunches with choices are particularly good value. The wine list is very well balanced and, for the quality on offer, inexpensive. • L££-££ Tues-Fri, D££-£££ Tues-Sat • Amex, MasterCard, Visa •

Comber   The Old Schoolhouse Inn

100 Ballydrain Road Comber Co Down BT23 6EA

HOTEL/RESTAURANT   Tel: 01238 541182   Fax: 01238 542583

Almost next door to Castle Espie, home to the largest collection of wildfowl in Ireland (50 species of birds), and exactly three miles out of town, this hostelry is best described as an auberge. Reminders of its former existence are still in evidence – old bike sheds in the car park under the arch for example. Just what an old fire engine is doing in front of the restaurant is anyone's guess, however, but it's that sort of place. Run by Avril (chef) and Terry (the genial host) Brown, it's a magnet for returning regulars, who are treated as long-lost friends.They enjoy the straightforward and traditional cooking (with a hint of modernism). For a main course you could choose crispy roast duckling with an orange and champagne sauce, poached fillet of salmon with a béarnaise sauce or an almost fillet steak Rossini. There's also a three-course £18 (£14 on Sunday) fixed-price menu, perhaps confit of duck, roast loin of pork and bread and butter pudding. The separate bedroom block is self-contained with its own breakfast room and honesty bar/lounge. Each of the twelve comfortable and well-furnished ensuite rooms are named after American presidents of Ulster descent. • Acc££ • D££ Mon-Sat, L£ Sun only • Open all year • Amex, Diners, MasterCard, Visa •

Crawfordsburn   Old Inn
15 Main Street Crawfordsburn Co Down BT19 1JH

HOTEL   Tel: 01247 853255   Fax: 01247 852775

The pretty village setting of this famous 16th century inn – the oldest in continuous use in all Ireland – belies its convenient location close to Belfast and its City Airport. Oak beams, antiques and gas lighting emphasise the natural character of the building, an attractive venue for business people (conference facilities for 100) and private guests alike. Individually decorated bedrooms vary in size and style, most have antiques, some have four-posters and a few have private sitting rooms. The Ulster Folk and Transport Museum and the Royal Belfast Golf Club are nearby. • Acc££ • Closed 25 Dec • Amex, Diners, MasterCard, Visa •

Donaghadee   Grace Neill's
33 High Street Donaghadee Co Down BT21 0AH

PUB/RESTAURANT   Tel: 01247 882533/884595   Fax: 01247 810930

Dating back to 1611, Grace Neill's lays a fair claim to be one of the oldest inns in all Ireland; Grace Neill herself was born when the pub was more than two hundred years old and died in 1916 at the age of 98. Extensions and improvements under the present ownership have been done with due sensitivity to the age and character of the original front bar, which has been left simple and unspoilt. The back of the building has been imaginatively developed in contemporary style, creating Bistro Bistro, a bright, high-ceilinged area. Food is along the lines of shredded duck & red onion tortillas with sundried tomato, rack of lamb with chargrilled vegetables and (a great favourite this) homemade pork sausage with mash potato & onion gravy; good desserts follow, all at very reasonable prices. Sunday Brunch is a speciality, with live jazz (unnecessarily amplified, it sounds better from the conservatory or, in fine weather, from tables which are set up outside the car park.) • Meals£-££ • MasterCard, Visa •

Downpatrick   The Hunt Club
19 English Street Downpatrick Co Down BT30 6AB

RESTAURANT   Tel: 01396 617886   Fax: 01396 617191

Sam and Jane McMeekin and chef Brian Donnelly run The Hunt Club restaurant in the restored Assembly Rooms in Downpatrick. They present differently priced menus according to the occasion but the style is ambitious and contemporary. A top-of-the-range menu (£24.50) offers luxurious dishes, including a starter of foie gras with grape chutney (£2 supplement) and main courses like pheasant (braised and served with a sweetcorn and chilli purée, potato rosti and a light thyme jus) and roast sea bass with baby fennel and fresh linguine. At the time of going to press they are catering only for parties of 10 or more, but they plan to open on Saturday evenings and for Sunday lunch from November 1st 1998, so a phone call to check is advised. • D & private parties £-££ • Amex, MasterCard, Visa •

Dundrum   The Buck's Head
77 Main Street Dundrum Co Down BT33 0LU

RESTAURANT   Tel: 01396 751868   Fax: 01396 751898

Situated on the main Belfast-Newcastle road, this attractive, welcoming place has developed over the years from a pub with bar food and a restaurant, to its present position as a restaurant with bar. Head chef Michael Mooney sources local produce, especially seafood, from Dundrum Bay – in starters like Dundrum seafood pie and Dundrum Bay oysters. Note that many dishes on the dinner menu, including foie gras, lobster, Dover sole and fillet steak, attract supplements. Desserts are tempting and a short but imaginative vegetarian menu is also offered. Good service under the direction of the proprietor Michael Crothers. • Meals£-££ • Amex, MasterCard, Visa •

Gilford

The Yellow Door

Banbridge Road Gilford Co Down BT63 6EP

RESTAURANT

Tel: 01762 831543   Fax: 01762 831180

Tucked away in the south of County Down, alongside the River Bann, is The Yellow Door, one of Ireland's best kept culinary secrets. Roisin Hendron and Simon Dougan's fine restaurant combines a real talent for cooking with warm hospitality and a genuine desire to please. The restaurant is in a series of rooms, creating a cottage-like atmosphere – offset by an element of contemporary style, especially in the comfortable, elegant reception room/bar area. Thoughtfully appointed tables with Irish linen table mats and napkins, fresh flowers and generous, gleaming wine glasses immediately suggest a serious restaurant, a feeling confirmed by Simon Dougan and head chef Michael Donnaghey's modern, international menus. Seven or eight choices are offered on each course at dinner, rather less at lunch; the cooking is contemporary. Well-balanced main courses include a strong vegetarian option – maybe a trio of dishes such as asparagus and red onion tart, mille feuille of vegetables & herbs and dressed salad leaves – and there might be a fine example of New Irish Cuisine in fillet of beef with potato and bacon cake, creamed leeks and crispy fried onions. Finish with farmhouse cheese or good desserts, including updated renditions of classic puddings such as chocolate bread and butter pudding with homemade vanilla ice cream. • L£ Tues-Fri & Sun, D££ Tues-Sat •Closed Mon • Amex, MasterCard, Visa •

* As the guide went to press we heard that The Yellow Door Deli & Patisserie is to open shortly at 6-8 Bridge Street, Portadown; open 9-6 Mon-Sat..

Groomsport

The Anchorage

49 Main Street Groomsport Co Down BT19 6JR

RESTAURANT

Tel: 01247 465757

A discreet brass plaque beside the door of one of the oldest buildings in the village of Groomsport identifies The Anchorage, Jenny McCrea and Michael Scott's restaurant. This unusual establishment is divided into two areas, with a different atmosphere on each side – one has a wooden floor, large mirrors and Scandinavian simplicity – while the other, which is carpeted, has a much more intimate atmosphere. The Anchorage has earned a great reputation in the locality for interesting menus in the modern idiom, good cooking and a relaxed atmosphere. • D£-££ Wed-Sat, L£ Sun only • MasterCard, Visa •

Groomsport

Islet Hill

21 Bangor Road Groomsport Co Down BT19 6JF

ACCOMMODATION

Tel/Fax: 01247 464435

Just outside the town of Bangor, Islet Hill is a lovely old farmhouse set in fields overlooking the North Channel. It is a comfortable place to stay but it is the hospitality offered by Denis and Anne Mayne that make it really special. Children are particularly welcome and can play safely in the lovely garden. Both bedrooms are suitable for family use – one has a double bed and a single, the other a kingsize bed and adjoining bunk room; and, in addition to en-suite showers, there's a shared guest bathroom on the landing. Short on rules and regulations and long on welcome, there is no set time for breakfast, guests can use the house at any time and there's a fire in the guests' private sitting room in winter. Children under 14 B&B £10, under 2s free. • Acc£ •

Hillsborough

Hillside Restaurant & Bar

21 Main Street Hillsborough Co Down BT26 6AE

PUB/RESTAURANT

Tel:01846 682765   Fax: 01846 689888

Peel off the Belfast-Dublin motorway when you see the Hillsborough sign and you'll soon find Diane Shields' Hillside Bar in the steep main street. Established in 1777, it's an attractive pub in fine country style, with a welcoming atmosphere, soothing natural colours and plenty of tables. Real ale is one of the major attractions of the Hillside (they run a Real Ale Festival in late July and have 20-30 real ales on tap) and so is the food. The Refectory (bar food) and restaurant are run independently, with separate kitchens. Colin Elder, head chef in the Refectory kitchen, presents lively international seasonal menus which change with the time of day and provide a wide selection of consistently interesting food throughout – everything from ploughman's with brie, cheddar, apple, chutney and wheaten bread to sweet chilli steak strips served in a pitta pocket. • Refectory/bar meals£ •

Restaurant

Albert Neely, executive chef in the evening restaurant upstairs, returned to cook in his home town in 1996 after gaining experience abroad. He is doing a fine job at the Hillside. Dark-walled and low-ceilinged, the restaurant is inviting, with antique mirrors, well-appointed tables and welcoming bowls of olives, tapenade and breads. Albert presents a compact dinner menu (£25) and an à la carte: world cuisine with a nod to Irish traditions. Main courses might include char-grilled halibut steak cooked with lemon, served on chilli couscous with an array of imaginative vegetables like baby potatoes, herby peperonata, champ, slivered carrots and mangetout. Pudding choices tend to be modernised traditional – caramelised rice pudding with marinated black cherries, perhaps. Plated farmhouse cheeses- Gubbeen, Cashel Blue, St Killian – are served attractively with a biscuit selection and butter balls. Good service and good value. Interesting, well-priced wine list; house wine (£8.95) • D££ Tues-Sat • Amex, Diners, MasterCard, Visa •

Hillsborough   The Plough Inn

3 The Square Main Street Hillsborough Co Down BT26 6AG
PUB/RESTAURANT   **Tel: 01846 682985**   **Fax: 01846 682472**

Established in 1752,this former coaching inn enjoys a fine position at the top of the hill. Since 1984 it has been owned by the Patterson family, who have built up a national reputation for hospitality and good food, especially seafood. Somehow they manage to run three separate food operations each day, so pleasing customers looking for a casual daytime meal and more serious evening diners. Derek Patterson, who has been head chef since 1989, creates menus offering a nicely judged combination of traditional food – bacon loin with champ & colcannon, for example – and the world cuisine which is currently so popular, such as Thai-style steamed mussels with lemongrass, chilli, ginger & coconut cream. The evening restaurant is in the old stables at the back of the pub and booking is required; here Derek creates his renowned seafood menus – assorted shellfish soup & crème fraiche, seared king scallops, semi-dried tomato & basil sauce, mediterranean seafood ragout rustic style, with seasalted garlic focaccia. Seafood certainly rules here, but carnivores and vegetarians are not completely ignored – a sprinkling of meat and poultry dishes will always include fine Angus steaks – a fillet with cracked peppercorn crust and Bushmills whiskey cream perhaps – and there's a vegetarian menu available. • Bar meals£, restaurant D££ • Amex, Diners, MasterCard, Visa • * The Pattersons have recently acquired another pub The Pheasant Inn, at Annahilt. Menus suggest less dedication to seafood but the overall approach – informal world cuisine – is similar.

Hillsborough   White Gables Hotel

14 Dromore Road Hillsborough Co Down
HOTEL   **Tel: 01846 682755**

The historic Georgian village of Hillsborough is some ten miles south of Belfast, off the A1 Dublin road. The hotel, designed for business travellers, is modern, though already somewhat dated. Uniform and practical bedrooms provide the usual facilities, and there are conference facilities for up to 150. • Acc£££ • Open all year •

Holywood   Bay Tree Coffee House

118 High Street Holywood Co Down BT18 9HW
CAFÉ   **Tel: 01232 421419**

Since 1988 Sue Farmer has been attracting people from miles around to her delightful craft shop and coffee house on the main street. The craft shop, which sells exclusively Irish wares, is a busy, colourful place specialising in pottery, with over two dozen Irish potters represented. There is also a gallery exhibiting the work of Irish artists and – perhaps best of all – Sue's delicious food. Baking is a strength, especially the cinnamon buns which are a house speciality. There's quite a strong emphasis on vegetarian dishes – soups, pates, main courses such as red bean & aubergine stew with spiced mash – and organic salads, especially in summer, when you can also eat out on a patio in fine weather. No reservations for lunch but they are required on Friday evenings, when the Bay Tree is open for dinner; it's then that Sue might augment her informal lunch time fare with more serious dishes such as crown of Irish lamb with garlic, redcurrant and rosemary. • Mon-Sat L£, Fri D££ •

Holywood

Culloden Hotel

HOTEL 🏨🏨

Bangor Road Holywood Co Down BT18 0EX
Tel: 01232 425223   Fax: 01232 426777
email: res.cull@hastingshotels.com   www.hastingshotels.com

Hasting Hotels' flagship property, on the main Belfast to Bangor road, is set in 12 acres of beautifully secluded gardens and woodland overlooking Belfast Lough and the County Antrim coastline. The building was originally the official palace for the Bishops of Down, and is a fine example of 19th-century Scottish Baronial architecture – though we do wonder what the bishops would have made of the glass cabinet containing yellow plastic ducks signed by visiting dignitaries. The elegant and luxurious surroundings include fine paintings, antiques, chandeliers, plasterwork ceilings, stained glass windows and an imposing staircase. The spacious bedrooms (most in a side extension, and including seven suites and the Presidential Suite with the best views) are lavishly furnished and decorated and offer the usual facilities, plus additional extras such as a bowl of fruit and biscuits. Bathrobes and fine toiletries feature in the splendidly equipped bathrooms. The hotel also has a fine health club, the 'Cultra Inn' (an informal bar and restaurant in the grounds), and an association with The Royal Belfast Golf Club, four minutes away by car (book the complimentary hospitality limousine). A variety of meeting rooms is offered, ranging from the air-conditioned Stuart Suite (500 theatre-style, 460 banqueting) to boardrooms that overlook the Lough.• Acc££££ • Open all year • Amex, Diners, MasterCard, Visa •

Holywood

Rayanne House

COUNTRY HOUSE

60 Demesne Road Holywood Co Down BT18 9EX
Tel: 01232 425859   Fax: 01232 423364

Situated almost next to the Holywood Golf Club and Redburn Country Park, and with views across to Belfast Lough, this is a tranquil spot in which to unwind and a fine alternative to 'faceless hotel syndrome'. Rayanne House has character and is a veritable treasure trove of arts and crafts, collectables and curios, many hand-painted by Ray himself. Some might consider it kitsch (in the nicest sense) – one of the bedrooms features cherubs, painted, wall-mounted, even outside on the window ledge! However, it's a wonderful and relaxing place, family-run and offering one of the best breakfasts in Ireland, with dishes such as prune soufflé and bacon, Stilton and avocado kedgeree, grilled kippers and baked fresh herring fillets tossed in oatmeal. Dinner is served Wed-Sat incl. and open to non-residents. • Acc££ • D££ Mon-Sat • Closed Xmas wk • Amex, MasterCard, Visa •

Establishment reports for Dublin City and Greater Dublin can be found on the Dublin Live section of The Irish Times On Line site (www.irish-times.com).

Holywood

Sullivans

RESTAURANT

Sullivan Place Holywood Co Down BT18 9JF
Tel: 01232 421000   Fax: 01232 426664

Chef-proprietor Simon Shaw's bright, friendly and informal restaurant off the main street has new opening hours and is now licensed. Before and after lunch you can pop in for tea or coffee and light snacks. The lunch menu, though somewhat shorter than the full à la carte offered in the evening, does include several substantial dishes, from a daily home-made soup (cream of celery perhaps) served with crusty bread to a pan-fried salmon fillet that comes with couscous and chili butter. Vegetarians are well catered for (Caesar salad with aged parmesan, buttery vegetable risotto, and tortellini with sundried tomatoes), and others will enjoy generous proportions of wild duck breast with carrot and parsnip purée or a warm salad of sugar snap peas and peppered chicken liver, followed by braised lamb shank with champ, sausages and mash with onion gravy, crispy duck confit with borlotti beans, or roast sea bass with fennel and olives. This is first-class cooking, confirmed by super desserts such as mango and lemon tart, summer fruit brûlée or pecan pie with maple syrup. Cheese lovers will enjoy a plate of Cashel Blue, served with pears. Excellent coffee, fair prices. • Daytime meals£, D££ Mon-Sun • Closed 1 wk Jan • Amex, MasterCard, Visa •

Newcastle   Burrendale Hotel & Country Club

51 Castlewellan Road Newcastle Co Down

HOTEL   **Tel: 013967 22599**   **Fax: 013967 22328**

Just outside the traditional seaside holiday town of Newcastle, and close to the championship links of the Royal County Down golf course, this area on the edge of the Mourne mountains has an isolated atmosphere yet is just an hour's drive from Belfast. Public areas in the hotel are spacious. They include the Cottage Bar with an open log fire, welcome on chilly days. Well-appointed accommodation includes rooms suitable for disabled guests, family rooms, non-smoking rooms and the recently built Ambassador Rooms, which offer suites and executive standard accommodation. Leisure facilities at the Country Club include a 12 metre pool and there's a range of rooms for conferences and banqueting. • Acc££ • Open all year • Amex, Diners, MasterCard, Visa •

Newcastle   Hastings Slieve Donard Hotel

Downs Road Newcastle Co Down BT33 0AH

HOTEL   **Tel: 013967 23681**   **Fax: 013967 24830**

email: gmsdh@hastingshotels.com   www.hastingshotels.com

This famous hotel stands beneath the Mournes in six acres of public grounds, adjacent to the beach and the Royal County Down Golf Links. The Victorian holiday hotel par excellence, the Slieve Donard first opened in 1897 and has been the leading place to stay in Newcastle ever since. Recent years have seen great improvements in both the public rooms and accommodation. Bedrooms – which include two suites, two junior suites and 14 non-smoking rooms – are finished to a high standard and all the bathrooms sport one of the famous yellow Hastings ducks! The nearby Tollymore Forest Park provides excellent walking on clearly marked trails, just one of the many outdoor pursuits that attract guests; should the weather be unsuitable, the Elysium health club has enough facilities to keep the over-energetic occupied for weeks. The hotel also offers a wide range of special breaks. • Acc£££ • Open all year • Amex, Diners, MasterCard, Visa •

Newtownards   Edenvale House

130 Portaferry Road Newtownards Co Down BT22 2AH

ACCOMMODATION   **Tel: 01247 814881**   **Fax: 01247 826192**

Diane Whyte's charming Georgian house is set peacefully in seven acres of garden and paddock, with views over Strangford Lough to the Mourne mountains and a National Trust wildfowl reserve. The house has been sensitively restored and modernised, providing a high standard of accommodation and hospitality. Guests are warmly welcomed and well fed, with excellent traditional breakfasts and afternoon tea with homemade scones. Evening meals can be arranged if required, or Diane directs guests to one of the local restaurants. Edenvale is close to the National Trust properties Mount Stewart and Castle Ward. • Acc££ • Closed Xmas wk • MasterCard, Visa •

Portaferry   The Narrows

8 Shore Road Portaferry Co Down BT22 1JY

ACCOMMODATION/RESTAURANT   **Tel: 012477 28148**   **Fax: 012477 28105**

email: the.narrows@dial.pipex.com

On the Portaferry waterfront, an archway in the middle of a primrose yellow facade attracts attention to the inspired eighteenth century courtyard development that is central to Will and James Browns' unusual guesthouse and conference facilities. The ground floor includes a cosy sitting room with an open fire and a spacious restaurant; the style throughout is light and bright, with lots of natural materials and local art. Minimalist bedrooms are all different and have a serene, almost oriental atmosphere; all are en-suite but only three have baths. For guests with special needs, all the shower rooms are wheelchair-friendly, eight are specially designed and there is a lift. There are two interconnecting rooms and two family rooms; children's tea is available at 5 pm. A fine room over the archway, opening onto a private balcony, provides banqueting/conference facilities for 40/50 respectively.

Restaurant

At lunch and dinner every day, head chef Danny Millar presents lively modern menus based on carefully sourced local ingredients – notably seafood, including lobster, but also local meats and organic vegetables and herbs from their own garden. Lunch menus tend to include some more homely dishes like sausages and mash with onion gravy. Will's wife Sara Brown, who specialises in baking, makes all the breads herself and also tutors a breadmaking course in their programme of off-season workshops. • Acc££ • L£ & D££ daily • Amex, MasterCard, Visa •

Portaferry

HOTEL

Portaferry Hotel

The Strand Portaferry Co Down BT22 1EP
Tel: 012477 28231   Fax: 012477 28999
email: potfery@iol.ie

Originally an 18th-century waterfront terrace, the Portaferry Hotel presents a neat, traditional exterior overlooking the Lough to the attractive village of Strangford and the National Trust property, Castleward, home to an opera festival each June. Extensions and refurbishment undertaken by John and Marie Herlihy, who have owned the hotel since 1980, have been sensitively done and the inn is now one of the most popular destinations in Northern Ireland – not least for its food. There's an excellent lunchtime bar menu (including 'Children's Choice') available every day except Sunday. Accommodation is of a high standard and most of the individually decorated en-suite bedrooms have views of the water.

Restaurant

The restaurant has been recently refurbished but not too noticeably so – its slightly cottagey style provides the perfect background for good unpretentious food. Local produce features prominently in prime Ulster beef, Mourne lamb and game from neighbouring estates – but it is, of course, the seafood from daily landings at the nearby fishing villages of Ardglass and Portavogie that take pride of place. Gerry Manley, head chef since early 1998, presents well-balanced table d'hôte lunch and dinner menus plus a short carte, providing plenty of choice although majoring on local seafood. • Acc££ • L£ & D££ daily • Closed 25-26 Dec • Amex, Diners, MasterCard, Visa •

Sketrick Island

PUB

Daft Eddy's

Sketrick Island Killinchy Co Down BT23 6QH
Tel/Fax: 01238 541615
email: cadew@aol.com

This well-known pub enjoys a stunning position on a small island, with views to Strangford Lough. It was taken over by the Stronge family in 1996 and virtually rebuilt in 1997. It is reached by a short causeway. To those with a sentimental attachment to the old pub it may now seem more ordinary; however it is an attractive building and serves its purpose well, with a split-level bar and a restaurant. The maritime decor reflects the pub's large sailing clientele, as well as its location. Head chef Gordon Potts prepares good bar food, which is strongest on fresh fish dishes. • Meals£ Mon-Sun • Diners, MasterCard, Visa •

FERMANAGH

Ireland is a watery place of many lakes, rivers and canals. So it's quite an achievement to be the most watery county of all, yet this is but one of Fermanagh's many claims to distinction. It is the only county in Ireland where you can travel the complete distance between its furthest extremities throughout the heart of its territory entirely by boat. For Fermanagh is divided – or linked if you prefer – throughout its length by the handsome waters of the River Erne. Southeast of Enniskillen, Upper Lough Erne is a myriad of small waterways. Northwest of the historic and characterful town, the riverway opens out into the broad spread of Lower Lough Erne, a magnificent inland sea set off against the spectacular heights of the Cliffs of Magho. Boating has always been central to life in Fermanagh, so much so that in ancient times the leading local family, the Maguires, reputedly had a fleet of pleasure craft on Lough Erne as long ago as the 12th Century. It's a stunningly beautiful county with much else of interest, including the Marble Arch caves, and the great houses of Castle Coole and Florence Court, the latter with its own forest park nestling under the rising heights of Cuilcagh (667m). And if you think lakes are for fishing rather than floating over, then in western Fermanagh the village of Garrison gives access to Lough Melvin, an angler's heaven.

Local Attractions and Information

Belleek	(porcelain & Explore Erne Exhibition) 013656 58866
Enniskillen	Castle 01365 325000
Enniskillen	Castle Coole 01365 322690
Enniskillen	Florence Court 01365 348249
Lough Erne Cruises	01365 322882
Marble Arch Caves	01365 348855
Newtownbutler	Crom Estate (National Trust conservation site) 01365 738174
Tourist Information	01365 323110

Enniskillen   Blakes of the Hollow

6 Church Street Enniskillen Co Fermanagh BT74 6JE
PUB   **Tel: 01365 322143**   **Fax: 01365 748491**
One of the great classic pubs of Ireland, Blakes has been in the same family since 1887 and, up to now, has always been one of the few places that could be relied upon to be unchanged. Not a food place, a pub. Maybe a sandwich, but mainly somewhere to have a pint and put the world to rights. It will be a great relief to Blakes' many fans all over the world that the building is listed both inside and out – because the big news, as we go to press, is that major changes are planned – to include three new bars, a café/wine bar and a restaurant. How will that be accomplished without changing the building? We shall all know by summer 1999. • Open all year •

Enniskillen   Killyhevlin Hotel

Dublin Road Enniskillen Co Fermanagh BT74 4AU
HOTEL   **Tel: 01365 323481**   **Fax: 01365 324726**
Just south of Enniskillen, on the A4, this pleasant modern hotel on the banks of the Erne has fishing and river cruising as particular local attractions in addition to other outdoor activities such as golf and horseriding. The hotel is spacious, with conference/banqueting facilities as well as a warm welcome and comfortable accommodation for private guests. Rooms, which include one suitable for disabled guests and one suite, have good amenities. There are also some holiday chalets in the grounds, with private jetties. • Acc££ • Amex, Diners, MasterCard, Visa •

Irvinestown   The Hollander Bar & Restaurant

5 Main Street Irvinestown Nr Enniskillen Co Fermanagh
RESTAURANT   **Tel: 013656 21231**
The Holland family's long-established town-centre restaurant draws locals and visitors alike, whether for popular bar food dishes with a special "home-made" touch or the house specialities (salmon en croute, beef Wellington) which are always on the evening menu. These can also be produced by arrangement at lunchtime for groups of four or more. Boating visitors can even be run back to the local marina after dinner. • Bar & restaurant meals£-££ • Closed Mon & Tues Sept-Jun •

Kesh

HOTEL

Lough Erne Hotel

Main Street Kesh Co Fermanagh

Tel: 01365 631275   Fax: 01365 631921

In a very attractive location on the banks of the Glendurragh River, this friendly town centre hotel has twelve comfortable rooms with en-suite bath/shower rooms, TV and tea/coffee facilities. The hotel is understandably popular for weddings, as the bar and function rooms overlook the river and have access to an attractive paved riverside walkway and garden. Popular for fishing holidays, it would also make a good base for a family break; there is plenty to do in the area, including golf, watersports and horseriding. • Acc££ • Closed 24-25 Dec • Amex, Diners, MasterCard, Visa •

LONDONDERRY

When its boundaries were first defined, this was the County of Coleraine, named for the busy little port on the River Bann a few miles inland from the Atlantic coast. It was an area long favoured by settlers, for Mountsandel on the salmon-rich Bann a mile south of the town is where the 9,000 year old traces of some of the oldest-known houses in Ireland have been found. Today, Coleraine is the main campus of the University of Ulster, with the vitality of student life spreading to the nearby coastal resorts of Portstewart and Portrush in the area known as the "Golden Triangle", appropriately fringed to the north by the three golden miles of Portstewart Strand. Southwestward from Coleraine the county – which was re-named after the City of Derry became Londonderry in 1613 – offers a fascinating variety of places and scenery, with large areas of fine farmland being punctuated by ranges of hills, while the rising slopes of the Sperrin Mountains dominate the County's southern boundary. The road from Belfast to Derry sweeps through the Sperrins by way of the stirringly-named Glenshane Pass, and from its heights you begin to get the first glimpses westward of the mountains of Donegal. This is an appropriate hint of the new atmosphere in the City of Derry itself. This lively place could reasonably claim to be the most senior of all Ireland's modern cities, as it can trace its origins back to a monastery of St Colmcille, otherwise Columba, founded in 546AD. Today, the city with up-dated port facilities, while preserving many aspects of its turbulent history, is nevertheless moving into a vibrant future in which it thrives on the energy drawn from its natural position as the focal point of a larger catchment area which takes in much of Donegal to the west in addition to Londonderry to the east.

Local Attractions and Information

Derry City	Tourist Information 01504 267284
Derry	Harbour Museum 01504 377331
Foyle Valley Railway Centre	
Magherafelt	Springhill (17th century furnished house) 016487 48210

Aghadowey — The Brown Trout Golf & Country Inn

Aghadowey Co Londonderry BT51 4AD

HOTEL/RESTAURANT   Tel: 01265 868209   Fax: 01265 868878

email: billohara@aol.com

Golf is the major attraction at this lively country inn, both on-site and in the locality. Newcomers will soon find friends in the convivial bar, where food is served from noon to 10 pm every day. Spacious en-suite rooms with plenty of space for golfing gear are all on the ground floor, arranged around a garden courtyard. At the time of going to press high specification cottages are under construction 100 yards from the main building, the first of this standard in Northern Ireland.

Restaurant

Up a steep staircase (with chair lift for the less able), the restaurant overlooks the garden end of the golf course. Jane O'Hara's good home cooking is based on fresh local ingredients – trout fillet with fresh herbs & lemon butter or sirloin steak with a Bushmills whiskey sauce. High Tea (very popular in this part of the country) is followed by an à la carte dinner menu.• Acc££ • Bar meals£ • Restaurant £ • Open all year • Amex, Diners, MasterCard, Visa •

Limavady — The Lime Tree

Limavady Co Londonderry BT49 9DB

RESTAURANT   Tel: 015047 64300

Stanley and Maria Matthews opened their restaurant on the main street of Limavady in June 1996. Limavady is a handsome, wide-streeted town in a beautiful and prosperous part of the country. There is a great sense of contentment about The Lime Tree; the room is pleasant but quite modest, Stanley is a fine chef and Maria a welcoming and solicitous hostess. Ingredients are carefully sourced, many of them local; menus are generous, with a classical base that Stanley works on to introduce new ideas, thus duck rilletes listed beside crab and prawn filo parcels with a chilli oil dressing; prime fillet steak with a green peppercorn sauce and breast of chicken with a couscous, almond and raisin filling served with a cumin scented sauce. In addition to set menus, they operate a very good à la carte lunch menu, with a dressier version in the evening. They also do theme nights "to try out different dishes and ideas". Good cooking and good value go hand in hand with warm hospitality at The Lime Tree. Limavady is lucky to have it. • L£ & D££ Wed-Sun • Closed 1 wk Mar, 1 wk Jul & 1 wk Nov • Amex, MasterCard, Visa •

Limavady   Streeve Hill

Limavady Co Londonderry BT49 0HP

COUNTRY HOUSE   Tel: 015047 66563   Fax: 015047 68285

Peter and June Welsh have welcomed guests to their lovely 18th century home since they moved here in 1996. It is a very charming house, with a Palladian facade of rose brick and fine views over parkland towards the Sperrin mountains – but there is also beauty closer to home, in and around the house itself and in the nearby gardens of their former home, Drenagh. The stylish country house accommodation at Streeve Hill is extremely comfortable and the food and hospitality exceptional. Although the maximum number they can accommodate is six, they are happy for guests to bring friends to dine (provided 24 hour notice is given). They also cater for private dinner parties. Breakfast is another high point and, in the event of fine summer weather, it can be even more enjoyable if served on the terrace outside the drawing room. • Acc££ • Closed Xmas wk • Amex, MasterCard, Visa •

Londonderry   Beech Hill Country House Hotel

32 Ardmore Road Londonderry Co Londonderry BT47 3QP

HOTEL   Tel: 01504 349279   Fax: 01504 345366

email: beechhill@nisecrets.com   www.nisecrets.com/beechhill

Beech Hill is just a couple of miles south of Londonderry, in a lovely setting of 42 acres of peaceful woodland, waterfalls and gardens. Built in 1729, the house has retained many of its original details. It has 17 excellent bedrooms which vary in size and outlook – many overlook the gardens – but all of which are very attractively furnished with antiques. Public rooms include a good-sized bar, a fine restaurant (in what was originally the snooker room) and an elegant room seating up to 20 for meetings or private parties. Banqueting/conference facilities for 100, with good business back-up services. • Acc££ • L££ & D££ • Closed 25 Dec • Amex, MasterCard, Visa •

Londonderry   Everglades Hotel

Prehen Road Londonderry Co Londonderry BT47 2PA

HOTEL   Tel: 01504 346722   Fax: 01504 349200

email: res.egh@hastingshotel.com   www.hastingshotels.com

Situated on the banks of the River Foyle, close to City of Derry airport and just a mile from the city centre, this modern hotel is well located for business and pleasure. Like all the Hastings Hotels, Everglades Hotel undergoes an ongoing system of refurbishment and upgrading, a policy which pays off in comfortable well-maintained bedrooms and public areas which never feel dated. Accommodation includes 3 suites and is all of a high standard, with good amenities including a spacious working desk area and, on request, female executive and no-smoking rooms. Conference and banqueting facilities include a purpose-built meeting, private dining and presentation room, the Keys Centre. The hotel is well located for golf, with the City of Derry course just a couple of minutes away and six other courses, including Royal Portrush, within driving distance. • Acc££ • Closed 24-25 Dec • Amex, Diners, MasterCard, Visa •

Magherafelt   Trompets

25 Church Street Magherafelt Co Londonderry BT45 6AP

RESTAURANT   ★   Tel: 01648 32257   Fax: 01648 34441

email: eclectic.trompets@dnet.co.uk   www.my-place.co.uk/trompets

After working abroad Noel McMeel made his name at Beech Hill Country House, Londonderry, before opening this smart little restaurant in the centre of Magherafelt in July 1997. Trompets uses limited space well and has a bright, minimalist bar/reception area leading into the restaurant, which is modestly furnished but has the well-appointed tables indicative of a dedicated chef. Restaurant manager Aidan Rooney is a welcoming host and, under his direction, everything runs like clockwork. Noel's stated philosophy is to use the highest quality ingredients, cooked in the simplest of ways. Local meats, organic produce and eels from the nearby fishery at Toomebridge feature in a selection of menus, changed fortnightly, including set lunch (2/3 course, £10/15), set dinner (2/3 course, £17.95/22.95) and a three course surprise menu (£19.95). Some dishes attract supplements. The style is "modern global" with a nod to New Irish Cuisine and a strong hint of the chef's regard for American cooking. Typical main courses might include cannon of lamb with ratatouille and basil & tomato infusion, or steamed turbot with roasted tomatoes, herbed couscous and parsley sauce. Dramatic desserts include Trompets eclectic white chocolate soup with a lime & walnut tuile and there's also a good selection of plated Irish cheeses, served with dried fruit and walnut bread. Noel is a good chef and his dishes work – his is a courageous stance for the area and deserves success. An enormous choice is offered for such a small restaurant. Nothing is too much trouble in this delightful restaurant – a positive attitude which, together with Noel's fine cooking, will gain Trompets many friends. The wine list offers good value, including eight house wines, £9.25-£15.95, but could benefit from some tasting notes. • L£-££ & D££ Tues-Sat & L Sun • Closed 1 wk Jan • Amex, MasterCard, Visa •

Upperlands   Ardtara House

8 Gorteade Road Upperlands Nr Maghera Co Londonderry BT46 5SA

COUNTRY HOUSE 🏛   Tel: 01648 44490   Fax: 01648 45080

Take the A29 to Maghera/Coleraine; follow the sign to Kilrea until reaching Ardtara, former home to the Clark linen milling family and now an attractive, elegantly decorated Victorian country house which, thanks to general manager Mary Breslin, has a genuinely hospitable atmosphere. Well-proportioned rooms have antique furnishings and fresh flowers. All the large, luxuriously furnished bedrooms enjoy views of the garden and surrounding countryside and have king size beds and original fireplaces, while bathrooms combine practicality with period details, some including freestanding baths and fireplaces. Breakfast is a high point, so allow time to enjoy it. Private parties catered. Tennis, woodland walk, golf practice tee. No dogs. • Acc£££ • Closed 25-26 Dec • Amex, MasterCard, Visa •

Restaurant

In a dining room converted from its previous use as a snooker room – still with full Victorian skylight and original hunting frieze – Patrick McLarnon, a committed supporter of seasonal and local ingredients, offers a choice of around four on each course at lunch, seven or eight at dinner, with game well represented in season. Main courses will usually include Sperrin lamb – roast leg, perhaps, served simply with its own juices – and Ardtara toasted oatmeal and whiskey brûlée may well be among the tempting desserts, or you could finish with two Irish cheeses and Ditty's oatcake. Dishes on the dinner menu are a bit dressier – the lamb, for example, might be peat-smoked and served on champ with rosemary gravy – but in the same admirably strong style and, in both cases, backed up by caring service – and good value too. It's worth noting that bookings are taken for lunch as well as dinner. • L£ Sun-Fri & D££ daily • Closed 25-26 Dec • Amex, MasterCard, Visa •

TYRONE

Tyrone is Northern Ireland's biggest county, so it is surprising for the traveller to discover that its geography appears to be largely dominated by a range of modestly high mountains of which nearly half seem to be in the neighbouring county of Londonderry. Yet such is the case with Tyrone and the Sperrins. The village of Sperrin itself towards the head of Glenelly may be in Tyrone, but the highest peak of Sawel (678 m), which looms over it, is actually right on the county boundary. But as well, much of the county is upland territory and moorland, giving the impression that the Sperrins are even more extensive than is really the case. In such a land, the lower country and the valleys gleam like fertile jewels, and there's often a vivid impression of a living – and indeed prosperity – being wrested from a demanding environment. It's a character-forming sort of place, so it's perhaps understandable that it was the ancestral homeland of a remarkable number of early American Presidents, and this connection is commemorated in the Ulster American Folk Park a few miles north of the county town of Omagh. Forest parks abound, but as well attractive towns like Castlederg and Dungannon, as well as villages such as those in the uplands and along the charming Clogher Valley, provide entertainment and hospitality for visitors refreshed by the wide open spaces of the moorlands and the mountains.

Local Attractions and Information

CO TYRONE
Omagh   Ulster-American Folk Park Tel 01662 243292

Clogher   Corick House

20 Corick Road Clogher Co Tyrone BT76 OB2
COUNTRY HOUSE   Tel: 016625 48216   Fax: 016625 49531

Corick House is a charming 17th century William and Mary House, a listed building overlooking the river Blackwater in the scenic Clogher Valley area of South Tyrone. The house is built on a grand scale, with large well-proportioned reception rooms and surrounded by fine gardens. After period conversion, extension and refurbishment by Jean Beacon, who took over the house in 1995, it was opened as a licensed country house with ten luxurious bedrooms (all individually decorated, with antiques – giving it a private house atmosphere) and a restaurant which is open to non-residents. All facilities are accessible to wheelchair users and one of the bedrooms is specially adapted for disabled guests. The romantic setting and good banqueting facilities (up to 250) makes it an excellent venue for weddings, but banqueting is kept separate from the rest of the house. The novelist William Carleton grew up in the area and an annual Summer School, which attracts some highly distinguished speakers, is held at Corick House to honour his memory. A number of special breaks are available. • Acc££ • Open all year • Amex, Diners, MasterCard, Visa •

Cookstown   Tullylagan Country House

40B Tullylagan Road Cookstown Co Tyrone BT80 8UP
HOTEL/RESTAURANT   Tel: 016487 65100   Fax: 016487 61715

Halfway between Dungannon and Cookstown, this impressive country house hotel is set in 30 acres of grounds, with the Tullylagan river flowing through the estate. The lovely setting enhances a hotel which is particularly notable for friendly and enthusiastic staff. The public areas include a spacious foyer/reception with a fine staircase leading up to a range of well-appointed bedrooms, which vary according to their position in the house (five are shower only). All attractively decorated in country house style and include two disabled rooms, two non-smoking rooms, a full suite and a junior suite. The hotel takes pride in its dining room and has recently added an extra dimension, the Tullylagan Wine Bar, situated in a separate building which is used for banqueting (open Friday-Sunday 7-12pm). The hotel is within 10 minutes drive of two golf courses, and equestrian activities and fishing are also available nearby; weekend and other special breaks offer good value. • Acc££ • L£ & D££ • Closed 25-26 Dec • Amex, MasterCard, Visa •

Dungannon   Grange Lodge

7 Grange Road Dungannon Co Tyrone BT71 1EJ
COUNTRY HOUSE   Tel: 01868 784212   Fax: 01868 723891

Norah and Ralph Brown's renowned Georgian retreat offers comfort, true family hospitality and extremely good food. The house is on an elevated site just outside

385

Dungannon, with about 20 acres of grounds; mature woodland and gardens (producing food for the table and flowers for the house) with views over lush countryside. Improvements over the years have been made with great sensitivity and the feeling is of gentle organic growth, culminating in the present warm and welcoming atmosphere. Grange Lodge is furnished unselfconsciously, with antiques and family pieces throughout. Bedrooms (and bathrooms) are exceptionally comfortable and thoughtful in detail. Norah's home cooking is superb and, although they no longer accept bookings from non-residents for dinner, they will cater for groups of 10-30. Grange Lodge is fully licensed and dinner menus change daily (in consultation with guests). Breakfasts are also outstanding, so allow time to indulge. • Acc££ • D££ • Open all year • MasterCard, Visa •

Omagh   Hawthorn House

72 Old Mountfield Road Omagh Co Tyrone BT79 7EN

RESTAURANT/ACCOMMODATION   **Tel: 01662 252005**

On the edge of the town, in a lovely part of the country at the foot of the Sperrin Mountains, Hawthorn House was only established in the autumn of 1997 and yet is already recognised as one of the leading guesthouses and restaurants in Ulster. Owner-manager Michael Gaine is putting years of experience in the hotel business to work in this fine venture supported by an excellent team. Bedrooms are large and comfortable, with all the amenities expected of top quality accommodation. Public areas are also furnished to a high standard. Warm hospitality and helpful staff ensure guests' comfort, in both the accommodation and the restaurant.

Restaurant

Donal Keane, previously head chef at the Portaferry Hotel in County Down, presents tempting modern menus for both lunch and dinner. Main courses might be mixed grill of turbot, salmon & sole with pesto, aioli and tapenade, with peach and amaretti trifle to finish perhaps. Sunday lunch offers a nicely judged combination of traditional and more adventurous dishes. • Acc£ • L£ & D££ • Closed 25-26 Dec • MasterCard, Visa •

Maps

Republic of Ireland

Central Dublin

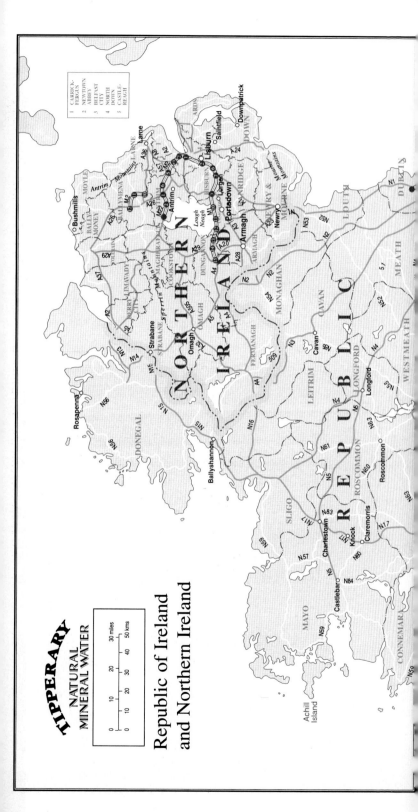

TIPPERARY
NATURAL
MINERAL WATER

Republic of Ireland
and Northern Ireland

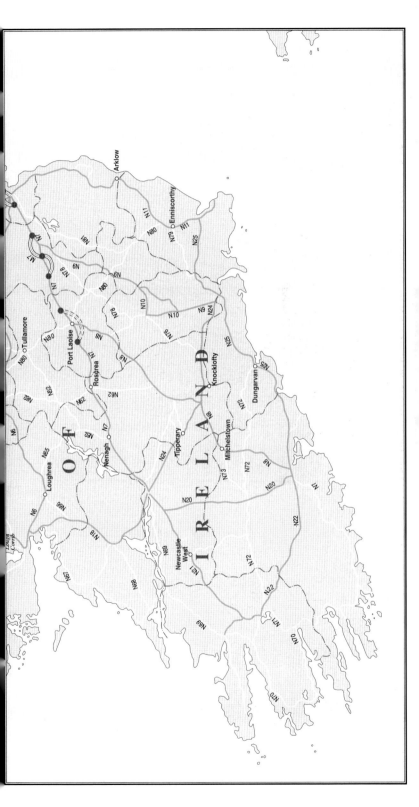

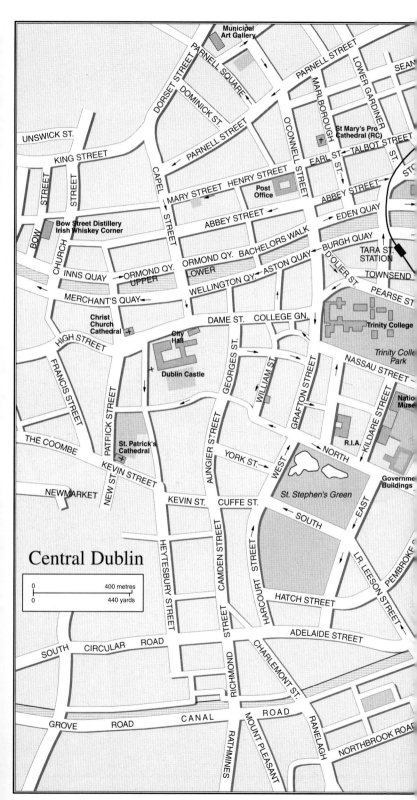

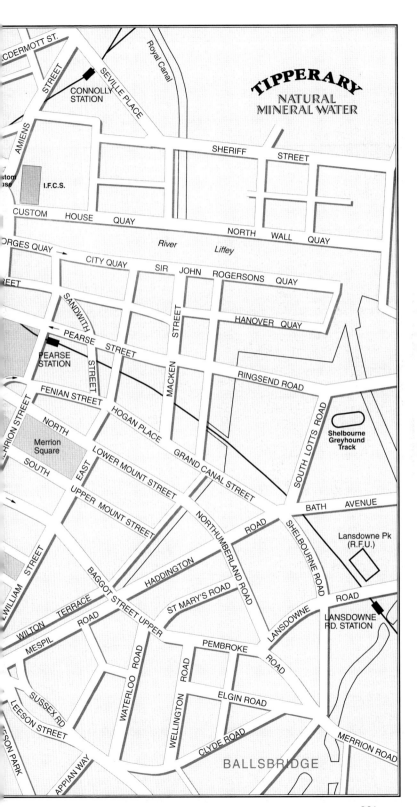

Index